EVIDENCE-BASED PRACTICE FOR NURSES

Appraisal and Application of Research

THE PEDAGOGY

Evidence-Based Practice for Nurses: Appraisal and Application of Research, *Second Edition* focuses on transitioning research into nursing practice through a variety of strategies that meet the learning needs of students while generating enthusiasm about evidence-based practice. This interactive approach addresses different learning styles, making the *Second Edition* the ideal text to ensure mastery of key concepts. The pedagogical aids that appear in most chapters include the following:

Chapter Objectives These objectives provide instructors and students with a snapshot of the key information they will encounter in each chapter. They can serve as a checklist to help guide and focus study.

Key Terms Found in a list at the beginning of each chapter and in bold within the chapter, these terms will create an expanded vocabulary in evidence-based practice. Visit **http://go.jblearning.com/schmidt** to see these terms in an interactive glossary and use flashcards and word puzzles to nail the definitions.

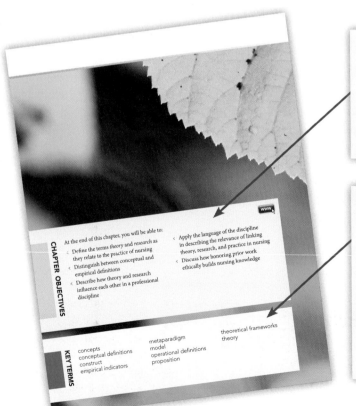

CHAPTER OBJECTIVES

At the end of this chapter, you will be able to:

‹ Define the terms *theory* and *research* as they relate to the practice of nursing
‹ Distinguish between conceptual and empirical definitions
‹ Describe how theory and research influence each other in a professional discipline

‹ Apply the language of the discipline in describing the relevance of linking theory, research, and practice in nursing
‹ Discuss how honoring prior work ethically builds nursing knowledge

KEY TERMS

concepts
conceptual definitions
construct
empirical indicators

metaparadigm
model
operational definitions
proposition

theoretical frameworks
theory

Critical Thinking An integral part of the learning process, critical-thinking scenarios and questions are presented by the authors to spark thought and provide insight into the situations you may face in practice. Visit **http://go.jblearning.com/schmidt** to complete your answer to each question.

CRITICAL THINKING EXERCISE 5-3

Reflect on your most recent patient encounter. When you assessed your patient, what theoretical assumptions guided your data collection? Were there questions you had about nursing needs or health circumstance that puzzled you? How did you go about addressing these questions? How might you assessed your future? Who might you involve in addressing questions? What did you do that worked when providing care for this patient? Would you use the approach with another patient? Why or why not?

is delivered, and if positive outcomes are achieved, the theory is validated. If outcomes are not positive, the theory is refuted and a new theory is created, resulting in a revised plan of care. Learning from each patient encounter is applied to new encounters. Case by case, the nurse learns about both the unique and universal characteristics of individuals.

Researchers engage in a similar process but from a different perspective. Nursing researchers systematically study individuals in groups to uncover knowledge about universal characteristics of individuals as they apply to their health. Knowledge from research assists nurses as they apply to their have a known probability of success. Although research findings help nurses predict what will be successful for the majority of individuals, outcomes cannot be predicted for an individual. When an individual does not respond like the majority of people, a nurse will rely more on clinical judgment and patient preferences.

Like researchers, theorists also work at a macro level building knowledge that can be universally applied. Theory provides understanding and guidance to the practice of nursing. It also provides language for describing nursing's work.

It is clear from the debate in the literature that nurses, researchers, and theorists can work more closely together and that such partnerships will be very fruitful for the development of nursing knowledge. Schmelzer (2006) encourages nurses to collaborate with researchers to find answers for practice problems. Waterman et al. (1995) also supports closer working relationships among nurses, researchers, and theorists. It is quite reasonable for nurses to be members of formal research teams as content experts. Another way to increase collaboration is for more researchers and theorists to engage in practice.

TEST YOUR KNOWLEDGE

Fill in the blanks:

1. A concept at the abstract level is comparable to a _____ at the operational level.
2. A _____ at the abstract level is comparable to a hypothesis at the operational level.
3. Quantitative research typically _____ theory, while qualitative research typically _____ theory.

True/False

4. Theory, research, and practice should be developed in isolation.
5. Nurses are encouraged to collaborate with researchers and theorists to expand nursing knowledge.
6. Concepts of the metaparadigm of nursing include: nursing, health, disease, social interaction, and persons.

How did you do? 1. variable, 2. proposition, 3. tests, builds, 4. F, 5. T, 6. F

Test Your Knowledge These questions serve as benchmarks for the knowledge you are acquiring as you move throughout the chapter.

5.2 Keeping It Ethical

At the end of this section, you will be able to:

‹ Discuss how honoring prior work ethically builds nursing knowledge

Students of any discipline are taught the body of knowledge that has been built over time, including the origins of the ideas that comprise that body of knowledge. As individuals contribute to the body of knowledge, credit should be given to those on whose work they are building.

Knowledge in a discipline is built in small steps that in time mark a long and fruitful journey of discovery. When reading the works of nurses, researchers, and theorists, students of the discipline should be able to trace the evolution of ideas. Credit must be given for ideas built on earlier work as well as for new ideas generated by challenging old ideas. This trail can be followed by examining references and reading the work of those who made

FYI

Credit must be given for ideas built on earlier work as well as for new ideas generated by challenging old ideas.

Keeping It Ethical Woven throughout the book, relevant ethical content concludes each chapter to ensure ethics are kept at the forefront of every step of the research process.

Rapid Review This succinct list at the end of the chapter compiles the most pertinent and key information for quick review and later reference.

Apply What You Have Learned With this outstanding feature, you will be challenged to apply your newly acquired knowledge to specific evidence-based practice scenarios and research studies. The "www" icon directs you to the companion website (**http://go.jblearning.com/schmidt**) to reference articles and blank grids to aid in fully understanding and implementing the research process.

5.1 How Are Theory, Research, and Practice Related?   135

TEST YOUR KNOWLEDGE

True/False
1. In the discipline of nursing, it is easy to follow how knowledge has developed since theorists have carefully provided citations for their ideas.
2. Giving credit to those who provide the basis for ideas is ethical practice.

How did you do? 1. F, 2. T

earlier contributions. Sadly, nurses have been poor at leaving such a trail. Few theorists cite the nurses who influenced their thinking. For example, Peplau (1952) gives credit to Adler, a psychologist, for influencing her thinking, but she makes no mention of nurses who may have influenced her thinking despite the fact that she published for nurses practicing in mental health areas. Likewise, Rogers (1970) does not credit the sources of her nursing knowledge even though she published a model for nurses in all settings. In other cases, an author may state that an idea came from another individual but does not provide a reference, or an author may use a secondary source for a quote when a primary source is available. Failure to honor the work of others creates problems for nurses trying to understand the evolution of nursing knowledge and practice.

When studying the writings of nurses who are contributors to disciplinary knowledge, it is important to look for the foundation of their ideas. Where information about these ideas is lacking, nurses should critically appraise claims that the work is a legitimate part of the disciplinary knowledge of nursing. To write as a contributor to the disciplinary body of knowledge without giving credit to those who provided the basis for the ideas is not just poor practice; it is unethical, and is, in fact, plagiarism.

FYI
To write as a contributor to the disciplinary body of knowledge without giving credit to those who provided the basis for the ideas is not just poor practice; it is unethical, and is, in fact, plagiarism.

RAPID REVIEW

- Theories are sets of concepts linked by propositions that explain phenomena. They provide a belief system to guide practice.
- Concepts are words or phrases conveying unique ideas or mental images. They are the building blocks of theories.

---

136   CHAPTER 5   Linking Theory, Research, and Practice

- The metaparadigm of nursing has four concepts: person, health, environment, and nursing.
- Propositions are statements describing relationships between two or more concepts.
- Constructs are properties that are inferred because they cannot be directly observed.
- Variables describe how concepts will be measured at the empirical level, and hypotheses are propositions that can be tested empirically.
- Concepts, propositions, variables, and hypotheses form theoretical frameworks that provide structure for research studies. Models are pictorial representations of theoretical frameworks.
- Conceptual definitions are like definitions found in dictionaries and are abstract in nature. Operational definitions specify how variables will be measured. Empirical indicators are the instruments used to measure variables.
- Deductive quantitative research is typically used to test theory, while inductive qualitative research can be used to build theory. Mixed methods can also contribute to the development of theory.

APPLY WHAT YOU HAVE LEARNED

A committee member tells you she has found two articles (Mark, Salyer, & Wan, 2003; Rich, 2005) that use a theoretical framework. She is excited about these and would like the committee to consider how these models might be useful to its work. As the chairperson, you are responsible for facilitating discussion. To prepare, you read the articles and consider the following questions.

1. The article by Mark and colleagues (2003) describes a study that uses a structural contingency theory. How does this framework influence the study?
2. In the article by Rich (2005), the corkscrew model of error reduction is discussed. How might this model be used as a framework for designing interventions that reduce medication errors?
3. Enter information about these two articles into the first and second columns of your grid on the companion website.

Case Examples Found in select chapters, these vignettes illustrate research questions and studies in actual clinical settings and provide critical-thinking challenges for students and follow-up discussion questions and answers.

CASE EXAMPLE 5-1

Early Methods of Resuscitation: An Example of Practice Based on Untested Theory

Throughout the past century, nursing students have been taught how to resuscitate patients who stop breathing. As early as 1912, students were taught a variety of methods for providing artificial respiration. It was theorized that moving air in and out of the lungs would be effective. One of these techniques was designed for resuscitating infants. Byrd's Method of Infant Resuscitation (Goodnow, 1919) directed the nurse to hold the infant's legs in one hand, and the head and back in the other. Then the nurse would double the child up by pressing the head and the knees against the chest. The nurse would then extend the knees to undouble the child. This would be repeated but "not too rapidly" (Goodnow, 1919, p. 305). At intervals, the nurse would dip the child into a mustard bath, in the hope that this would also stimulate respiration. The nurse would continue this until help arrived.

Other methods of artificial respiration taught included Sylvester's method for adults (Goodnow, 1919). The patient was placed flat on his back. The nurse would grasp his elbows, and press them close to his sides, pushing in the ribs to expel air from the chest. The arms would then be slowly pulled over the head allowing the chest to expand. The arms would be lowered to put pressure on the chest, and the cycle was then repeated. This was to be done at the rate of 18 to 20 cycles per minute.

By 1939, postmortem examinations after unsuccessful resuscitations showed veins to be engorged while the arteries were empty (Harmer & Henderson, 1942). Although this evidence indicated other factors needed to be considered, resuscitation techniques continued to focus only on the respiratory system. The same methods of resuscitation that were in use in 1919 were still being taught in 1942. Although students were still being taught the Sylvester method, they were also learning the new "Schäfer method" (Harmer & Henderson, 1942, p. 941). This method involved placing the patient in a prone position. The nurse would straddle the thighs, facing the patient's head, and alternatively apply and remove pressure to the thorax.

Eventually, it was noted that what was believed to be best practice was not effective. Results of postmortem examinations indicated that something was missing in the techniques, and therefore research was begun to determine best practice. Today, nursing students are taught cardiopulmonary resuscitation techniques based on updated research and theories.

CRITICAL THINKING EXERCISE 5-1

In your nursing program, how are the concepts of the metaparadigm defined? Is there a model or theory that is used?

Concepts are individual building blocks joined together in statements to create propositions. A *proposition* is a statement about the relationship between two or more concepts. For example, Nightingale (1969) linked a concept from the environment, sunlight, to the concept of health when she wrote:

> It is the unqualified result of all my experience with the sick, that second only to their need of fresh air is their need of light . . . not only light, but direct sunlight they want . . . People think the effect is upon the spirits only . . . we must admit that light has quite as real and tangible effects upon the human body. (p. 84)

Nightingale's proposition is that exposure to sunlight promotes healing and recovery in the person. Knowing this, nurses will expose people to sunlight to promote health.

Another important word in the language of theory is *construct*. A construct is a property that is neither directly nor indirectly observed. It is a word or phrase to communicate a specific, key idea to others. One example of a construct is social support. Social support cannot actually be seen, but it can be inferred through assessment of other observable attributes. To assess social support, nurses could count the number of people in a patient's circle of family and friends or could assess the quality of social support by asking patients about their perceptions of the support they receive.

The Importance of Testing Theory

Nurses look to research to develop and test ideas that may be useful and also look to researchers to address practice questions for which there are no answers. Nursing researchers are responsible for developing and testing knowledge to guide nursing practice (Butcher, 2006). There are important distinctions to note in order to understand what is and what is not relevant for practice, either at the level of basic research or at the level of applied research. Some researchers claim their work is nursing research because the researcher is a nurse or because the researcher studied nurses. But it is the focus on nursing practice

KEY TERMS

Proposition: A statement about the relationship between two or more concepts

Construct: A word or phrase used to communicate a specific, key idea to others

FYI

Nursing research provides results that are relevant to and expand or enhance practice. For research to be considered nursing research, the focus is on nursing practice, rather than research that happens to be conducted by a nurse.

FYI Quick tidbits and facts are pulled out in chapter margins to highlight important aspects of the chapter topic.

SECOND EDITION

EVIDENCE-BASED PRACTICE FOR NURSES

Appraisal and Application of Research

Edited by

NOLA A. SCHMIDT, PhD, RN, CNE
Associate Professor
College of Nursing
Valparaiso University
Valparaiso, Indiana

JANET M. BROWN, PhD, RN
Dean and Professor
College of Nursing
Valparaiso University
Valparaiso, Indiana

JONES & BARTLETT
LEARNING

World Headquarters
Jones & Bartlett Learning
40 Tall Pine Drive
Sudbury, MA 01776
978-443-5000
info@jblearning.com
www.jblearning.com

Jones & Bartlett Learning Canada
6339 Ormindale Way
Mississauga, Ontario L5V 1J2
Canada

Jones & Bartlett Learning International
Barb House, Barb Mews
London W6 7PA
United Kingdom

Jones & Bartlett Learning books and products are available through most bookstores and online booksellers. To contact Jones & Bartlett Learning directly, call 800-832-0034, fax 978-443-8000, or visit our website, www.jblearning.com.

Substantial discounts on bulk quantities of Jones & Bartlett Learning publications are available to corporations, professional associations, and other qualified organizations. For details and specific discount information, contact the special sales department at Jones & Bartlett Learning via the above contact information or send an email to specialsales@jblearning.com.

The authors, editor, and publisher have made every effort to provide accurate information. However, they are not responsible for errors, omissions, or for any outcomes related to the use of the contents of this book and take no responsibility for the use of the products and procedures described. Treatments and side effects described in this book may not be applicable to all people; likewise, some people may require a dose or experience a side effect that is not described herein. Drugs and medical devices are discussed that may have limited availability controlled by the Food and Drug Administration (FDA) for use only in a research study or clinical trial. Research, clinical practice, and government regulations often change the accepted standard in this field. When consideration is being given to use of any drug in the clinical setting, the health care provider or reader is responsible for determining FDA status of the drug, reading the package insert, and reviewing prescribing information for the most up-to-date recommendations on dose, precautions, and contraindications, and determining the appropriate usage for the product. This is especially important in the case of drugs that are new or seldom used.

Production Credits
Publisher: Kevin Sullivan
Associate Editor: Patricia Donnelly
Editorial Assistant: Rachel Shuster
Production Editor: Amanda Clerkin
Associate Marketing Manager: Meagan Norlund
V.P., Manufacturing and Inventory Control: Therese Connell
Composition: Publishers' Design and Production Services, Inc.
Cover Design: Scott Moden
Cover Image: © loriklaszio/ShutterStock, Inc.
Printing and Binding: Courier Kendallville
Cover Printing: Courier Kendallville

To order this product, use ISBN: 978-1-4496-2407-1

Library of Congress Cataloging-in-Publication Data
Evidence-based practice for nurses : appraisal and application of research / editors, Nola A. Schmidt, Janet M. Brown. — 2nd ed.
    p. ; cm.
  Includes bibliographical references and index.
  ISBN 978-0-7637-9467-5
  1. Nursing—Research. 2. Evidence-based nursing.   I. Schmidt, Nola A. II. Brown, Janet M. (Janet Marie), 1947-
  [DNLM: 1. Nursing Research—methods. 2. Evidence-Based Nursing. WY 20.5]
  RT81.5.E95 2012
  610.73072—dc22
                                                                              2010040551

6048

Printed in the United States of America
15 14 13 12   10 9 8 7 6

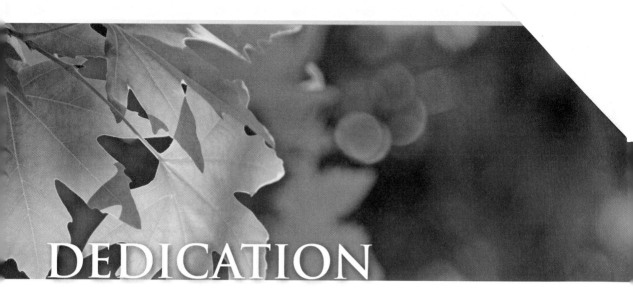

DEDICATION

For Mom, whose love and support are endless.

N. A. S.

To my husband, my children, and my granddaughters,
who enrich my life in every way.

J. M. B.

CONTENTS

UNIT 3 Persuasion 141

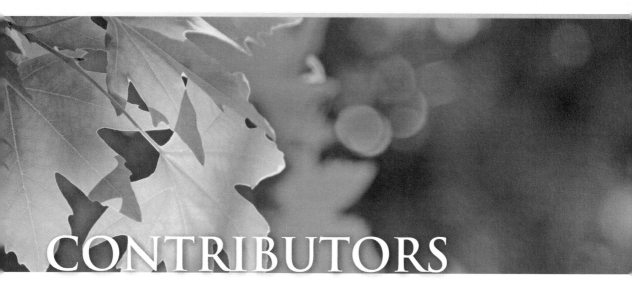

CONTRIBUTORS

Susie Adams, PhD, RN, PMHNP, FAANP
Professor and Director
Program School of Nursing
Vanderbilt University
Nashville, Tennessee

Janet M. Brown, PhD, RN
Dean and Professor
College of Nursing
Valparaiso University
Valparaiso, Indiana

Jan Dougherty, MS, RN
Director
Family and Community Services
Banner Alzheimer's Institute
Phoenix, Arizona

Moira Fearncombe
Associate Professor
The Illinois Institute of Art
Schaumburg, Illinois

Diane McNally Forsyth, PhD, RN
Professor
College of Nursing and Health Sciences
Winona State University
Rochester, Minnesota

Emily Griffin, MN, RN, FNP-C
Family Nurse Practitioner
UI Quick Care, University of Iowa Health Care
Iowa City, Iowa

Elisabeth Jensen, PhD, RN
Associate Professor
School of Nursing
York University
Toronto, Ontario

Carol O. Long, PhD, RN, FPCN
Principal
Capstone Healthcare Group
Phoenix, Arizona

Kristen L. Mauk, PhD, DNP, RN, CRRN,
    GCNS-BC, GNP-BC, FAAN
Professor Kreft Endowed Chair for the
    Advancement of Nursing Science
College of Nursing
Valparaiso University
Valparaiso, Indiana

Patricia Mileham, MA
Associate Professor of Library Services, Director
    of Public Service
Christopher Center for Library & Information
    Resources
Valparaiso University
Valparaiso, Indiana

Rosalind M. Peters, PhD, RN
Associate Professor
College of Nursing
Wayne State University
Detroit, Michigan

Kathleen A. Rich, PhD, RN, CCNS-CSC, CNN
Cardiovascular Clinical Specialist
La Porte Regional Health System
La Porte, Indiana

Cynthia L. Russell, PhD, RN, ACNS-BC
Associate Professor
Sinclair School of Nursing
University of Missouri
Columbia, Missouri

Nola A. Schmidt, PhD, RN, CNE
Associate Professor
College of Nursing
Valparaiso University
Valparaiso, Indiana

Marita G. Titler, PhD, RN, FAAN
Associate Dean, Office of Practice and Clinical
    Scholarship
Rhetaugh G. Dumas Endowed Chair
University of Michigan School of Nursing
Ann Arbor, Michigan

Ann H. White, PhD, MBA, RN, NE-BC
Associate Dean and Professor
College of Nursing and Health Professions
University of Southern Indiana
Evansville, Indiana

Maria Young, PhD, RN, APRN-BC
Cardiovascular Clinical Nurse Specialist
St. Elizabeth Regional Health
West Lafayette, Indiana

REVIEWERS

Carol Beltz, MSN, RN
Kent State University
Kent, Ohio

Susan Weber Buchholz, PhD, RN
Assistant Professor of Nursing
Purdue University Calumet
Hammond, Indiana

Nathania A. Bush, MSN, APRN, BC
Assistant Professor of Nursing
Morehead State University
Morehead, Kentucky

Janie Canty-Mitchell, PhD, RN
University of North Carolina—Wilmington
Wilmington, North Carolina

Kim Clevenger, MSN, RN
Assistant Professor of Nursing
Morehead State University
Morehead, Kentucky

Suzanne Edgett Collins, PhD, RN, MPH, JD
Associate Professor
Department of Nursing
University of Tampa
Tampa, Florida

Marianne Curia, PhD, MSN, RN
Assistant Professor
University of St. Francis College of Nursing and
    Allied Health
Joliet, Illinois

Maureen B. Doyle, PhD, APRN
Assistant Professor
Fairleigh Dickinson University
Henry P. Becton School of Nursing and Allied
    Health
Teaneck, New Jersey

Catherine M. Jennings, RN, MSN, APN-C
Felician College
Lodi, New Jersey

Jane Kapustin, PhD, CRNP
University of Maryland—Baltimore
Baltimore, Maryland

Cathy Leahy, MSN, MEd, RN
Department of Nursing
Xavier University
Cincinnati, Ohio

Cheryl Martin, PhD
BSN Programs Director
Associate Professor
University of Indianapolis
Indianapolis, Indiana

Mary A. Megel, PhD, RN
Associate Professor
College of Nursing
Family & Systems Department
University of Nebraska Medical Center
Omaha, Nebraska

Arlene Morris, EdD, RN, CNE
Associate Professor
Department of Nursing
Auburn University Montgomery School of
    Nursing
Montgomery, Alabama

Iris Mullins, PhD, RN
Assistant Professor
School of Nursing
New Mexico State University
Las Cruces, New Mexico

Jenenne P. Nelson, PhD, RN, CNS
Associate Professor and Kaiser Permanente
    Professorship in Nursing
Beth-El College of Nursing and Health Sciences
Colorado Springs, Colorado

Katherine Peck, MSN, RN, CNS
Instructor
New Mexico State University
Las Cruces, New Mexico

Michael Perlow, DNS, RN
Murray State University
Murray, Kentucky

Ginger Raterink, DNSc, ANP-C
School of Nursing
University of Colorado
Denver, Colorado

Jacquelyn Reid, EdD
Associate Professor
School of Nursing
Indiana University Southeast
New Albany, Indiana

Linda S. Rieg, PhD, RN
Associate Professor
Xavier University
Cincinnati, Ohio

Kandy K. Smith, DNS, RN
Associate Professor
College of Nursing
University of South Alabama
Mobile, Alabama

Claudette Spalding, PhD, ARNP, CNAA
Associate Dean for Graduate Education
Associate Professor
Barry University School of Nursing
Miami Shores, Florida

Nancy Wilk, DNS, WHNP
St. John Fisher College
Rochester, New York

PREFACE

Baccalaureate prepared nurses, given the emphasis on leadership, critical thinking, and communication in their curricula, are ideally positioned to advance best practices. Therefore, nursing faculty must create educational strategies for students that develop a lifelong commitment to critically examine nursing practice in light of scientific advances. While there are many texts and references dealing with the principles, methods, and appraisal of nursing research, few sources address the equally important aspect of integrating evidence into practice. Because there is a growing expectation by accrediting bodies that patient outcomes are addressed through best practice, it is imperative that books be available to prepare nurses for implementing best practices. This nursing research textbook provides substantive strategies to assist students with applying evidence to the point of care.

The American Association of Colleges of Nursing (AACN) charges nursing programs to prepare baccalaureate nurses with the basic understanding of the processes of nursing research. This book includes content related to methods, appraisal, and utilization, which is standard in many other texts. Furthermore, AACN expects BSN prepared nurses to apply research findings from nursing and other disciplines into their clinical practice. The framework for this text is the model of diffusion of innovations (Rogers, 2003), which gives readers a logical and useful means for creating an evidence-based practice. Readers are led through a step-by-step process using the innovation-decision process (IDP) to examine the nursing practice problem of medication errors. It is recommended that faculty use this text with students to guide them through assignments that hold the potential of affecting actual change in patient care at a healthcare facility. Schmidt and Brown (2007) describe this teaching strategy more fully elsewhere. Because students typically express that research content is uninteresting and lacks application to real life, we have tried to create a textbook that is less foreboding and more enjoyable through the use of friendly language and assignments to make content more pertinent for students.

The primary audience for this textbook is baccalaureate undergraduate nursing students and their faculty in an introductory nursing research course. All baccalaureate nursing programs offer an introductory research course for which this text would be useful.

In this second edition, input from students and feedback from faculty are incorporated. We are most grateful for their time and thoughtful critique. This edition continues to follow the five steps of the IDP: knowledge, persuasion, decision, implementation, and confirmation. This organizational approach allows the research process to be linked with strategies that promote progression through the IDP. The chapters follow a consistent format: key terms, objectives, major content, test your knowledge, rapid review, case study, and reference lists. Critical thinking exercises and user-friendly tables and charts are interspersed throughout each chapter to allow readers to see essential information at a glance. Textbook users will be pleased to find that efforts to provide consistency between chapters have been made. A glossary has been added for convenience. The evidence pyramid and questions to consider when appraising nursing studies have been printed inside the back cover for easy reference. The chapter about quantitative design in the previous edition was divided into two chapters to make content more manageable.

The case study continues to be a significant feature of this textbook. More recent evidence has been provided to challenge students to make decisions about practice related to the elimination of medication errors. The case study unfolds in a manner that integrates chapter content with the associated steps of the IDP. Concrete strategies, in the form of exemplars and checklists, allow readers to master competencies needed to perform these activities in the clinical setting.

Another unique feature of this textbook is the integration of ethical content throughout the chapters. Organizing content in this manner assisted students to integrate ethical principles into each step of the research process.

As a learning strategy, chapters are subdivided so that content is presented in manageable "bites." Students commented that they liked this feature. New to this edition, chapters begin with a complete of list of all objectives addressed in the chapter. Objectives are repeated for each subsection, followed by content, and ending with a section called Test Your Knowledge. Multiple choice and true and false questions, including an answer key, reinforce the objectives and content. Chapters also include critical thinking exercises that challenge readers to make decisions based on the content. New to this edition are call-outs involving definitions of key terms, which should reinforce learning. Users will find significant alterations to the companion website that is available to readers at **http://go.jblearning.com/schmidt**. It includes updated articles for the case study about medication errors. Templates needed to progress through the IDP model are also included. PowerPoint resources for faculty can also be obtained at this site.

We hope that the variety of strategies incorporated in this textbook meet your learning needs and generate enthusiasm about EBP. We wish you the best as you begin your professional career as an innovator who provides care based on best practices.

REFERENCES

Rogers, E. M. (2003). *Diffusion of innovations* (5th ed.). New York: Free Press.

Schmidt, N. A., & Brown, J. M. (2007). Use of the innovation-decision process teaching strategy to promote evidence based practice. *Journal of Professional Nursing, 23*, 150–156.

ACKNOWLEDGMENTS

A s with every endeavor, there are many individuals who make accomplishing the goal a reality. We wish to begin by expressing our gratitude to the contributors who shared our vision to create a text that can excite undergraduate nurses about evidence-based practice. The efforts of Karen Stacy and Patti Reid to protect sacred writing times were instrumental in allowing us to meet deadlines. Without their help and understanding, writing sessions would not have been as productive as they were. Special thanks are in order for Jones & Bartlett Learning staff. Tricia Donnelly, Wendy Swanson, and Amanda Clerkin offered invaluable editorial assistance. Kevin Sullivan believed in our vision of the text and facilitated our work. Finally, we are indebted to our families who afforded us the time to complete this book. They provided invaluable support throughout the process.

Introduction to Evidence-Based Practice

Without evidence, clinical practice cannot advance scientifically.

UNIT 1

At the end of this chapter, you will be able to:

< Define evidence-based practice (EBP)

< List sources of evidence for nursing practice

< Identify barriers to the adoption of EBP and pinpoint strategies to overcome them

< Explain how the process of diffusion facilitates moving evidence into nursing practice

< Define research

< Discuss the contribution of research to EBP

< Categorize types of research

< Distinguish between quantitative and qualitative research approaches

< Describe the sections found in research articles

< Describe the cycle of scientific development

< Identify historical occurrences that shaped the development of nursing as a science

< Identify factors that will continue to move nursing forward as a science

< Discuss what future trends may influence how nurses use evidence to improve the quality of patient care

< Identify four unethical studies involving the violation of the rights of human subjects

abstract
applied research
barriers
basic research
cycle of scientific development
deductive reasoning
definitions research
discussion section
early adopters
empirical evidence
evidence-based practice (EBP)

explanatory research
inductive reasoning
innovation
introduction
Jewish Chronic Disease Hospital Study
laggards
list of references
methods section
model of diffusion of innovations
Nazi experiments
Nuremberg Code

predictive research
pyramid of evidence
qualitative research
quantitative research
research
research utilization
results section
review of literature
theoretical framework
theory
Tuskegee study
Willowbrook studies

CHAPTER 1

What Is Evidence-Based Practice?

Nola A. Schmidt and Janet M. Brown

It is not uncommon for students to question the need to study a textbook such as this. To many students, it seems much more exciting and important to be with patients in various settings. As a beginning practitioner, it is often hard to appreciate the value of learning the research process and the importance of evidence in providing patient care. To appreciate the importance of *evidence*, imagine that a family member required nursing care. Would it not be much more desirable to have care based on evidence rather than on tradition, trial and error, or an educated guess? To be competent, a nurse must have the ability to provide care based on evidence. A journey through this textbook will assist you with developing your skills and talents for providing patients with care based on evidence so that the best possible outcomes can be achieved.

1.1 EBP: What Is It?

At the end of this section, you will be able to:

< Define evidence-based practice (EBP)
< List sources of evidence for nursing practice
< Identify barriers to the adoption of EBP and pinpoint strategies to overcome them
< Explain how the process of diffusion facilitates moving evidence into nursing practice

Nurses' unique perspective of patient care obliges nurses to build their own body of evidence through scientific research. There are a variety of sources of evidence for nursing research, some of which build a stronger case than others.

KEY TERMS

Evidence-based practice (EBP): Practice based on the best available evidence, patient preferences, and clinical judgment

Research utilization: Changing practice based on the results of a single research study

Overview of EBP

When examining the literature about *EBP*, one will find a variety of definitions. Most definitions include three components: research-based information, clinical expertise, and patient preferences. Ingersoll's (2000) definition succinctly captures the essence of EBP, defining it as, "the conscientious, explicit, and judicious use of theory-derived, research-based information in making decisions about care delivery to individuals or groups of patients and in consideration of individual needs and preferences" (p. 152). What does this mean? EBP is a process involving the examination and application of research findings or other reliable evidence that has been integrated with scientific theories. For nurses to participate in this process, they must use their critical thinking skills to review research publications and other sources of information. After the information is evaluated, nurses use their clinical decision-making skills to apply evidence to patient care. As in all nursing care, patient preferences and needs are the basis of care decisions and therefore essential to EBP.

EBP has its roots in medicine. Archie Cochrane, a British epidemiologist, admonished the medical profession for not critically examining evidence (Cochrane, 1971). He contended that individuals should pay only for health care based on scientific evidence (Melnyk & Fineout-Overholt, 2005), and he believed that random clinical trials were the "gold standard" for generating reliable and valid evidence. He suggested that rigorous, systematic reviews of research from a variety of disciplines be conducted to inform practice and policy making. As a result of his innovative idea, the Cochrane Center established a collaboration "dedicated to making up-to-date, accurate information about the effects of health care readily available worldwide. It [the Cochrane Center] produces and disseminates systematic reviews of healthcare interventions and promotes the search for evidence in the form of clinical trials and other studies of interventions" (The Cochrane Collaboration, n.d.). Others built on Dr. Cochrane's philosophy, and the definition of EBP in medicine evolved to include clinical judgment and patient preferences (Sackett, Rosenberg, Gray, Haynes, & Richardson, 1996; Straus, Richardson, Glasziou, & Haynes, 2005).

During this time, nursing was heavily involved in trying to apply research findings to practice, a process known as *research utilization*. This process involves changing practice from the results of a single research study (Barnsteiner & Prevost, 2002). Nursing innovators recognized that shifting from this model to an EBP framework would be more likely to improve patient outcomes and provide more cost-effective methods of care (Ingersoll, 2000; Melnyk, 1999; Youngblut & Brooten, 2001). Why? Many nursing questions cannot be answered by a single study, and human conditions are not always amenable to clinical trials. Also, the research utilization process does not appreciate the importance of clinical decision making, nor is it noted for being patient focused.

CRITICAL THINKING EXERCISE 1-1

Look carefully at the steps in each EBP model cited in Table 1-1. Are you reminded of a similar process?

These innovators recognized that the EBP framework allows for consideration of other sources of evidence relevant to nursing practice.

There are many different models for EBP. Three models that are especially well known in nursing are shown in **Table 1-1**. While each is unique, they have commonalities. For example, each one begins with a question or need for the identification of acquiring knowledge about a question. All involve appraisal of evidence and making a decision about how to use evidence. These models conclude by closing the loop through evaluation to determine that the practice change is actually meeting the expected outcomes.

Sources of Evidence

Over the years, a variety of sources of evidence have provided information for nursing practice. While it would be nice to claim that all nursing practice is based on substantial and reliable evidence, this is not the case. Evidence derived from tradition, authority, trial and error, personal experiences, intuition, borrowed evidence, and scientific research are all used to guide nursing prac-

TABLE 1-1 Models of EBP

ACE Star Model of Knowledge Transformation	Iowa Model of EBP	Model of Diffusion of Innovation
1. Discovery	1. Ask clinical question	1. Acquisition of knowledge
2. Summary	2. Search literature	2. Persuasion
3. Translation	3. Critically appraise evidence	3. Decision
4. Integration	4. Implement practice change	4. Implementation
5. Evaluation	5. Evaluate	5. Confirmation
Stevens, 2004	Titler et al., 2001	Rogers, 2003

tice. Just as you know from your own life, some sources are not as dependable as others. Tradition has long been an accepted basis for information. Consider this: Why are vital signs taken routinely every 4 hours on patients who are clinically stable? The rationale for many nursing interventions commonly practiced is grounded in the phrase, "This is the way we have always done it." Nurses can be so entrenched in practice traditions that they fail to ask questions that could lead to changes based in evidence. Consistent use of tradition as a basis for practice limits effective problem solving and fails to consider individual needs and preferences. How often have you heard the phrase, "Because I said so!"? This is an example of authority. There are various sources of authority such as books, articles, Web pages, and individuals and groups. These are perceived as being meaningful sources of reliable information; yet in reality, the information provided may be based in personal experience or tradition rather than scientific evidence. Authority has a place in nursing practice as long as nurses ascertain the legitimacy of the information provided. Trial and error is another source of evidence. While we all use this approach in our everyday problem solving, it is often not the preferred approach for delivering nursing care. Because trial and error is not based on a systematic scientific approach, patient outcomes may not be a direct result of the intervention. For example, in long-term care the treatment of decubitus ulcers is often based on this haphazard approach. Nurses frequently try a variety of approaches to heal ulcers. After some time, they settle on one approach that is more often than not effective. This approach can lead to reduced critical thinking and wasted time and resources. Nurses often make decisions about patient care based on their personal experiences. While previous experience can help to build confidence and hone skills, experiences are biased by perceptions and values that are frequently influenced by tradition, authority, and trial and error. Personal intuition has also been identified as a source of evidence. It is not always clear what is meant by intuition and how it contributes to nursing practice. Intuition is defined as "quick perception of truth without conscious attention or reasoning" (Read et al., 2005, p. 668). While on very rare occasions a "gut feeling" may be reliable, most patients would prefer health care that is based on stronger evidence. Thus, intuition is not one of the most advantageous sources of evidence for driving patient care decisions because nurses are expected to use logical reasoning as critical thinkers and clinical decision makers.

Because of the holistic perspective used in nursing and the collaboration that occurs with other healthcare providers, it is not uncommon for nurses to borrow evidence from other disciplines. For example, pediatric nurses rely heavily on theories of development as a basis for nursing interventions. Borrowed evidence can be useful because it fills gaps that exist in nursing science, provides a basis on which to build new evidence, and can be a stronger type of evidence than sources that are not based on theory and science. When using borrowed evidence, it is important for nurses to consider its fit with the nursing phenomenon. Because nursing offers a unique perspective to patient care, nurses cannot rely solely on borrowed evidence and must build their own body of evidence through scientific research. Scientific research is considered to yield the best source of evidence. There are many different research methods that can be used to describe, explain, and predict phenomena that are central to nursing care. To have an EBP, nurses must emphasize the use of *theory*-derived, research-based information over the use of evidence. obtained through tradition, authority, trial and error, personal experience, and intuition whenever possible.

Not all scientific research is equal. Some types of studies are designed in ways that yield results that nurses can use with confidence. For example, experiments are considered more strongly designed than studies that use surveys. When multiple studies have been conducted about a particular topic, the findings of the studies can be combined into a synthesis. Syntheses provide results that can be used with even more confidence. To rank evidence from strongest to weakest, nurses refer to the *pyramid of evidence*. A figure of the pyramid of evidence is located on the inside front cover of this book. You will find the need to frequently refer to this figure as you learn about appraising evidence and research designs.

Adopting an Evidence-Based Practice

One would think that when there is compelling scientific evidence, findings would quickly and efficiently transition to practice. However, most often this is not the case. Many *barriers* complicate the integration of findings into practice. In fact, it can take as many as 200 years for an innovation to become a standard of care. Consider the history of controlling scurvy in the British Navy.

> In the early days of long sea voyages, scurvy killed more sailors than did warfare, accidents, and other causes. In 1601 an English sea captain, James Lancaster, conducted an experiment to evaluate the effectiveness of lemon juice in preventing scurvy. He commanded four ships that sailed from England on a voyage to India. Three teaspoonfuls of lemon juice were served

KEY TERMS

Theory: A set of concepts linked through propositions to provide an explanation of a phenomenon

Pyramid of evidence: Ranking of evidence from strongest to weakest

Barriers: Factors that limit or prevent change

CRITICAL THINKING EXERCISE 1-2

Consider your last clinical experience. How much was your practice based on scientific research? What other sources of evidence did you use? Divide a circle into sections (like a pie chart) to show how much influence each of the sources of evidence had on the patient care you provided.

every day to the sailors in one of his four ships. These men stayed healthy. The other three ships constituted Lancaster's "control group," as their sailors were not given any lemon juice. On the other three ships, by the halfway point in the journey, 110 out of 278 sailors had died from scurvy.

The results were so clear that one would have expected the British Navy to promptly adopt citrus juice for scurvy prevention on all ships. But it did not become accepted practice. In 1747, about 150 years later, James Lind, a British Navy physician who knew of Lancaster's results, carried out another experiment on the *HMS Salisbury*. To each scurvy patient on this ship, Lind prescribed either two oranges and one lemon, or one of five other supplements. The scurvy patients who got the citrus fruits were cured in a few days and were able to help Dr. Lind care for the other patients.

Certainly, with this further solid evidence of the ability of citrus fruits to combat scurvy, one would expect the British Navy to have quickly adopted this innovation for all ships' crews on long sea voyages. Yet it took another 48 years for this to become standard practice, and scurvy was finally wiped out.

Why were the authorities so slow to adopt the idea of citrus for scurvy prevention? Other competing remedies for scurvy were also being proposed, and each cure had its champions. For example, the highly respected Captain Cook reported that during his Pacific voyages there was no evidence that citrus fruits cured scurvy. In contrast, the experimental work by Dr. Lind, who was not a prominent figure in the field of naval medicine, did not get much attention. This leads one to wonder if the British Navy was typically hesitant to adopt new innovations. But, while it resisted scurvy prevention for years, other innovations, such as new ships and new guns, were readily accepted. (Adapted from Rogers, 2003, p. 7, with permission from Free Press, a division of Simon & Schuster.)

Even when the benefits and advantages of an ***innovation*** have been made evident, adoption can be slow to occur. Even today, studies demonstrate that nurses do not use nursing research in their practice. Recently, a large survey of registered nurses (RNs) from across the United States was conducted. Of the clinical nurses who responded to the survey, more than 54% were not familiar with the term *EBP*. The typical source of information for 67% of these nurses was a colleague. Alarmingly, 58% of the respondents had never used research articles to support clinical practice. Only 18% had ever used a hospital library. Additionally, 77% had never received instruction in the use of electronic resources (Pravikoff, Tanner, & Pierce, 2005).

Overcoming Barriers

Studies demonstrate that the reasons nurses do not draw on research are related to individual and organizational factors. Individual factors are those characteristics that are inherent to the nurse. Organizational factors are related to administration, resources, facilities, and culture of the system. Barriers such as nurses not valuing research, being resistant to change, or lack of time and resources to obtain evidence (Pravikoff et al., 2005) are major reasons nurses do not use research findings at the point of care. In addition, the communication gap between researcher and clinician (Brown, 1995), organizational culture, as well as the inability of individuals to evaluate nursing research have been identified by registered nurses, healthcare administrators, midwives, and oncology nursing staff (Barta, 1995; Carroll et al., 1997; Funk, Champagne, Tornquist, & Wiese, 1995; Funk, Champagne, Wiese, & Tornquist, 1991; Kajermo, Nordstrom, Krusebrant, & Bjorvell, 2000; Meah, Luker, & Cullum, 1996; Pettengill, Gillies, & Clark, 1994; Rutledge, Ropka, Greene, Nail, & Mooney, 1998).

Strategies that do not overcome these barriers do little to promote EBP. To overcome barriers related to individual factors, strategies need to be aimed at instilling an appreciation for EBP, increasing knowledge, developing necessary skills, and changing behaviors. Strategies to overcome organizational barriers must be directed toward creating and maintaining an environment where EBP can flourish. Research has focused on strategies to overcome both individual and organizational factors to bring about change (Camiah, 1997; Caramanica et al., 2002; Dufault, 2001; Janken, Dufault, & Yeaw, 1988; Maljanian, Caramanica, Taylor, MacRae, & Beland, 2002). Practical strategies for successfully overcoming these barriers are summarized in **Table 1-2**.

TABLE 1-2 Strategies for Overcoming Barriers to Adopting an EBP

Barrier	Strategy
Time	
	‹ Devote 15 minutes per day to reading evidence related to a clinical problem.
	‹ Sign up for e-mails that offer summaries of research studies in your area of interest.
	‹ Use a team approach when considering policy changes to distribute the workload among members.
	‹ Bookmark websites having clinical guidelines to promote faster retrieval of information.
	‹ Evaluate available technologies (i.e., PDA) to create time-saving systems that allow quick and convenient retrieval of information at the bedside.
	‹ Negotiate release time from patient care duties to collect, read, and share information about relevant clinical problems.
	‹ Search for already established clinical guidelines because they provide synthesis of existing research.

Barrier	Strategy
Research in practice not valued	
	< Make a list of reasons why healthcare providers should value research, and use this list as a springboard for discussions with colleagues.
	< Invite nurse researchers to share why they are passionate about their work.
	< When disagreements arise about a policy or protocol, find an article that supports your position and share it with others.
	< When selecting a work environment, ask about the organizational commitment to EBP.
	< Link measurement of quality indicators to EBP.
	< Participate in EBP activities to demonstrate professionalism that can be rewarded through promotions or merit raises.
	< Provide recognition during National Nurses Week for individuals involved in EBP projects.
Lack of knowledge about EBP and research	
	< Take a course or attend a continuing education offering on EBP.
	< Invite a faculty member to a unit meeting to discuss EBP.
	< Consult with advanced practice nurses.
	< Attend conferences where clinical research is presented and talk with presenters about their studies.
	< Volunteer to serve on committees that set policies and protocols.
	< Create a mentoring program to bring novice and experienced nurses together.
Lack of technological skills to find evidence	
	< Consult with a librarian about how to access databases and retrieve articles.
	< Learn to bookmark important websites that are sources of clinical guidelines
	< Commit to acquiring computer skills.
Lack of resources to access evidence	
	< Write a proposal for funds to support access to online databases and journals.
	< Collaborate with a nursing program for access to resources.
	< Investigate funding possibilities from others (i.e., pharmaceutical companies, grants).

Barrier	Strategy
Lack of ability to read research	
	‹ Organize a journal club where nurses meet regularly to discuss the evidence about a specific clinical problem.
	‹ Write down questions about an article and ask an advanced practice nurse to read the article and assist in answering the questions.
	‹ Clarify unfamiliar terms by looking them up in a dictionary or research textbook.
	‹ Use one familiar critique format when reading research.
	‹ Identify clinical problems and share them with nurse researchers.
	‹ Participate in ongoing unit-based studies.
	‹ Subscribe to journals that provide uncomplicated explanations of research studies.
Resistance to change	
	‹ Listen to people's concerns about change.
	‹ When considering an EBP project, select one that interests the staff, has a high priority, is likely to be successful, and has baseline data.
	‹ Mobilize talented individuals to act as change agents.
	‹ Create a means to reward individuals who provide leadership during change.
Organization does not embrace EBP	
	‹ Link organizational priorities with EBP to reduce cost and increase efficiency.
	‹ Recruit administrators who value EBP.
	‹ Form coalitions with other healthcare providers to increase the base of support for EBP.
	‹ Use EBP to meet accreditation standards or gain recognition (i.e., Magnet Recognition).

To overcome barriers to using research findings in practice, it can be helpful to use a model to assist in understanding how new ideas come to be accepted practice. The *model of diffusion of innovations* (Rogers, 2003) has been used in the nursing literature for this purpose (Barta, 1995; Carroll et al., 1997; Schmidt & Brown, 2007). You are already familiar with the concept of diffusion. From studying chemistry you know that diffusion involves the movement of molecules from areas of higher concentration

KEY TERM

Model of diffusion of innovations: Model to assist in understanding how new ideas come to be accepted practice to lower concentration. In the same way, innovative nursing practices frequently begin in a small number of institutions and eventually spread or diffuse, becoming standard practice everywhere. The model includes four major concepts: innovation, communication, time, and social system. Rogers (2003) defines diffusion as "the process by which (1) an *innovation* (2) is *communicated* through certain *channels* (3) over *time* (4) among the members of a *social system*" (p. 11). An innovation is an idea, practice, or object that is perceived as new by an individual or other unit of adoption. Before adopting an innovation, individuals seek information about its advantages and disadvantages.

Initially, only a minimal number of individuals, known as *early adopters*, embrace the innovation. With time, early adopters who are opinion leaders, through their interpersonal networks, become instrumental as the diffusion progresses through the social system. Those individuals who are slow or fail to adopt the innovation are known as *laggards*. In the scurvy example, it took about 200 years for the innovation to diffuse throughout the British Navy. You may also be surprised to see how long it has taken other things we take for granted to diffuse throughout American households (**Figure 1-1**).

FIGURE 1-1 Spread of Products to a Quarter of the Population

Product	Year Invented	Years to Spread
Electricity	1873	48
Telephone	1876	35
Automobile	1896	55
Airplane	1903	64
Radio	1906	22
Television	1926	26
VCR	1952	34
Microwave oven	1953	30
PC	1975	16
Cellular phone	1983	13
Internet	1991	7

Source: Adapted from Federal Reserve Bank of Dallas (1996).

CRITICAL THINKING EXERCISE 1-3

Remembering the scurvy example, identify communication channels and social system barriers to the adoption of citrus fruits as a treatment for scurvy. Now, consider how the model of diffusion of innovations could be applied to this situation. How could the physicians have overcome the barriers you identified and convince others to become early adopters so that citrus became accepted practice for the treatment of scurvy?

TEST YOUR KNOWLEDGE 1-1

1. EPB involves all of the following except:
   a. clinical expertise
   b. nursing research
   c. organizational culture
   d. patient preferences

2. Strategies to promote EBP must address (select all that apply):
   a. lack of commitment to EBP
   b. lack of computer skills
   c. lack of time
   d. research in practice not valued

How did you do? 1. c; 2. a, b, c, d

1.2 What Is Nursing Research?

At the end of this section, you will be able to:

< Define research
< Discuss the contribution of research to EBP
< Categorize types of research
< Distinguish between quantitative and qualitative research approaches
< Describe the sections found in research articles

Research: Systematic study that leads to new knowledge and/or solutions to problems or questions

FYI

Research can be categorized as descriptive, explanatory, or predictive; basic or applied; and quantitative or qualitative. Nursing research concerns persons, health, nursing practice, and environment and can be used to generate new knowledge or validate and refine existing knowledge that directly or indirectly influences nursing practice.

Research is a planned and systematic activity that leads to new knowledge and/or the discovery of solutions to problems or questions (Polit & Beck, 2004). Simply stated, research means to search again. But the search must be deliberate and organized as relevant questions are examined. It is essential that established steps be followed.

Following a systematic approach (**Table 1-3**) is more likely to yield results that can be used with confidence. Through research, scientists aim to describe, explain, and predict phenomena. But isn't science supposed to prove that things are true? Sometimes you may hear the phrase "research proves" by others or in the media; however, the use of the word "prove" is inaccurate. Research findings "support" a particular approach or view, because the possibility of error exists in every research study. This underscores why a planned, systematic approach is necessary and why replication studies are important.

Nurses use research to generate new knowledge or validate and refine existing knowledge that directly or indirectly influences nursing practice. In nursing research, the phenomena of interest are persons, health, nursing, and environment. Nurses study patient outcomes, attitudes of nurses, effectiveness of administrative policy, and teaching strategies in nursing education. Nursing research contributes to the development and refinement of theory. But most important, as a baccalaureate-prepared nurse, you will use research as a foundation for EBP. Without research, nursing practice would be based on tradition, authority, trial and error, personal experiences, intuition, and borrowed evidence. This is why you must have the skills to read, evaluate, and apply nursing research so that as an early adopter you can be instrumental in moving an innovation to the point of care.

TABLE 1-3 Steps of the Research Process

1. Identify the research question.
2. Conduct a review of the literature.
3. Identify a theoretical framework.
4. Select a research design.
5. Implement the study.
6. Analyze data.
7. Draw conclusions.
8. Disseminate findings.

Types of Research

There are a variety of terms used to describe the research conducted by scientists. Research can be categorized as *descriptive*, *explanatory*, or *predictive*; *basic* or *applied*; and *quantitative* or *qualitative*. These categories are not necessarily mutually exclusive. For example, a study may be descriptive, applied, and qualitative. While this sounds very complicated, when you understand the definitions, it will become clear.

One way to classify research is by its aims. Descriptive research answers, "What is it?" This category of research is concerned with providing accurate descriptions and can involve observation of a phenomenon in its natural setting. The goal of the explanatory category is to identify the relationships a phenomenon has with individuals, groups, situations, or events. Explanatory studies address "why" or "how" phenomena are related. Predictive research aims to forecast precise relationships between dimensions of phenomena or differences between groups. This category of research addresses "when" the phenomena will occur. **Table 1-4** provides an example of how these different types helped nurses to better understand the phenomenon of pain during chest tube removal.

Another way to classify research is to consider whether findings can be used to solve real world problems. Basic research, sometimes known as bench research, seeks to gain knowledge for the sake of gaining that knowledge. This knowledge may or may not become applicable to practical issues or situations. It may be years before a discovery becomes useful when it is combined with other discoveries. For example, vitamin K was studied for the sake of learning more about its properties. Years later, the knowledge gained about its mechanism of action during coagulation formed the foundation for vitamin K becoming an accepted treatment for bleeding disorders. In contrast, the aim of applied research is to discover knowledge that will solve a clinical problem. The findings typically have immediate application to bring about changes in practice, education, or administration.

Quantitative and *qualitative* are terms that are also used to distinguish among types of research. Philosophical approach, research questions, designs, and data all provide clues to assist you to differentiate between these two methods of classification. Quantitative research views the world as objective. This implies that researchers can separate themselves from phenomena being studied. The focus is on collecting *empirical evidence*, in other words, evidence gathered through the five senses. Researchers quantify observations by using numbers to obtain precise measurements that can later be statistically analyzed. Many quantitative studies test hypotheses. In contrast, the premise of qualitative research is that the world is not objective. There can be multiple

KEY TERMS

Descriptive research: Research concerned with providing accurate descriptions about phenomena

Explanatory research: Research concerned with identifying relationships among phenomena

Predictive research: Research that forecasts precise relationships between dimensions of phenomena or differences between groups

Basic research: Research to gain knowledge for the sake of gaining knowledge

Applied research: Research to discover knowledge that will solve a clinical problem

Quantitative research: Research that uses numbers to obtain precise measurements

Qualitative research: Research that uses words to describe human behaviors

Empirical evidence: Verifiable by experience through the five senses

TABLE 1-4 An Example of Building Knowledge in Nursing Science: Pain and Chest Tube Removal (CTR)

Study	Aim of Research	Findings
Gift, Bolgiano, & Cunningham (1991)	Describe	Individuals reported burning pain and pulling with CTR. Women reported pain more frequently than men.
Puntillo (1994)	Describe	Compared CTR pain with endotracheal suctioning. Patients reported less pain with suctioning than with CTR. "Sharp" was the most frequent adjective for CTR pain.
Carson, Barton, Morrison, & Tribble (1994)	Explain	Patients were assigned to one of four groups for treatment with pain medications: IV morphine, IV morphine and subfascial lidocaine, IV morphine and subfascial normal saline solution, and subfascial lidocaine. There were no significant differences in pain alleviation.
Puntillo (1996)	Predict	Patients were assigned to either placebo normal saline interpleural injection or bupivacaine interpleural injection. There was no significant difference in pain reports.
Houston & Jesurum (1999)	Explain	Examined effect of Quick Release Technique (QRT), a form of relaxation using a breathing technique, during CTR. Patients were randomly assigned to either an analgesic only group or an analgesic with QRT. Combination of QRT with analgesic was not more effective than analgesic alone in reducing pain.
Puntillo & Ley (2004)	Predict	Patients were randomly assigned to one of four combinations of pharmacological and nonpharmacological interventions to reduce pain: 4 mg IV morphine with procedural information, 30 mg IV ketorolac and procedural information, 4 mg IV morphine with procedural and sensory information, and 30 mg IV ketorolac with procedural and sensory information. There were no significant differences between the groups regarding pain intensity, pain distress, or sedation levels.

TABLE 1-5 **Comparisons Between Quantitative and Qualitative Approaches**

Attribute	Quantitative	Qualitative
Philosophical Perspective	One reality that can be objectively viewed by the researcher	Multiple realities that are subjective, occurring within the context of the situation
Type of Reasoning	Primarily deductive	Primarily inductive
Role of Researcher	Controlled and structured	Participative and ongoing
Strategies	< Control and manipulation of situations < Analysis of numbers with statistical tests < Larger number of subjects	< Naturalistic; allows situations to unfold without interference < Analysis of words to identify themes < Smaller numbers of participants
Possible Designs	< Nonexperimental < Correlational < Quasiexperimental < Experimental	< Phenomenology < Ethnography < Grounded Theory < Historical

realities because the context of the situation is different for each person and can change with time. The emphasis is on verbal descriptions that explain human behaviors. In this type of research, the focus is on providing a detailed description of the meanings people give to their experiences. **Table 1-5** provides a comparison of these two approaches.

Another important point about quantitative and qualitative approaches is that there are two styles of reasoning associated with them. *Deductive reasoning*, primarily linked with quantitative research, is reasoning that moves from the general to the particular. For example, researchers use a theory to help them reason out a hunch. If the researcher believes that the position of the body affects circulation, then the researcher could deduce that blood pressure readings taken while lying down will be different from those measured while standing. In contrast, *inductive reasoning* involves reasoning that moves from the particular to the general and is associated with qualitative approaches. By using inductive reasoning, researchers are able to take particular ideas and express an overall general summary about the phenomenon. (**Figure 1-2**).

KEY TERM

Deductive reasoning: Thinking that moves from the general to the particular

Inductive reasoning: Thinking that moves from the particular to the general

FIGURE 1-2   **Ways of Reasoning**

What Makes Up a Research Article?

The development of EBP requires careful attention to research already published. Therefore, it is essential for nurses to identify research studies from among the many other types of articles seen in the literature. The trick is knowing what sections are contained in a research article.

Typically, an *abstract* is the first section of a research article and is usually limited to 100–150 words. The purpose of the abstract is to provide an overview of the study, but the presence of an abstract does not necessarily mean that it is a research article. Because abstracts can frequently be found online, it is usually helpful to read them before printing or requesting a copy of the article. Careful attention to abstracts can avoid wasted time and effort retrieving articles that are not applicable to the clinical question.

The *introduction*, which follows the abstract, contains a statement of the problem and a purpose statement. The problem statement identifies the problem in a broad and general way. For example, a problem statement may read, "falls in hospitalized patients can increase length of stay." Authors usually provide background information and statistics about the problem to convince readers that the problem is significant. The background information provided should set the stage for the purpose statement that describes what was examined in the study. For example, a purpose statement may read, "the purpose of this study was to examine the relationship between time of evening medication administration and time of falls." A good introduction will convince readers that the study was worthy of being conducted.

The third section is the *review of literature*. An unbiased, comprehensive, synthesized description of relevant, previously published studies should be presented. The purpose, sample, design, and significant findings are discussed for each study included in the review. The review should focus on the most recent work in the field but may include older citations if they are considered to be landmark studies. A complete citation is provided for each article so that readers can retrieve them if desired. A well written literature review concludes with a summary of what is known about the problem and identifies gaps in the knowledge base to show readers how the study will add to existing knowledge.

In the research article, there should be a discussion of the *theoretical framework*, which may be a separate section or combined with the review of literature. A theoretical framework often describes the relationships among general concepts and provides linkages to what is being measured in the study. Authors frequently use a model or diagram to explain their theoretical framework.

A major portion of a research article is the *methods section*, which includes a discussion about study design, sample, and data collection. In most cases, authors will explicitly describe the type of design selected to answer the research question. In this section, it is important for the authors to describe the target population and explain how the sample will be obtained. Procedures for collecting data, including the types of measures that will be used, should also be outlined. Throughout this section, authors will provide rationale for decisions made regarding how the study was implemented.

The *results section* is frequently considered to be the most difficult to understand. Here, authors describe the methods used to analyze their data, and the characteristics of the sample are reported. In quantitative studies, data tables are frequently included for interpretation, and authors indicate which findings were significant and which were not. In qualitative studies, themes

KEY TERMS

Theoretical framework: The structure of a study that links the theory concepts to the study variables

Methods section: Major portion of a research article describing the study design, sample, and data collection

Results section: Component of a research article that reports the methods used to analyze data and characteristics of the sample

TEST YOUR KNOWLEDGE 1-2

True/False

1. When reading a quantitative research article, you would expect to see words being analyzed as data.

2. The purpose of research is to prove something is true.

3. It is possible for a descriptive, qualitative study to be applied to practice.

How did you do? 1. F; 2. F; 3. T

KEY TERM

Discussion section:
Portion of a research
article that interprets
results and how
findings extend the
body of knowledge

List of references:
Information for each
article cited in a
research report

are presented that are supported by quotes from participants. After reading the results section, the reader should be confident that the researchers selected the appropriate analysis for the data collected.

The body of a research article concludes with a *discussion section*. Authors provide an interpretation of the results and discuss how the findings extend the body of knowledge. Results should be linked to the review of the literature and theoretical framework. Limitations of the study design are discussed, and sometimes possible solutions are suggested to address them in future studies. Implications for practice, research, and education are proposed. Often it is helpful to read this section after reading the abstract and introduction because it provides clarity by giving you an idea of what is to come.

The article concludes with the *list of references* that are cited in the article. While styles vary, many journals adhere to the guidelines provided in the *Publication Manual of the American Psychological Association*. Because it is often helpful to refer to the original works listed in the reference section, it is wise to obtain a copy of the entire article, including the reference list.

1.3 How Has Nursing Evolved as a Science?

At the end of this section, you will be able to:

‹ Describe the cycle of scientific development
‹ Identify historical occurrences that shaped the development of nursing as a science

Nursing has been described as both an art and a science. Historically, the emphasis was more on the art than the science. But as nursing has developed, the emphasis has shifted. We propose that nursing is the artful use of science to promote the health and well-being of individuals, families, and communities. Thus, nursing is based on scientific evidence that provides the framework for practice. The art of nursing is the blending of science with caring to create a therapeutic relationship in which holistic care is delivered. The profession of nursing is entering a new era in which the emphasis is on EBP, therefore reaffirming the importance of science in nursing.

Cycle of Scientific Development

To fully appreciate nursing as a science, an understanding of the history of research in nursing is necessary. While a grasp of history is important, it can be confusing when one focuses on a list of events and dates to memorize. By focusing on the "what" and "why" of historical occurrences, instead of the "when," the evolution of nursing as a science will be clearer. Nursing has developed in a similar fashion to other sciences. **Figure 1-3** depicts the *cycle of scientific development*. Scientists begin by developing grand theories to explain phenomena. A grand theory is a broad generalization that describes, explains, and predicts occurrences that take place around us. Research is then conducted to test these theories and to discover new knowledge. Conferences and publications result from the need to disseminate research findings. Findings are applied to patient care resulting in changes in practice and are used to refine established theories and propose new ones. This cycle repeats itself, building the science as new discoveries are made. Political and social factors are central to the cycle in that they channel research priorities, funding, and opportunities for dissemination of findings.

FYI

In the early 1900s, nursing research was primarily focused on education preparation.

KEY TERM

Cycle of scientific development: A model of the scientific process

A Glimpse of the Past

Before 1900

Florence Nightingale is considered by most to be the first nurse researcher. One could say that, as an innovator, she was the first nurse to create an EBP. Through the systematic collection and analysis of data, she identified factors that contributed to the high morbidity and mortality rates of British soldiers during the Crimean War (1853–1856). Health reforms, based on her evidence, significantly reduced these rates. Her observations during the war led her to theorize that environmental factors were critical influences on the health of individuals. In 1859 she disseminated her ideas in *Notes on Nursing: What It Is, and What It Is Not* (1946), which continues to be in print today. Even though Nightingale was an innovator in nursing research, it was another 40 years before nursing research reemerged as relevant to nursing practice.

1900–1929

During the first quarter of the 20th century, the focus of nursing research was closely aligned with the social and political climate. Women were empowered by the suffragette movement, thus increasing women's interest in higher education. Nursing education

FIGURE 1-3   **Cycle of Scientific Development**

became the focus of nursing research. The work of nursing leaders such as Lavinia Dock, Adelaide Nutting, Isabel Hampton Robb, and Lillian Wald was instrumental in reforming nursing education. Similarly, the Goldmark Report (1923) identified many inadequacies in nursing education and recommended that advanced educational preparation for nurses was essential. As a result, Yale University School of Nursing became the first university-based nursing program in the United States. Also during this time, the first nursing doctoral program in education was started at Teachers College at Columbia University (1924). These events were important because aligning programs of nursing with universities provided the environment for the generation and dissemination of nursing research.

During this era, nursing was prominent in community health, addressing clinical problems such as pneumonia, infant mortality, and blindness. Because nursing research was still in its infancy, descriptive studies focusing on morbidity and mortality rates of these problems were typically conducted. During this time, the first nursing journal, *American Journal of Nursing*, was published (1900) and the American Nurses Association was established (1912). As a result, nursing was organized and promoted as a profession.

1930–1949

This era was influenced by the Great Depression, which was followed by World War II. During the depression, families did not have money to provide a university education for their children. Consequently, university-based nursing education did not flourish, and nursing research did not advance. As a result of the war, the demand for nurses was so great that nursing education continued to be primarily in hospital-based diploma programs because this was the quickest way to prepare individuals for the workforce. Nurses continued to focus their research on educational issues, and their studies began to be published in the *American Journal of Nursing*. At the close of this era, the Brown Report (1948) was published. Like the Goldmark Report published 25 years earlier, the Brown Report recommended that nurses be educated in university settings. These events illustrate how the social system can impede the diffusion of an innovation as accepted practice.

1950–1969

In the 1950s, significant events occurred that advanced the science of nursing. The innovation of moving nursing education into universities began to become accepted. Through the work of the Western Interstate Commission for Higher Education (1957), nursing research began to be incorporated into graduate curricula, which provided a structure for the advancement of nursing science. Several nursing research centers, including the Institute of Research and Service in Nursing Education at Teachers College (1953), the American Nurses Foundation (1955), the Walter Reed Institute of Research (1957), and the National League for Nursing Research for Studies Service (1959), were established. The availability of funds from government and private foundations increased awards for nursing research grants and predoctoral fellowships.

During the 1950s, the focus of nursing research shifted from nursing education to issues such as the role of the nurse in the healthcare setting and characteristics that made the ideal nurse. Early nursing theories described the nurse–patient relationship (Peplau, 1952) and categorized nursing activity according to human needs (Henderson, 1966). To accommodate the growth of nursing science, journals were needed to disseminate findings. In response, *Nursing Research* (1952) and *Nursing Outlook* (1953) were published, and the *Cumulative Index to Nursing Literature* (CINL) became more prominent.

The scholarly work done by nurses during the 1960s propelled nursing science to a new level. Nursing's major organizations began to call for a shift to research that focused on clinical problems and clinical outcomes. Grand nursing theories began to develop in an attempt to explain the relationships among nursing, health, persons, and environment (King, 1964, 1968; Levine, 1967; Orem, 1971; Rogers, 1963; Roy, 1971). As in the evolution of any science, nursing began to conduct research to test these theories. Because of the volume of nursing scholarship, it became necessary to have new avenues for dissemination of information. Conferences for the sole purpose of exposing nurses to theory and research were organized. For example, in 1965 the American Nurses Association began to sponsor nursing research conferences. Worldwide dissemination became possible with the addition of international journals, such as the *International Journal of Nursing Research* (1963), thus increasing the interest in nursing research.

1970–1989

The hallmark of the 1970s and 1980s was the increased focus on the application of nursing research. The Lysaught Report (1970) confirmed that research focusing on clinical problems was essential but that research on nursing education was still indicated. It was recommended that findings from studies on nursing education be used to improve nursing curricula. During this era, there was a significant increase in the number of nurses with earned doctorates and the availability of funding for research fellowships. The scholarship generated by these doctoral-prepared nurses increased the demand for additional journals. Journals, such as *Advances in Nursing Science* (1978), *Research in Nursing and Health* (1978), and *Western Journal of Nursing Research* (1979), contained nursing research reports and articles about theoretical and practice issues of nursing. In 1977, CINL expanded its scope to include allied health journals, thus changing its name to the *Cumulative Index of Nursing and Allied Health Literature* (CINAHL), which allowed individuals in other disciplines to be exposed to nursing research.

On the national scene, much attention was being given to ethical implications of research involving human subjects. The first regulations to protect human subjects were proposed by the Department of Health, Education, and Welfare in 1973. The formation of institutional review boards to approve all studies was an important result of this regulation. Work regarding ethics in research continued throughout the decade with publication of the Belmont Report (1979). This report identified ethical principles that are foundational for the ethical treatment of individuals participating in studies funded by the federal government. Because the focus of nursing research on clinical problems involving patients was growing, nursing research was being held to the same standards as other clinical research. Thus, the protection of human subjects became an important issue for nurse researchers.

Despite the abundance of research produced during the 1960s and 1970s, little change was occurring in practice. Because nurses recognized a gap between research and practice, the emphasis in the 1980s was on closing this gap. The term *research utilization* was coined to describe the application of nursing research to practice. Activities to move nursing science forward included the Conduct and Utilization Research in Nursing Project. Through this project, current research findings were disseminated to practicing nurses, organizational changes were facilitated, and collaborative clinical research was supported.

The social and political climate of the 1980s included a major change in the financing of health care with the introduction of Diagnosis-Related Groups (DRGs). As a result, significant changes in the way health care was reimbursed occurred. Nurse researchers began to respond to the social and political demand for cost containment by conducting studies on the cost-effectiveness of nursing care. Another important social and political influence on nursing research was the establishment of the National Center for Nursing Research (NCNR) at the National Institutes of Health (1986). This was significant because nursing was awarded a place among other sciences, such as medicine, for guaranteed federal funding.

Activities that took place in the 1980s are consistent with the maturing of nursing as a science. As the body of knowledge grew, specialty organizations popped up allowing individuals to share their expertise in various clinical areas. In addition, the demand for places to publish research continued, and *Applied*

Nursing Research (1988), *Scholarly Inquiry for Nursing Practice* (1987), *Nursing Science Quarterly* (1988), and *Annual Review of Nursing Research* (1983) were started. In 1984, the CINAHL database became electronic. As nursing researchers became more sophisticated in research methods, approaches new to nursing, such as qualitative methods, were embraced. New theories (Benner, 1984; Leininger, 1985; Watson, 1979) that used caring as an important concept were especially amenable to emerging research methods.

1990–1999

In the 1990s, organizations began setting research agendas compatible with the social and political climate. For example, public concerns about the inequities of healthcare delivery were at the forefront. Nursing research that addressed access to health care, issues of diversity, patient outcomes, and the goals of Healthy People 2000 were made priorities. Because nursing research was gaining respect for its contributions to patient care, opportunities for interdisciplinary research became available. In 1993 the NCNR was promoted to full institute status within the National Institutes of Health and was renamed the National Institute of Nursing Research. This was significant because the change in status afforded a larger budget that allowed more nurses to conduct federally funded research. Furthermore, with increased funding, nurse researchers designed more complex studies and began to build programs of research by engaging in a series of studies on a single topic. The knowledge explosion created by technological advances vastly influenced nursing research. Electronic databases provided rapid access for retrieval of nursing literature, and in 1995, CINAHL became accessible to individuals through the Internet. Through email, nursing researchers were able to communicate quickly with colleagues. Software programs to organize and analyze data became readily available, allowing researchers to run more sophisticated analyses. Practice guidelines, from organizations such as the Centers for Disease Control and Prevention, were easily obtained on the Internet. *The Online Journal of Knowledge Synthesis for Nursing* (1993) was the first journal to take advantage of this technology by offering its content in an electronic format. In previous eras, the focus was on the application of findings from a single study to nursing practice. In the early to mid-1990s, the emphasis was on research utilization. The Iowa model of nursing utilization (Titler et al., 1994) and the Stetler model for research utilization (Stetler, 1994) were introduced to facilitate the movement of findings from one research study into nursing practice. In the late 1990s, it became apparent that multiple sources of evidence were desirable for making practice changes. Thus, EBP gained popularity over research utilization, and these models were adapted to fit with the EBP movement (Stetler, 2003; Titler et al., 2001).

2000–Present

In the new millennium, nursing research continues to be influenced by social and political factors. Healthcare reform in the United States, while considered a political priority, remained elusive throughout the decade. While the H.R.3962—Affordable Health Care for America Act was passed, significant changes have yet to be implemented. Nurses will be able to glean potential research questions as changes in health care come about.

Globalization has also been an important influential factor during this decade. With the ease of retrieving information has come the ability to share research findings internationally. Nurses can now access articles about research conducted in a variety of other countries. Nurses in other countries have become more equipped to conduct research as well. Sigma Theta Tau International has significantly broadened its membership to include more chapters in other countries. Globalization also has raised new concerns that provide nurses with opportunities for research. For example, globalization has contributed to an increasing threat of pandemic. Nurses are in an excellent position to study ways to effectively prevent the spread of diseases or contribute to the implementation of strategies to care for infected populations.

During this decade, there has been a renewed focus on patient safety and outcomes. The American Nurses Association has been instrumental in creating the National Database of Nursing Quality Indicators (NDNQI). The purpose of this database is to collect and evaluate unit-specific nurse-sensitive data from hospitals in the United States. Participating facilities receive unit-level comparative data reports to use for quality improvement purposes. Refer to **Table 1-6** for a listing of the current NDNQI Measures. Many of these measures are used by hospitals that have received Magnet Recognition for nursing excellence.

Another challenge being faced in the new millennium is a nursing shortage. Topics such as nurse–patient ratios and interventions to decrease length of stay are priorities for research. Other changes have occurred in nursing education. For example, the Doctor of Nursing Practice degree has been recommended

CRITICAL THINKING EXERCISE 1-4

Ten years from now nursing students will study how historical occurrences have shaped the evolution of nursing as a science. Discuss four current events that will be considered to have influenced the development of nursing science.

TABLE 1-6 2010 NDNQI Measures

Nursing Staff Skill Mix
Nursing Hours per Patient Day
Assault/Injury Assault Rates
Catheter-Associated Urinary Tract Infection Rate
Central Line-Associated Bloodstream Infection Rate
Fall/Injury Fall Rates
Hospital/Unit Acquired Pressure Ulcer Rates
Nurse Turnover Rate
Pain Assessment/Intervention/Reassessment Cycles Completed
Peripheral IV Infiltration Rate
Physical Restraint Prevalence
RN Education/Certification
RN Survey
Practice Environment Scale
Job Satisfaction
Ventilator-Associated Pneumonia Rate

Source: Adapted from ANA, 2010.

TEST YOUR KNOWLEDGE 1-3

True/False

1. Nursing research popular in the 1950s involved the study of nursing students.

2. Grand nursing theories were first introduced in the 1980s.

3. In the 1980s, DRGs were a driving force by focusing nursing research on cost-effectiveness.

4. Technological advances created a knowledge explosion that has vastly influenced nursing research.

5. Each historical era contributed to the development of nursing science.

How did you do? 1. T; 2. F; 3. T; 4. T; 5. T

as the minimal educational requirement for those entering advanced practice nursing. Nurses who are prepared at the doctoral level and practice in clinical settings can serve as leaders in EBP.

1.4 What Lies Ahead?

At the end of this section, you will be able to:

< Identify factors that will continue to move nursing forward as a science
< Discuss what future trends may influence how nurses use evidence to improve the quality of patient care

The factors similar to those who have propelled nursing research forward through history will continue to be influential into the future. In the 21st century, nursing research will grow in importance as EBP becomes more widely established and patient outcomes come under increased scrutiny. Nursing research agendas will be driven by social and political influences.

The cycle of scientific development must continue in order to expand the body of nursing knowledge and for nurses to be recognized for their contributions to health care. Midrange and practice theories that are more useful in clinical settings need to be developed. Nursing research must include studies that replicate previous studies with different populations to confirm prior findings. Studies that demonstrate nursing's contribution to positive health outcomes will be especially important. A commitment to the continued preparation of nurses as scientists is vital to achieve excellence in nursing research. It will be increasingly important for nurses to advocate for monies and draw on new funding sources. Interdisciplinary and international research will become increasingly important as complex health problems are addressed. Technology will continue to provide innovative ways to communicate research findings to a broader audience. Research topics that are most likely to be priorities are listed in **Table 1-7**.

Nursing will continue to be challenged to bridge the gap between research and practice. EBP offers the greatest hope of moving research findings to the point of care. Nursing education must prepare nurses to appreciate the importance of basing patient care on evidence. Educators need to create innovative strategies that teach students to identify clinical problems, use technology to retrieve evidence, read and analyze research, weigh evidence, and implement change (Schmidt & Brown, 2007). Nurses must accept responsibility for creating their own EBP and collaborating with others to improve patient care.

FYI

The Doctor of Nursing Practice degree has been recommended as the minimal educational requirement for those entering advanced practice nursing. Nurses who are prepared at the doctoral level and practice in clinical settings can serve as leaders in EBP.

TABLE 1-7 **Nursing Research Priorities**

Bioterrorism
Chronic illness
Cultural and ethnic considerations
End of life/palliative care
Genetics
Gerontology
Healthcare delivery systems
Health disparities
Health promotion
HIV/AIDS
Management of pandemics/natural disasters
Mental health
Nursing informatics
Patient outcomes/quality of care
Safe administration of medications
Symptom management

Nurses who work in clinical settings and are prepared at the doctoral level, are especially well positioned to move EBP forward. It will be expected that healthcare facilities embrace EBP to achieve Magnet Recognition (see p. 47). International collaborations, such as The Joanna Briggs Institute, will be essential so that when best practices are identified they can be easily shared.

The Challenge

Make a commitment to be an innovator when it comes to EBP! You are already well on your way to having the knowledge and skills needed to overcome barriers that laggards often cite as reasons for not adopting EBP. As you learn

CRITICAL THINKING EXERCISE 1-5

Recall a question you encountered during your last clinical experience. How might you have answered that question using an EBP approach?

TEST YOUR KNOWLEDGE 1-4

1. Nurses who use EBP are best described as:
   a. change agents
   b. early adopters
   c. innovators
   d. laggards

True/False

2. As the cycle of science continues, more mid-range and practice theories will emerge that will be useful in clinical settings.

How did you do? 1. B; 2. T

more through studying this text, don't go through the pages just to pass an exam. Learn the material so you can carry it with you throughout your career. To fulfill your commitment, begin with your next clinical assignment by adopting one or two of the strategies suggested in Table 1-1. Over the course of your career, your actions will convince laggards that EBP really does create excellence in patient care.

1.5 Keeping It Ethical

At the end of this section, you will be able to:

‹ Identify four unethical studies involving the violation of the rights of human subjects

While scientific research has made significant contributions to the good of society and the health of individuals, these contributions have not come without cost. In the past, studies have been conducted without regard for the rights of human subjects. It is surprising to learn that even after national and international guidelines were established, unethical scientific research continued. Four major studies that have been noted for their unethical conduct are: 1) the Nazi experiments, 2) the Tuskegee study, 3) the Jewish Chronic Disease Hospital study, and 4) the Willowbrook studies.

During World War II, physicians conducted medical studies on prisoners in Nazi concentration camps (National Cancer Institute, n.d.). Most of the *Nazi experiments* were aimed at determining the limits of human endurance and learning ways to treat medical problems faced by the German armed forces. For example, physicians exposed prisoners of war to mustard gas, made them drink seawater, and exposed them to high altitude experiments. People were frozen or nearly frozen to death so that physicians could study the body's response to hypothermia. They infected prisoners with diseases so that the natural course of disease processes could be followed. Physicians also continued Hitler's genocide program by sterilizing Jewish, Polish, and Russian prisoners through X-ray and castration. The War Crimes Tribunal at Nuremberg indicted 23 physicians, many of whom were leading members of the German medical community. They were found guilty for their willing participation in conducting "crimes against humanity." Seven physicians were sentenced to death, and the remaining 23 were imprisoned. As a result, the *Nuremberg Code*, a section in the written verdict, outlined what constitutes acceptable medical research, forming the basis for codes of ethical conduct internationally. The experiments conducted were so horrific that debate continues about whether the findings from these Nazi studies, or other unethical studies, should be published or even used (Luna, 1997; McDonald, 1985; Miller & Rosenstein, 2002), and professional organizations, such as the American Medical Association (AMA), have published position papers about this dilemma (AMA, 1998).

In the 1930s, the *Tuskegee study* was initiated to examine the natural course of untreated syphilis (National Cancer Institute, n.d.). In this study conducted by the United States Public Health Service, black men at Tuskegee were recruited to participate. Informed consent was not obtained, and many of the volunteers were led to believe that procedures, such as spinal taps, were free special medical care. Approximately 400 men with syphilis were compared to about 200 men without syphilis. Within 6 years, it was apparent that many more of the infected men had complications when compared to uninfected men, and by 10 years, the death rate was twice as high in the infected men as compared to the uninfected men. Even when penicillin was found to be effective for the treatment of syphilis in the 1940s, the study continued until 1972, and subjects were neither informed about nor offered treatment of penicillin.

 FYI

In the past research as conducted with human subjects who were not fully informed of the purpose and/or methods of the study. Today, students must be reviewed to assure that human subjects are protected.

KEY TERMS

Nazi experiments: An example of unethical research using human subjects during WWII

Nuremberg Code: Ethical code of conduct for research that uses human subjects

Tuskegee study: A study during which subjects were denied treatment so that the effects of the disease could be studied.

CRITICAL THINKING EXERCISE 1-6

Do you think that the findings from unethical studies should be published? Why or why not?

KEY TERM

Jewish Chronic Disease Hospital study: An unethical injection of cancer cells to subjects without their consent

Willowbrook studies: An unethical study involving coercion of parents to allow their children to participate in the study in exchange for admission to a long-term care facility

In 1963, the *Jewish Chronic Disease Hospital study* began and involved the injection of foreign, live cancer cells into hospitalized patients with chronic diseases (National Cancer Institute, n.d.). The purpose of the study was to examine whether the body's inability to reject cancer cells was due to cancer or the presence of a debilitating chronic illness. Because earlier studies indicated that injected cancer cells were rejected, researchers hypothesized that debilitated patients would reject the cancer cells at a substantially slower rate than healthy participants. When discussing the study with potential subjects, researchers failed to inform them about the injection of cancer cells because researchers did not want to frighten them. Although researchers obtained oral consent, they did not document the consent, claiming the documentation was unnecessary because it was a standard of care to perform much more dangerous procedures without consent forms. Researchers also failed to inform physicians caring for the patients about the study. At a review conducted by the Board of Regents of the State University of New York, researchers were found guilty of scientific misconduct, including fraud and deceit.

Also in the 1960s, a series of studies was conducted to observe the natural course of infectious hepatitis by deliberately infecting children admitted to the Willowbrook State School, an institution for mentally disabled children (National Cancer Institute, n.d.). During the *Willowbrook studies*, administrators claimed overcrowded conditions and stopped admitting patients; however, children could be admitted to the facility if they participated in the hepatitis program. Because places to care for children with mental disabilities were limited, many parents found themselves unable to obtain care for their children and fell victim to being coerced to allow their children to participate in the study.

TEST YOUR KNOWLEDGE 1-5

Match the following

1. Nazi Medical Experiments

2. Tuskegee Study

3. Jewish Chronic Disease Hospital Study

4. Willowbrook Study

a. infected subjects with cancer cells

b. coerced parents to allow children in study

c. exposed subjects to cold

d. failed to treat subjects with penicillin

How did you do? 1. c; 2. d; 3. a; 4. b

RAPID **REVIEW**

 EBP involves: 1) practice grounded in research evidence integrated with theory, 2) clinician expertise, and 3) patient preferences.

 Tradition, authority, trial and error, personal experiences, intuition, borrowed evidence, and scientific research are sources of evidence.

 Individual and organizational barriers can prevent adoption of EBP.

 Innovations are adopted by the diffusion of the innovation over time through communication channels among the members of a social system.

 Research is a planned and systematic activity that leads to new knowledge and/or the discovery of solutions to problems or questions.

 Scientific research offers the best evidence for nursing practice.

 Nurses use the pyramid of evidence to rank evidence from strongest to weakest.

 Research can be categorized as descriptive, explanatory, or predictive; basic or applied; and quantitative or qualitative.

 By analyzing words, qualitative research focuses on the meanings individuals give to their experiences. Quantitative research views the world as objective and focuses on obtaining precise measurements that are later analyzed.

 Most research articles include an abstract, introduction, review of literature, theoretical framework, and methods, results, and discussion sections, and conclude with a list of references.

 The cycle of scientific development involves theory, research, dissemination, and application. Social and political factors are central to the cycle.

 The cycle of scientific development can be seen in each historical era.

 Social and political factors will continue to influence nursing research.

 For nurses to use EBP to improve patient care, they must be committed to being early adopters of innovations.

 NDNQI is a national database that involves measurement and reporting of nursing sensitive outcomes.

 Four studies are recognized for their gross violation of human rights: Nazi medical experiments, the Tuskegee study, the Jewish Chronic Disease Hospital study, and the Willowbrook studies.

APPLY WHAT YOU HAVE LEARNED

On the companion website that accompanies this textbook, there is a collection of materials that will help you apply what you are learning. Articles, checklists, policies, and templates are included. There are two articles for this chapter that you can use to reinforce what you have learned. Locate the link for Chapter 1. You will find an article by Pipe et al. (2008) and another article by Flanagan, Carroll, and Hamilton (2010). One of these articles used qualitative methods and the other used quantitative methods. Identify which is which. After you have done that, for each article identify the various sections that make up a research article. You may want to share these articles with nurses during your next clinical experience and consider ways the recommendations can be incorporated into practice.

REFERENCES

American Medical Association. (1998). *CEJA Report 5—A-98 Information from unethical experiments*. Retrieved August 15, 2010, from http://www.ama-assn.org/ama1/pub/upload/mm/369/ceja_5a98.pdf

American Nurses Association. (2010). National Database of Nursing Quality Indicators: Guidelines for Data Collection on the American Nurses Association's National Quality Forum Endorsed Measures: Nursing Care Hours per Patient Day, Skill Mix, Falls, Falls with Injury. Retrieved September 14, 2010 from https://www.nursingquality.org/

Barnsteiner, J., & Prevost, S. (2002). How to implement evidence-based practice. Some tried and true pointers. *Reflections on Nursing Leadership, 28*(2), 18–21.

Barta, K. M. (1995). Information-seeking, research utilization, and barriers to research utilization of pediatric nurse educators. *Journal of Professional Nursing, 11*, 49–57.

Benner, P. (1984). *From novice to expert: Excellence and power in clinical nursing practice*. Menlo Park, CA: Addison-Wesley.

Brown, G. D. (1995). Understanding barriers to basing nursing practice upon research: A communication model approach. *Journal of Advanced Nursing, 21*, 154–157.

Camiah, S. (1997). Utilization of nursing research in practice and application strategies to raise research awareness amongst nurse practitioners: A model for success. *Journal of Advanced Nursing, 26*, 1193–1202.

Caramanica, L., Maljanian, R., McDonald, D., Taylor, S. K., MacRae, J. B., & Beland, D. K. (2002). Evidence-based nursing practice, part 1: A hospital and university collaborative. *JONA, 32*, 27–30.

Carroll, D. L., Greenwood, R., Lynch, K. E., Sullivan, J. K., Ready, C. H., & Fitzmaurice, J. B. (1997). Barriers and facilitators to the utilization of nursing research. *Clinical Nurse Specialist, 11*, 207–212.

Carson, M. M., Barton, D. M., Morrison, L. G., & Tribble, C. G. (1994). Managing pain during mediastinal chest tube removal. *Heart & Lung, 23*, 500–505.

Cochrane, A. L. (1971). *Effectiveness and efficiency. Random reflections on health services.* Abingdon, Berks: Nuffield Provincial Hospitals Trust.

Dufault, M. A. (2001). A program of research evaluating the effects of a collaborative research utilization model. *The Online Journal of Knowledge Synthesis for Nursing, 8*(3).

Federal Reserve Bank of Dallas. (1996). *The economy at light speed: Technology and growth in the information age—and beyond.* Retrieved August 15, 2010, from http://www.dallasfed.org/fed/annual/1999p/ar96.pdf

Flanagan, J. M., Carroll, D. L., & Hamilton, G. A. (2010). The long-term lived experience of patients with implantable cardioverter defibrillators. *MED-SURG Nursing, 19*, 113–119.

Funk, S. G., Champagne, M. T., Tornquist, E. M., & Wiese, R. A. (1995). Administrators' views on barriers to research utilization. *Applied Nursing Research, 8*, 44–49.

Funk, S. G., Champagne, M. T., Wiese, R. A., & Tornquist, E. M. (1991). Barriers to using research findings in practice: The clinician's perspective. *Applied Nursing Research, 4*, 90–95.

Gift, A. G., Bolgiano, C. S., & Cunningham, J. (1991). Sensations during chest tube removal. *Heart & Lung, 20*, 131–137.

Henderson, V. (1966). *The nature of nursing.* New York: Macmillan.

Houston, S., & Jesurum, J. (1999). The quick relaxation technique: Effect on pain associated with chest tube removal. *Applied Nursing Research, 12*, 196–205.

Ingersoll, G. L. (2000). Evidence-based nursing: What it is and what it isn't. *Nursing Outlook, 48*, 151–152.

Janken, J. K., Dufault, M. A., & Yeaw, E. M. S. (1988). Research round tables: Increasing student/staff nurse awareness of the relevancy of research to practice. *Journal of Professional Nursing, 4*, 186–191.

Kajermo, K. N., Nordstrom, G., Krusebrant, A., & Bjorvell, H. (2000). Perceptions of research utilization: Comparisons between health care professionals, nursing students and a reference group of nurse clinicians. *Journal of Advanced Nursing, 31*(1), 99–109.

King, I. M. (1964). Nursing theory: Problems and prospects. *Nursing Science, 1*, 394–403.

King, I. M. (1968). A conceptual frame of reference for nursing. *Nursing Research, 17*(1), 27–31.

Leininger, M. (1985). Transcultural care diversity and universality: A theory of nursing. *Nursing and Health Care, 6*, 209–212.

Levine, M. E. (1967). The four conservation principles of nursing. *Nursing Forum, 6*, 45–59.

Luna, F. (1997). Vulnerable populations and morally tainted experiments. *Bioethics, 11*, 256–264.

Maljanian, R., Caramanica, L., Taylor, S. K., MacRae, J. B., & Beland, D. K. (2002). Evidence-based nursing practice, part 2: Building skills through research roundtables. *JONA, 32*(2), 85–90.

McDonald, A. (1985). Ethics and editors: When should unethical research be published? *Canadian Medical Association Journal, 133,* 803–805.

Meah, S., Luker, K. A., & Cullum, N. A. (1996). An exploration of midwives' attitudes to research and perceived barriers to research utilisation. *Midwifery, 12,* 73–84.

Melnyk, B. M. (1999). Building a case for evidence-based practice: Inhalers vs. nebulizers. *Pediatric Nursing, 25*(1), 102–104.

Melnyk, B. M., & Fineout-Overholt, E. (2005). Making the case for evidence-based practice. In B. M. Melnyk & E. Fineout-Overholt (Eds.), *Evidence-based practice in nursing and healthcare: A guide to best practice* (pp. 3–37). Philadelphia: Lippincott Williams & Wilkins.

Miller, F. G., & Rosenstein, D. L. (2002). Reporting of ethical issues in publications of medical research. *The Lancet, 360,* 1326–1328.

National Cancer Institute. (n.d.). *Human participant protections education for research teams.* Retrieved June 9, 2007, from http://cme.cancer.gov/ clinical-trials/learning/humanparticipant-protections.asp

Nightingale, F. (1946). *Notes on nursing: What it is, and what it is not.* London: Harrison.

Orem, D. E. (1971). *Nursing: Concepts of practice.* New York: McGraw-Hill.

Peplau, H. E. (1952). *Interpersonal relations in nursing: A conceptual frame of reference for psychodynamic nursing.* New York: Putnam.

Pettengill, M. M., Gillies, D. A., & Clark, C. C. (1994). Factors encouraging and discouraging the use of nursing research findings. *Journal of Nursing Scholarship, 26,* 143–147.

Pipe, T. B., Kelly, A., LeBrun, G., Schmidt, D., Atherton, P., & Robinson, C.. (2008). A prospective descriptive study exploring hope, spiritual well-being, and quality of life in hospitalized patients. *MEDSURG Nursing, 17,* 247–257.

Polit, D. F., & Beck, C. T. (2004). *Nursing research: Principles and methods* (7th ed.). Philadelphia: Lippincott Williams & Wilkins.

Pravikoff, D. S., Tanner, A. B., & Pierce, S. T. (2005). Readiness of U.S. nurses for evidence-based practice. *AJN, 105*(9), 40–51.

Puntillo, K. A. (1994). Dimensions of procedural pain and its analgesic management in critically ill surgical patients. *American Journal of Critical Care, 3,* 116–122.

Puntillo, K. A. (1996). Effects of interpleural bupivacaine on pleural chest tube removal pain: A randomized control trial. *American Journal of Critical Care, 5,* 102–108.

Puntillo, K., & Ley, S. J. (2004). Appropriately timed analgesics: Control pain due to chest tube removal. *American Journal of Critical Care, 13,* 292–301.

Read, A. W., et al. (Eds.). (2005). *Funk & Wagnalls new international dictionary of the English language* (comprehensive millennium edition, Vol. 1). Naples, FL: Typhoon International.

Rogers, E. M. (2003). *Diffusion of innovations* (5th ed.). New York: Free Press.

Rogers, M. E. (1963). Some comments on the theoretical basis of nursing practice. *Nursing Science, 1*(1), 11–13, 60–61.

Roy, C. (1971). Adaptation: A basis for nursing practice. *Nursing Outlook, 19*, 254–257.

Rutledge, D. N., Ropka, M., Greene, P. E., Nail, L., & Mooney, K. H. (1998). Barriers to research utilization for oncology staff nurses and nurse managers/clinical nurse specialists. *Oncology Nursing Forum, 25*, 497–506.

Sackett, D. L., Rosenberg, W. M. C., Gray, J. A. M., Haynes, R. B., & Richardson,

W. S. (1996). Evidence based medicine: What it is and what it isn't. *British Medical Journal, 312*, 71–72.

Schmidt, N. A., & Brown, J. M. (2007). Use of the innovation-decision process teaching strategy to promote evidence based practice. *Journal of Professional Nursing, 23*, 150–156.

Stetler, C. B. (1994). Refinement of the Stetler/Marram model for application of research findings to practice. *Nursing Outlook, 42*, 15–25.

Stetler, C. B. (2003). Role of the organization in translating research into evidence-based practice. *Outcomes Management, 7*, 97–105.

Stevens, K. R. (2004). ACE Star model of EBP: knowledge transformation. *Academic Center for Evidence-based Practice.* Retrieved August 15, 2010, from http://www.acestar.uthscsa.edu/Learn_model.htm

Straus, S. E., Richardson, W. S., Glasziou, P., & Haynes, R. B. (2005). *Evidence-based medicine. How to practice and teach EBM* (3rd ed.). Edinburgh, Scotland: Churchill Livingstone.

The Cochrane Collaboration. (n.d.). *What is* The Cochrane Collaboration? Retrieved September 7, 2006, from http://www.cochrane.org/docs/ descrip. htm? version

Titler, M. G., Kleiber, C., Steelman, V., Goode, C., Rakel, B., Barry-Walker, J., . . . Buckwalter, K. (1994). Infusing research into practice to promote quality care. *Nursing Research, 43*, 307–313.

Titler, M. G., Kleiber, C., Steelman, V. J., Rakel, B. A., Budreau, G., Everett, L. Q., Buckwalter, K. C., . . . Goode, C. J. (2001). The Iowa model of evidence-based practice to promote quality care. *Critical Care Nursing Clinics of North America, 13*, 497–509.

Watson, J. (1979). *Nursing: The philosophy and science of caring.* Boston: Little, Brown.

Youngblut, J. M., & Brooten, D. (2001). Evidence-based nursing practice: Why is it important? *AACN Clinical Issue, 12*, 468–476.

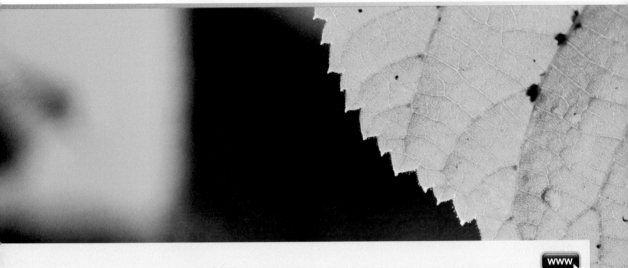

www

CHAPTER OBJECTIVES

At the end of this chapter, you will be able to:

< Discuss contributions to evidence-based practice (EBP) made by nurses practicing in various roles

< Examine organizational strategies that facilitate EBP

< Describe regional resources that foster collaborative EBP

< Identify national resources committed to EBP

< List international organizations that are committed to the promotion of EBP

< Discuss international and national initiatives designed to promote ethical conduct

< Describe the rights that must be protected and the three ethical principles that must be upheld when conducting research

< Explain the composition and functions of institutional review boards (IRBs) at the organizational level

< Discuss the nurse's role as patient advocate in research situations

KEY TERMS

autonomous
Belmont Report
beneficence
Declaration of Helsinki
exempt
expedited review
full review
human rights
individual nurse level

informed consent
institutional review boards
international level
justice
minimal risk
model of EBP levels of
   collaboration
national level
obligations

organizational level
regional level
research imperative
respect for persons
therapeutic imperative
translational research
   model

CHAPTER 2

Using Evidence Through Collaboration to Promote Excellence in Nursing Practice

Emily Griffin and Marita G. Titler

2.1 The Five Levels of Collaboration

At the end of this section, you will be able to:

- < Discuss contributions to EBP made by nurses practicing in various roles
- < Examine organizational strategies that facilitate EBP
- < Describe regional resources that foster collaborative EBP
- < Identify national resources committed to EBP
- < List international organizations that are committed to the promotion of EBP

In the late 1800s, Florence Nightingale followed many of the principles of EBP. Principles of EBP have been present for many years; however, until recently this process was not called EBP nor was EBP fully acknowledged as having an important impact on patient care. A culture of EBP is emerging within nursing through collaborative efforts by nurses and healthcare organizations, as well as by regional, national, and international entities. Nurses need to collaborate at these five levels. **Figure 2-1** illustrates the *model of EBP levels of collaboration*.

FYI

A culture of EBP is emerging within nursing through collaborative efforts by nurses and healthcare organizations, as well as by regional, national, and international entities. Nurses need to collaborate at these five levels.

FIGURE 2-1 **Model of EBP Levels of Collaboration**

In the model, the five levels are intertwined with one another. An international entity can be a resource for staff nurses, and they can reciprocate and contribute to EBP nationally and internationally. Nurses or organizations may use regional-level resources to help move EBP projects forward. In return, nurses or organizations assist regional or national resources to advance EBP. For example, a staff nurse may use the Joanna Briggs Institute to find evidence to support an EBP project. When the project is complete, the staff nurse disseminates her work by publishing the project and presenting at an annual Sigma Theta Tau International (STTI) EBP conference. At the conference, the nurse educates other nurses so that best practices can be adopted at their organizations.

Individual Nurse Level

At the *individual nurse level*, nurses play an integral role in advancing EBP. While it takes a team approach to be successful with EBP, each nurse has a unique set of skills to contribute that helps to advance EBP. Identifying clinical issues, education approaches, and implementation strategies are examples of some contributions that nurses can make to the team. Nurses can assume various roles for the team such as project leader, opinion leader, and mentor.

Staff nurses are an important link between research and the point of care. They are clinical experts and know how to access unit resources. They can contribute by problem solving, collaborating with the team, and acting as change champions. Because staff nurses are integral to EBP, many organizations provide performance criteria for promoting best practices. For example, performance criteria for staff nurses may include critical thinking, continual questioning of practice, participating in making EBP practice changes, serving as leaders of change in their site of care delivery, and participating in evaluating evidence-based changes in practice (Titler, 2006; see **Table 2-1**).

TABLE 2-1 Sample EBP Performance Criteria for Nursing Roles

Staff Nurse (RN)
- Questions current practices
- Participates in implementing changes in practice based on evidence
- Participates as a member of an EBP project team
- Reads evidence related to one's practice
- Participates in quality improvement (QI) initiatives
- Suggests resolutions for clinical issues based on evidence

Nurse Manager (NM)
- Creates a microsystem that fosters critical thinking
- Challenges staff to seek out evidence to resolve clinical issues and improve care
- Role models EBP
- Uses evidence to guide operations and management decisions
- Uses performance criteria about EBP in evaluation of staff

Advanced Practice Nurse (APN)
- Serves as coach and mentor in EBP
- Facilitates locating evidence
- Synthesizes evidence for practice
- Uses evidence to write/modify practice standards
- Role models use of evidence in practice
- Facilitates system changes to support use of EBPs

Nurse Executive
- Ensures the governance reflects EBP if initiated in councils and committees
- Assigns accountability for EBP
- Ensures explicit articulation of organizational and department commitment to EBP
- Modifies mission and vision to include EBP language
- Provides resources to support EBPs by direct care providers
- Articulates value of EBP to chief executive officer and governing board
- Role models EBP in administrative decision making
- Hires and retains NMs and APNs with knowledge and skills in EBP
- Provides learning environment for EBP
- Uses evidence in leadership decisions

Source: Adapted from Titler, 2006, p. 472.

FYI

APNs are ideally positioned to be opinion leaders and change champions. To promote consistent practice changes, this core group of nurses should include nurses across different shifts to facilitate practice changes.

Nurse managers are also essential to EBP. Their aim is to "get their units on board" with practice changes. They help to set unit expectations by discussing projects with staff and other healthcare providers. Managers facilitate progress by rewarding nurses involved in EBP and assisting noncompliant nurses to improve their performances. "The nurse manager's commitment is critical to project success and can make a significant impact on project outcomes" (Cullen, 2006, p. 471).

Advanced practice nurses (APNs) are EBP experts who facilitate appraisal and synthesis of the literature for the purpose of improving nursing practice. They often are mentors and are thus important to the advancement of EBP in the clinical setting (Shirey, 2006). They help with problem solving, planning, leading, and coaching. As clinical experts, APNs are ideally positioned to be opinion leaders and change champions. Opinion leaders are experts in their fields who facilitate adoption of an innovation through modeling and peer influence. Their sphere of influence is broad, usually encompassing several units or departments (Doumit, Gattellari, Grimshaw, & O'Brien, 2007). Change champions are also experts in their fields and facilitate change by persistence. They often work with a core group of nurses who are also working toward making EBP changes. To promote consistent practice changes, this core group of nurses should include nurses across different shifts to facilitate practice changes.

Nurse executives are responsible for establishing the culture for EBP. They create a culture where making evidence-based decisions and changing practice are valued. It is important for nursing leaders to create a vision that includes EBP and identify methods to sustain this vision. Shirey (2006) states that there is an expectation that nurse leaders will work to maximize the capabilities of the staff and partner with key professional organizations with goals to advance EBP.

Table 2-1 provides examples of performance criteria that may be expected at the individual nurse level (Titler, 2006). It is important to remember that each nurse is part of a team that is moving EBP forward. Specific advantages to teamwork include division of workload, comprehensive problem solving, building "buy-in," and expanding expertise. Overall, teamwork builds a more comprehensive plan for EBP.

Organizational Level

National initiatives and accrediting bodies are supporting EBP and urging healthcare systems to base patient care on evidence. At the *organizational level*, healthcare systems are finding increased interest from nurses wanting to practice from a research base, needing time to explore EBP, and desiring to develop excellence in the profession. "The goal of achieving excellence requires development of an organizational capacity, culture, and vision for evidence-based practice" (Cullen, Greiner, Greiner, Bombei, & Comried, 2005, p. 127). Healthcare organizations with a vision to provide excellence in nursing need to have an infrastructure that accommodates what is needed to implement EBP. As organizations restructure to focus on EBP, a culture of EBP is embraced. This culture sets a tone so that nurses know what is valued within the organization. One method for developing this culture is adding value statements about EBP to organizational mission or vision statements. For example, at the University of Iowa Hospitals and Clinics (UIHC), the mission statement is, "to provide high quality patient care based on our strong commitments to practice, education, research, innovation, and collaboration" (UIHC Department of Nursing, 2007). This statement outlines expectations for nursing care at this organization. Other factors that build a culture for EBP include setting performance expectations for individual nurses, integrating EBP into governance structures, and providing recognition and rewards for involvement in EBP. To help build organizational capacity for EBP, it is recommended that responsibility be designated to at least one committee (Cullen et al., 2005). One recommendation is to create four committees: an EBP steering committee, an EBP committee, specialty focus teams, and nursing policy and procedure committees. The EBP steering committee would oversee the other three committees, allocate the resources, and provide support and direction for the work involved with adopting EBP (Hudson, 2005).

At the organizational level, the focus is not only about developing a capacity for EBP to take place but also facilitating the adoption of individual EBP protocols. As a social system, organizations can facilitate or impede change. The *translational research model* (**Figure 2-2**), which is based on Rogers's model on diffusion of innovation (Rogers, 2003), provides specific strategies that organizations can use to improve adoption of an evidence-based innovation (Titler, 2006; Titler & Everett, 2001). Specific components of this model describe how characteristics of the innovation, communication process, social system, and users lead to the adoption of innovations. Organizational characteristics that influence the use of EBP include providing expectations that policies are evidence based, access to clinical researchers, authority to change practice, and support from peers, administrators, and other disciplines (Titler & Everett, 2001).

There are four specific interventions described in this model that social systems can use to promote excellence in nursing and move EBP forward. These interventions include modifying policies and standards, modifying medical record forms, senior administrator education and support, and orientation of new staff members.

FYI

Librarians are important resources for EBP, making them critical partners. They are experts in searching databases such as the *Cumulative Index of Nursing and Allied Health* (CINAHL) and PubMed, and many healthcare librarians specialize in searching for evidence in nursing and medicine.

KEY TERMS

Organizational level: When nurses in an organization affect practice changes

Translational research model: Provides specific strategies organizations can use to improve adoption of an evidence-based innovation

FIGURE 2-2 **Translational Research Model**

*Based on Rogers's model of Diffusion of Innovation.
Source: Titler, M.G., & Everett, L.Q. (2001). Translating Research into Practice: Considerations for Critical Care Investigators. *Critical Care Nursing Clinics of North America, 13*(4), 587–604. Reproduced with permission from Marita G. Titler, PhD, RN, FAAN; for permission to use and/or reproduce the model, please contact Dr. Titler.

The first intervention is for organizations to include EBP within policies and standards (Titler & Everett, 2001). Policies should be based on evidence, and there should be an attached bibliography with each policy identifying the evidence. For example, the UIHC developed a set of grading schema for each statement within a policy. There is a corresponding article from the bibliography included with each policy. To indicate the type of evidence available, each statement is assigned an R, N, E, or L that corresponds to research article, national guideline, expert opinion, or literature review. Staff nurses, nurse managers, and APNs serve on committees to develop policies and procedures and collaborate to see them implemented.

Modifying medical record forms or electronic documentation, the second intervention, is an excellent way to help integrate evidence into care (Titler & Everett, 2001). Reassessment of pain after an intervention is an example of a recommended best practice that may not always be followed. A medical record form or electronic documentation field could be modified to include a place for nurses to document pain reassessment, thus increasing compliance with this standard of care. A clinical reminder can be set up within some computerized documentation systems to prompt nurses to reassess patient pain levels.

The third intervention recommended involves supporting education of senior administrators (Titler & Everett, 2001). It is important for leaders to receive frequent updates on EBP activities within the organization. Updates could be given through e-mail or a narrative summary or through rounds with a project team. While it is essential for senior administrators to develop the vision and the organizational culture, they also need to be kept up to date with changes that are being made. Keeping nurse leaders updated enhances the EBP culture while keeping the organization accountable.

The fourth intervention that a social system can implement involves orienting new staff and travel staff (Titler & Everett, 2001). The orientation should send a message that EBP is valued at the organization. New staff members should be made aware of how policies and standards are developed in the organization so they can participate in the process.

Regional Level

At the *regional level*, collaboration is very important for the advancement of EBP. Using the skills of a local librarian, collaborating with a local program of nursing, and using resources from regional centers of excellence are examples of using regional collaboration.

KEY TERM

Regional level: When nurses from a large geographic area collaborate to change practice

CRITICAL THINKING EXERCISE 2-1

Consider the facilities that you have been to for clinical experiences. Which facilities appear to have embraced EBP? Why do you think that is the case? How are individual nurses involved?

It is critical to partner with a local librarian when trying to find the evidence. Many healthcare librarians specialize in searching for evidence in nursing and medicine. Librarians are an important resource for EBP because they are experts in searching databases such as CINAHL, PubMed, and Ovid (DiCenso, 2003). At the University of Iowa, the health sciences library has a program called "housecalls" whereby a librarian comes to your office to facilitate a literature search.

Programs of nursing are another regional resource available for collaboration. It is helpful to use the expertise of faculty to find, synthesize, and appraise the evidence. Some hospital systems match staff nurses with students or professors to appraise literature. Nursing professors can join organizational committees such as research committees, evidence-based planning committees, or quality outcomes committees.

Shirey (2006) identified four EBP regional resource centers of excellence (see **Table 2-2**). These regional centers resource provide resources for nurses and organizations incorporating best practices. Resources include toolkits, intensive training programs, conferences, and specific guidelines that are available for purchase. Most of these centers of excellence provide experts who are available by phone and e-mail to answer questions and guide nurses and organizations through the EBP process.

National Level

On the *national level*, several entities have made considerable contributions to nursing research and EBP. The Agency for Healthcare Research and Quality (AHRQ) launched an initiative in 1997 to establish EBP centers around the United States. These centers review scientific literature about specific topics and publish technology assessments and evidence reports. The National Guideline Clearinghouse (NGC) is another initiative of AHRQ that maintains a comprehensive database of EBP guidelines. The NGC website provides abstracts of practice guidelines and access to full-text publications (AHRQ, 2007). The National Institute of Nursing Research (NINR) has also significantly contributed to the development of nursing research. NINR is a federal agency that allocates funds for clinical and basic research and research training (NINR, 2007). Funded areas of research are based on social and political factors involving health and illness across the lifespan. Nursing research generated as a result of NINR funding is disseminated for the purpose of improving patient outcomes. Specialty nursing societies, such as the Oncology Nursing Society (ONS) and Association of Women's Health, Obstetric and Neonatal Nurses (AWHONN), are other examples of national organizations that facilitate the generation, dissemination, and use of new knowledge. ONS

TABLE 2-2 Regional Resource Centers of Excellence

RRC	Region	Website
University of North Carolina at Chapel Hill	Eastern	http://www.ahrq.gov/clinic/epc/rti-unc.htm
Arizona State University at Tempe	Western	http://nursing.asu.edu/caep/index.htm
University of Iowa Hospitals and Clinics at Iowa City	Midwestern	http://www.uihealthcare.com/depts/nursing/rqom/evidencebasedpractice/index.html
University of Texas at San Antonio	Southern	http://www.acestar.uthscsa.edu/resources_www.htm

has an EBP area on its website. This resource area provides information for starting an EBP project. It provides topic reviews as well as a toolkit with more resources (ONS, 2007). AWHONN regularly publishes EBP guidelines in its journal and website (AWHONN, 2002). The National Nursing Practice Network (NNPN) is committed to the promotion and implementation of EBP through a collaborative model designed to encourage shared learning and participation. The mission of the NNPN is to foster exceptional health-care outcomes, advance professional nursing practice through application of evidence, support nursing leadership development for EBP, and increase understanding of mechanisms and strategies that foster the use of evidence (NNPN, 2007). The vision of the NNPN is to be a national exemplar of nursing practice excellence, innovation, translation science, and promotion of EBP (NNPN, 2007). The American Nurses Credentialing Center (ANCC) has developed the Magnet Recognition Program to recognize healthcare organizations that provide nursing excellence. This program includes 14 forces of magnetism that are criteria required for organizations to become nationally recognized as Magnet Recognition Program healthcare facilities. Initiatives involving nursing research and EBP must be present to earn Magnet Recognition. For example, the organization must be able to demonstrate a culture that embraces EBP and nursing research. Structures and processes, such as committees, resources, and release time for research endeavors, must be evident. Nurses in direct care are expected to be involved in EBP, quality assurance, and nursing research. This national recognition has increased awareness about the importance of EBP at the individual nurse and organizational levels (ANCC, 2010).

KEY TERM

International level:
Changes that result
from collaboration
among nurses from
different countries

International Level

Efforts to enhance EBP are also conducted at the *international level*. Dr. Archie Cochrane (1971) criticized the medical profession for not providing systematic reviews of evidence from existing studies. In response to this criticism, the Cochrane Center was established 20 years later in Oxford, England. One year after that, The Cochrane Collaboration was established. This international not-for-profit organization is dedicated to making up-to-date, accurate healthcare information available worldwide. The purpose of this establishment is to offer healthcare providers current systematic reviews of medical interventions and treatments. These summary reports are essential because mass media and the Internet provide an abundance of information, making it difficult for practitioners to stay current (The Cochrane Collaboration, 2007). STTI is a leader in the development and dissemination of knowledge to improve nursing practice. This organization has published a position statement on evidence-based nursing and strives to provide nurses with the most current comprehensive resources to assist them with translating evidence into nursing research, education, administration, policy, and practice. STTI presents awards to honor nurses that have demonstrated excellence in research and EBP. For example, the Founder's Award is given for excellence in research. Several specific research awards for research dissemination in nursing and research utilization are also given (STTI, 2007). The Joanna Briggs Institute is an international research and development unit of the Royal Adelaide Hospital, which is located in Adelaide, the capital city of

TEST YOUR KNOWLEDGE 2-1

Match the following:

1. APN

2. Joanna Briggs Institute

3. Policy committee

4. AHRQ

5. Librarian

6. NINR

7. Staff nurse

    a. Individual nurse level

    b. Organizational level

    c. Regional level

    d. National level

    e. International level

How did you do? 1. a; 2. e; 3. b; 4. d; 5. c; 6. d; 7. a

South Australia (Joanna Briggs Institute, 2010). The Institute was established in 1995 and fully operationalized in 1996; it aims to improve the effectiveness of nursing practice and healthcare outcomes. Some initiatives include conducting systematic reviews, collaborating with expert researchers to facilitate development of practice information sheets, and designing, promoting, and delivering short courses about EBP.

2.2 Keeping It Ethical

At the end of this section, you will be able to:

< Discuss international and national initiatives designed to promote ethical conduct
< Describe the rights that must be protected and the three ethical principles that must be upheld when conducting research
< Explain the composition and functions of IRBs at the organizational level
< Discuss the nurse's role as patient advocate in research situations

Ethical research exists because international, national, organizational, and individual factors are in place to protect the rights of individuals. Without these factors, scientific studies, such as the Nazi experiments, could proceed unchecked. Many factors, which evolved in response to unethical scientific conduct, are aimed at protecting human rights. *Human rights* are "freedoms, to which all humans are entitled, often held to include the right to life and liberty, freedom of thought and expression, and equality before the law" (Houghton Mifflin Company, 2007). Rights cannot be claimed unless they are justified in the eyes of another individual or group of individuals (Haber, 2006). When individuals have rights, others have *obligations*, that is, they are required to act in particular ways. This means that when nursing research is being conducted, subjects participating in studies have rights, and all nurses are obligated to protect those rights.

International and National Factors: Guidelines for Conducting Ethical Research

One of the earliest international responses to unethical scientific conduct was the Nuremberg Code. This code was contained in the written verdict given by those presiding at the trial of the German Nazi physicians accused of torturing prisoners during medical experiments. Writers of the Nuremberg Code

KEY TERMS

Human rights:
Freedoms to which all humans are entitled

Obligations:
Requirements to act in particular ways

KEY TERM

Declaration of Helsinki: An international standard providing physicians guidelines for conducting biomedical research

(**Table 2-3**) identified that voluntary consent was absolutely necessary for participation in research. Conduct avoiding harm, producing results that benefit society, and allowing participants to withdraw at will was deemed ethical. The Nuremberg Code became the standard for other codes of conduct.

Another example of an international standard is the *Declaration of Helsinki*, which was adopted by the World Medical Association (WMA) in 1964. Last amended in 2006, the declaration provides guidelines for physi-

TABLE 2-3 Articles of the Nuremberg Code

1. The voluntary consent of the human subject is absolutely essential.

2. The experiment should be such as to yield fruitful results for the good of society, unprocurable by other methods or means of study, and not random and unnecessary in nature.

3. The experiment should be so designed and based on the results of animal experimentation and a knowledge of the natural history of the disease or other problem under study that the anticipated results will justify the performance of the experiment.

4. The experiment should be so conducted as to avoid all unnecessary physical and mental suffering and injury.

5. No experiment should be conducted where there is an a priori reason to believe that death or disabling injury will occur; except, perhaps, in those experiments where the experimental physicians also serve as subjects.

6. The degree of risk to be taken should never exceed that determined by the humanitarian importance of the problem to be solved by the experiment.

7. Proper preparations should be made and adequate facilities provided to protect the experimental subject against even remote possibilities of injury, disability, or death.

8. The experiment should be conducted only by scientifically qualified persons. The highest degree of skill and care should be required through all stages of the experiment of those who conduct or engage in the experiment.

9. During the course of the experiment the human subject should be at liberty to bring the experiment to an end if he has reached the physical or mental state where continuation of the experiment seemed to him to be impossible.

10. During the course of the experiment the scientist in charge must be prepared to terminate the experiment at any stage, if he has probably [sic] cause to believe, in the exercise of the good faith, superior skill and careful judgment required of him that a continuation of the experiment is likely to result in injury, disability, or death to the experimental subject.

Source: U.S. Department of Health and Human Services. (n.d.). *IRB guidebook. Appendix 6* (pp. 7–8). Retrieved August 29, 2010, from http://www.hhs.gov/ohrp/irb/irb_guidebook.htm

cians conducting biomedical research (WMA, 2004). *Informed consent* is considered to be the hallmark requirement for the conduct of ethical research (National Cancer Institute, n.d.). The 32 articles and two clarifications included in the document address issues such as protecting the health of all patients, obtaining informed consent, and conducting research with the aim of benefiting science and society (WMA, 2004). The Declaration of Helsinki offers more specific detail about what constitutes ethical scientific research than does the Nuremberg Code.

Like the WMA, the American Nurses Association (ANA) was ahead of the federal government in establishing codes of scientific conduct. In 1968, *The Nurse in Research: ANA Guidelines on Ethical Values* was approved by the ANA board of directors (Haber, 2006). The ANA established the Commission on Nursing Research, whose report emphasized the rights of human subjects in three ways: 1) right to freedom from harm, 2) right to privacy and dignity, and 3) right to anonymity. The ANA (1985) published six ethical guidelines for nurses (**Table 2-4**). As a result of these guidelines, all nurses are charged

KEY TERM

Informed consent: Voluntary participation by research subjects who have been informed of possible risks and benefits

TABLE 2-4 **ANA Guidelines for Protecting the Rights of Human Subjects**

Rights/Guidelines	Obligations
Right to Self-Determination	‹ Employers must inform nurses in writing if participating as a subject in research is a condition of employment. ‹ Potential subjects must be advised of risks and benefits of participation.
Right to Freedom From Risk or Harm	‹ Nurses must ensure freedom from harm. ‹ Researchers must monitor vulnerable or captive subjects to reduce potential risk of injury.
Scope of Application	‹ All nurses must ensure that all human subjects enjoy protection of their rights.
Responsibilities to Support Knowledge Development	‹ All nurses must support the development of scientific knowledge.
Informed Consent	‹ Nurses must ensure that informed consent from potential subjects (or legal guardians) protects right to self-determination.
Participation on IRB	‹ Nurses should support inclusion of nurses on IRB. ‹ Nurses have an obligation to serve on IRB.

Source: Adapted from ANA (1985).

with the responsibility of protecting the rights of all subjects in their care. Similar guidelines have also been created by professional nursing organizations (Ketefian, Bays, Draucker, Herrick, & Lee, 2002).

It was not until the 1970s that federal guidelines about the ethical treatment of human subjects were formulated (National Cancer Institute, n.d.). In 1973, the Department of Health, Education, and Welfare published the first set of proposed regulations about the protection of human rights. One of the most important regulations to emerge was the mandated implementation of *institutional review boards* to review and approve all studies. The National Commission for the Protection of Human Subjects of Biomedical and Behavioral Research was established in 1974 when the National Research Act was passed. One of the first charges to the commission was to identify basic ethical principles that are foundational to the conduct of ethical scientific research involving human subjects. The commission was also charged with developing guidelines to ensure that medical research was conducted in a manner consistent with the principles it identified. The result was the *Belmont Report*, issued in 1979. In the report, three major principles were identified: 1) respect for persons, 2) beneficence, and 3) justice. These same principles provide the foundation for present codes of conduct in many disciplines that conduct research with human subjects.

Respect for Persons

In the Belmont Report (U.S. Department of Health and Human Services [USDHHS], n.d.), *respect for persons* is based on two ethical convictions. The first conviction is that individuals should be treated as *autonomous*, that is, having the ability to make decisions. An autonomous person can deliberate about personal goals and act in accordance with those goals. Nurses are obligated to show respect for the autonomy of others. When they elicit and act upon the opinions of others, nurses are fulfilling their obligations. The second conviction related to the ethical principle of respect for persons is the recognition that persons with diminished autonomy are entitled to protection (USDHHS, n.d.). Individuals with diminished autonomy, often referred to as vulnerable, include children, individuals with mental disabilities, and prisoners. Some past research studies have violated this right. During the Nazi experiments, individuals were not allowed to refuse participation. In the Jewish Chronic Disease Hospital studies, subjects were not able to make deliberate decisions because the information about the injection of cancer cells was not shared. Researchers conducting the Willowbrook studies did not allow parents free choice, but rather they used admission to the facility in return for enrolling children in the study.

Beneficence

Beneficence is the principle of doing good. In the Belmont Report, two rules were formulated: 1) to do no harm, and 2) to maximize possible benefits and minimize possible harm (USDHHS, n.d.). Individuals may face risk of harm while participating in research because in order to learn what is harmful, subjects risk being harmed. Therefore, researchers are obligated to identify and reduce possible risks as much as possible. Furthermore, the risks must be justified in light of the possible benefits that may result from the research. The principle of beneficence was not upheld in a number of earlier studies. In the Willowbrook studies, injection of live hepatitis virus created a monumental risk for harm that was not justified by the rationale provided by researchers that children were at risk for infection because they were institutionalized. Furthermore, learning about the natural course of the disease was not an outcome that could be justified by the high risk for harm. Individuals were also harmed in the Tuskegee studies. Men with syphilis were not offered penicillin even when it was known that it was an effective treatment.

Justice

The principle of *justice* is concerned with equity or fairness in the distribution of burdens and benefits. In this third principle identified in the Belmont Report, the main consideration is that individuals ought to be treated equally (USDHHS, n.d.). Nurses and other healthcare providers are obligated to ensure that some groups of subjects, such as ethnic minorities or institutionalized individuals, are not being selected for studies because they are easily available or in compromised positions. Individuals cannot be denied treatment because they decline to participate in research. Subjects cannot receive less than the standard of care. Furthermore, outcomes of publicly funded research need to be reported. Unfair treatment of individuals has been a problem in past studies. In the Tuskegee study, African American men were singled out and were not provided standard of care. Vulnerable subjects were also targeted in the Jewish Chronic Disease Hospital study and Willowbrook studies.

KEY TERMS

Beneficence: The principle of doing good

Justice: The principle of equity or fairness in the distribution of burdens and benefits

FYI

Individual nurses are accountable for ensuring that the rights of subjects are protected, which means they must be familiar with international, national, and organizational standards.

CRITICAL THINKING EXERCISE 2-2

What vulnerable groups of individuals were targeted in the Jewish Chronic Disease Hospital study and the Willowbrook studies? Can you think of other groups of individuals who may be at risk for unjust selection?

Organizational Factors: The IRB

There are also mechanisms in place for the protection of human subjects at the organizational level. The primary mechanism is the IRB. Although the structure and functions of IRBs are federally mandated, organizations are held accountable. Hospitals, nursing homes, and universities commonly have established IRBs because these are organizations that typically have employees conducting research. Organizations without established IRBs or organizations with established IRBs that do not hold researchers accountable for upholding ethical standards are not eligible for federal funds to conduct research. Furthermore, conducting research without IRB approval is illegal. In 1991, a statutory framework was enacted, and these laws resulted in standards set forth in the Code of Federal Regulations 45 C.F.R. 46 (National Cancer Institute, n.d.). Research involving animals, food and drug testing, or others kinds of research that do not involve human subjects is not reviewed by an IRB. Components and areas of concern that are reviewed by the IRB are listed in **Table 2-5**.

Federal guidelines stipulate membership of the IRB (USDHHS, n.d.; National Cancer Institute, n.d.). Members are appointed or invited to participate

TABLE 2-5 Components and Areas of Concern Appraised by IRB

Component	Areas of Concern
Risk/Benefit Analysis	
	‹ Are possible risks and benefits identified, evaluated, and described?
	‹ Are risks greater than minimal risk?
	‹ Have attempts been made to minimize risks?
	‹ Will the risk/benefit ratio be reassessed as the study progresses?
	‹ Are subjects receiving less than the standard of care?
Informed Consent	
	‹ Does the study involve vulnerable subjects?
	‹ Is the language appropriate for the subjects?
	‹ Who will explain the study to potential subjects?
	‹ Do subjects need to be reinformed about the purpose of the study periodically?
	‹ Is a waiver of consent justified?

Component	Areas of Concern
Selection of Subjects	
	‹ Does the burden of participating in research fall (most likely) on those who will benefit from the findings?
	‹ Does the research require using the proposed population?
	‹ Are there groups of people who will be more susceptible to risk?
	‹ Have vulnerable subjects been overprotected?
Privacy and Confidentiality	
	‹ Does the research involve intrusion?
	‹ How will information be kept private?
	‹ Should permission be sought for records?
	‹ Should documentation of consent be waived to protect confidentiality?
	‹ Are procedures compliant with Health Insurance Portability and Accountability Act (HIPAA) rules?
Monitoring and Observation	
	‹ How will data be recorded and maintained?
	‹ Who will have access to the data?
	‹ Can information be provided to the IRB should unexpected results be discovered?
Additional Safeguards	
	‹ Are recruitment procedures designed to ensure that informed consent is given freely?
	‹ Does the nature of the disease or behavioral issue permit free consent?
Incentives for Participation	
	‹ Are offered incentives reasonable?
	‹ Should the IRB monitor subject recruitment to ensure that coercion is not a problem?
Continuing Review	
	‹ Are the actual risks and benefits as anticipated?
	‹ Has any subject been seriously harmed?
	‹ Have any unforeseen accidents or problems occurred?

Source: Adapted from USDHHS (n.d.).

by the organization that is establishing the IRB. They are selected because they have knowledge of and experience in working with people of vulnerable populations because the major purpose of the IRB is to protect the rights of vulnerable populations. Knowledge of the research process and the ethical and legal regulations of research are also expected of members. There must be a minimum of five members. Their expertise must vary because all members cannot practice in the same discipline. At least one member of the IRB must be employed in a scientific area, and at least one member, often a clergy member residing in the community, must be employed in a nonscientific area. There must be at least one member of the IRB who is not affiliated with the organization and has no family member who is affiliated with the organization. Membership must include both men and women. When conflicts of interest arise, members must not participate in the review. For example, if a researcher who is a member of the IRB has submitted a proposal, that researcher is excused from the deliberations about that specific study. Each IRB has a chairperson who is accountable for leading the IRB and who can make decisions about how applications are reviewed.

There are two kinds of review: full and expedited. A *full review* is necessary when vulnerable populations are involved or when risks are not minimal. Prior to the meeting, members of the IRB read proposals. Members then convene to discuss whether protocols meet the requirements of the Code of Federal Regulations (**Table 2-6**). A vote is taken whether or not to approve the studies, and recommendations for changes may be made to researchers. Proposals may be eligible for an *expedited review* when there is minimal risk to human subjects (USDHHS, n.d.). *Minimal risk* means that the probability and magnitude of harm or discomfort anticipated in the research are not greater in and of themselves than those ordinarily encountered in daily life or during the performance of routine physical or psychological examinations or tests. Examples of research qualifying for expedited review include:

< Collection of hair and nail clippings
< Collection of excreta and external secretions
< Recording data on subjects 18 years or older using noninvasive routine clinical procedures
< Voice recordings
< Study of existing documents, data, records, and specimens

Proposals of studies qualifying for expedited reviews are read by the chairperson of the IRB, who confirms that expedited review is appropriate and determines whether the standards of the Code of Federal Regulation are being met.

TABLE 2-6 Key Points of the *Code of Federal Regulations*

1. Risks to subjects are minimized.
2. The risks to subjects are reasonable in relation to anticipated benefits.
3. The selection of subjects is equitable.
4. Informed consent must be sought from potential subjects or their legal guardians.
5. Informed consent must be properly documented.
6. When appropriate, research plans monitor data collection to ensure subject safety.
7. When appropriate, privacy of subjects and confidentiality of data are maintained.
8. Safeguards must be in place when subjects are vulnerable to coercion.

Source: Adapted from National Cancer Institute (n.d.).

Certain low-risk studies can be considered *exempt* from obtaining consent from individuals. These studies still need IRB approval. There are six exempt categories of research (**Table 2-7**). These exemptions do not apply to prisoners, pregnant women, fetuses, newborns, and most children (National Cancer Institute, n.d.). Researchers should never assume that their proposals qualify for exempt status, but rather they must follow the policies specified in their organizations. Most policies require that another person, usually the IRB chairperson, review proposals to ensure that they qualify for exempt status.

It is becoming more common for the IRB to require review of EBP projects. The reason is because personal data, for example demographic information or

KEY TERM

Exempt: Certain studies may be low enough risk not to require consent from individuals

CRITICAL THINKING EXERCISE 2-3

A physician comes to the unit and states that she is working in the lab and needs some blood to run a lab test for her research study. The physician asks the nurse to assist with drawing some blood. The physician and nurse enter the room of one of the physician's patients. Without a parent present, the physician asks the 17 year old if she can draw some blood. The adolescent seems reluctant but agrees to the procedure. The physician and nurse draw the blood, and the physician leaves the unit without documenting the procedure. The nurse feels uncomfortable and talks with the charge nurse about the situation. What principles are being violated? How did the nurse fail to act as a patient advocate? What should the nurse have done to protect the rights of the adolescent? What should the charge nurse recommend?

TABLE 2-7 Six Categories Of Exempt Research

1. Research conducted in established or commonly accepted educational settings, involving normal educational practices.

2. Research involving the use of educational tests (i.e., cognitive, diagnostic, aptitude, achievement), survey procedures, interview procedures, or observation of public behavior, unless:
   a) Information obtained is recorded in such a manner that human participants can be identified, directly or through identifiers linked to them.
   b) Any disclosure of the human participant's responses outside the research could reasonably place the participant at risk of criminal or civil liability or be damaging to the participant's financial standing, employability, or reputation.

3. Research involving the use of educational tests (i.e., cognitive, diagnostic, aptitude, achievement), survey procedures, interview procedures, or observation of public behavior that is not exempt under item (2) of this list, if:
   a) The participants are elected or appointed public officials or candidates for public office.
   b) Federal statute(s) require(s) without exception that the confidentiality of the personally identifiable information be maintained throughout the research and thereafter.

4. Research involving the collection or study of existing data, documents, records, pathological specimens, or diagnostic specimens, if these sources are publicly available or if the information is recorded by the researcher in such a manner that participants cannot be identified, directly or through identifiers linked to them.

5. Research and demonstration projects conducted by or subject to the approval of Federal department or agency heads and designed to study, evaluate, or otherwise examine public health benefit or service programs.

6. Taste and food-quality evaluation and consumer acceptance studies.

Source: National Cancer Institute (n.d.).

patient outcomes, may be collected to be shared publically. Because there is growing interest in EBP, data from such projects are being shared at conferences and in publications. Sometimes it is not until the end of a project that nurses consider the possibility of publically sharing their findings. At this point, it may be unethical to present findings, especially if personal data were collected without consent. Therefore, it is wise for nurses who are initiating EBP projects to obtain IRB approval prior to implementing data collection even when they do not anticipate publically sharing findings.

In many organizations, there are other factors that ensure ethical research. Many hospitals also have nursing research committees that review research proposals. These committees are usually composed of staff nurses, nurse managers, advanced practice nurses, and the director of nursing research if there is such a person in the organization.

Individual Factors: Nurses as Patient Advocates

Individual nurses are accountable for ensuring that the rights of subjects are protected. The ANA has charged nurses to be patient advocates. Thus, nurses must be familiar with international, national, and organizational standards to be effective in their roles as patient advocates. Nurses must be able to distinguish between advocacy and science. Nurses have both a duty to care and duty to advance nursing knowledge. This means that the *research imperative* must be weighed against the *therapeutic imperative*. When there is doubt, the therapeutic imperative must take precedence over the research imperative. Nurses can act as patient advocates in a variety of ways. Nurses should be certain that subjects never receive treatment that is less than the standard of care and that participation in research is chosen freely by subjects. Ensuring that HIPAA guidelines are followed when data are collected advocates for the privacy of patients and confidentiality of information. When subjects express the desire to withdraw from a study, nurses can assist by contacting the researcher. If unethical behaviors are observed, nurses should report them to chairpersons of the IRBs at their institutions. Nurses can also contribute by participating on IRBs and nursing research committees.

KEY TERMS

Research imperative: An ethical rule stating that nurses should advance the body of knowledge

Therapeutic imperative: An ethical rule stating that nurses should perform actions that benefit the patient

TEST YOUR KNOWLEDGE 2-2

True/False

1. Informed consent is the hallmark of the Declaration of Helsinki.

2. The Belmont Report identified four ethical principles: respect for persons, nonmaleficence, beneficence, and justice.

3. IRB approval must be obtained for studies involving animals, foods, or drugs.

4. A qualitative study of adults that only involves tape recording interviews would likely receive an expedited review.

5. When there is a conflict, the therapeutic imperative takes precedence over the research imperative.

How did you do? 1. T; 2. F; 3. F; 4. T; 5. T

It is imperative that nurses recognize that IRB approval does not guarantee that ethical dilemmas will not arise. Unanticipated events can lead to unethical conduct, either intentionally or unintentionally. Nurses must use their own ethical frameworks for judging whether their actions, or the actions of others, are in the best interest of patients and nursing science.

RAPID REVIEW

- The model of EBP levels of collaboration has five levels: individual nurse level, organizational level, regional level, national level, and international level.

- Nurses, in a variety of roles, contribute to creating EBP. They can identify clinical problems, participate in EBP changes, serve as change agents or opinion leaders, or establish a vision for the organization.

- Organizational factors that build a culture for EBP include setting performance expectations for individual nurses, integrating EBP into governance structures, and providing recognition and rewards for involvement in EBP.

- Interventions that social systems can use to promote excellence in nursing and move EBP forward include modifying policies and standards, modifying medical record forms, senior administrator education and support, and orientation of new staff members.

- Regional interventions include using skills of a local librarian, collaborating with a local program of nursing, and using resources from regional centers.

- Many national and international entities have made considerable contributions to nursing research and EBP.

- The Nuremberg Code and the Declaration of Helsinki are international factors aimed at protecting the rights of human subjects.

- Federal laws have been enacted to protect subjects participating in research. National organizations have created codes of conduct for researchers.

- The Belmont Report identified three ethical principles for guiding research: respect for persons, beneficence, and justice.

- IRBs are federally mandated organizational structures that review research proposals to ensure that the rights of human subjects are protected. Nursing research committees can also be involved in the protection of human subjects.

APPLY WHAT YOU HAVE LEARNED

The National Cancer Institute offers a free web-based course about protecting the rights of human subjects. Many researchers complete this tutorial as a requirement for obtaining federal funds. Visit the National Cancer Institute website at http://cme.cancer.gov/clinicaltrials/learning/humanparticipant-protections.asp. Sign in, take the tutorial, and print your certificate. Successfully completing the tutorial means that you can qualify to be a research assistant over the next 2 years!

 Nurses are expected to act as patient advocates by ensuring that their rights are upheld. Nurses are also expected to facilitate the development of scientific knowledge in nursing.

REFERENCES

Agency for Healthcare Research and Quality. (2007). *AHRQ home.* Retrieved August 15, 2010, from http://www.ahrq.gov

American Nurses Association. (1985). *Guidelines for nurses in clinical and other research.* Kansas City, MO: Author.

American Nurses Credentialing Center. (2010). *Nursing excellence. Your journey. Our passion.* Retrieved August 15, 2010, from http://www. nursecredentialing.org

Association of Women's Health, Obstetric and Neonatal Nurses. (2002). *Evidence-based clinical practice guidelines.* Retrieved April 20, 2007, from http://www.awhonn.org/awhonn/?pg=873-5580

Cochrane, A. L. (1971). *Effectiveness and efficiency. Random reflections on health services.* Abingdon, Berks: Nuffield Provincial Hospitals Trust.

Cullen, L. (2006). Evidence-based practice: Strategies for nursing leaders. In D. Huber (Ed.), *Leadership and nursing care management* (3rd ed., pp. 461–478). Philadelphia: Saunders Elsevier.

Cullen, L., Greiner, J., Greiner, J., Bombei, C., & Comried, L. (2005). Excellence in evidence-based practice: Organizational and unit exemplars. *Critical Care Nursing Clinics of North America, 17,* 127–142.

DiCenso, A. (2003). Evidence-based nursing practice: How to get there from here. *Nursing Leadership, 16*(4), 20–26.

Doumit, G., Gattellari, M., Grimshaw, J., & O'Brien, M. A. (2007). Local opinion leaders: Effects on professional practice and health care outcomes. *Cochrane Database of Systematic Reviews 2007,* Issue 1. Art. No.: CD000125. DOI: 10.1002/14651858.CD000125.pub3.

Haber, J. (2006). Legal and ethical issues. In G. LoBiondo-Wood & J. Haber (Eds.), *Nursing research: Methods and critical appraisal for evidence-based practice* (6th ed., pp. 295–321). St. Louis, MO: Mosby.

Houghton Mifflin Company. (2007). *American heritage dictionary of the English language* (4th ed.). Boston: Author.

Hudson, K. (2005). From research to practice on the magnet pathway. *Nursing Management, 36*(3), 33–37.

Joanna Briggs Institute. (2010). *Home.* Retrieved August 15, 2010, from http://www.joannabriggs.edu.au/about/home.php

Ketefian, S., Bays, C., Draucker, C., Herrick, L., & Lee, R. K. (2002). *Guidelines for scientific integrity* (2nd ed.). Wheat Ridge, CO: Midwest Nursing Research Society. Retrieved August 15, 2010, from http://www.mnrs.org/files/public/MNRSGuidelinesforScientificIntegrity.pdf

National Cancer Institute. (n.d.). *Human participant protections education for research teams.* Retrieved June 9, 2007, from http://cme.cancer.gov/clinical-trials/learning/humanparticipant-protections.asp

National Institute of Nursing Research. (2007). *Nursing research: Changing practice, changing lives.* Retrieved February 20, 2007, from http://www.ninr.nih.gov

National Nursing Practice Network. (2007). *Welcome to the National Nursing Practice Network.* Retrieved March 1, 2007, from http://www.nnpnetwork.org

Oncology Nursing Society. (2007). *ONS home.* Retrieved August 15, 2010, from http://www.ons.org

Rogers, E. (2003). *Diffusion of innovations* (5th ed.). New York: Free Press.

Shirey, M. (2006). Evidence-based practice: How nurse leaders can facilitate innovation. *Nursing Administration Quarterly, 30*, 252–265.

Sigma Theta Tau International Honor Society of Nursing. (2007). *Home.* Retrieved August 15, 2010, from http://www.nursingsociety.org

The Cochrane Collaboration. (2007). *Home.* Retrieved August 15, 2010, from http://www.cochrane.org/index.htm

Titler, M. (2006). Developing an evidence-based practice. In G. LoBiondo-Wood & J. Haber (Eds.), *Nursing research: Methods and critical appraisal for evidence-based practice* (6th ed., pp. 439–481). St. Louis, MO: Mosby Elsevier.

Titler, M., & Everett, L. (2001). Translating research into practice: Considerations for critical care investigators. *Critical Care Nursing Clinics of North America, 13*, 587–604.

U.S. Department of Health and Human Services. (n.d.). *IRB guidebook.* Retrieved August 15, 2010, from http://www.hhs.gov/ohrp/irb/irb_guidebook.htm

University of Iowa Hospitals and Clinics Department of Nursing. (2007). *Mission, vision, and philosophy of nursing.* Retrieved August 15, 2010, from http://www.uihealthcare.com/depts/nursing/about/mission.html

World Medical Association. (2004). *World Medical Association declaration of Helsinki: Ethical principles for medical research involving human subjects.* Retrieved August 15, 2010, from http://www.wma.net/en/30publications/10policies/b3/index.html

Acquisition of Knowledge

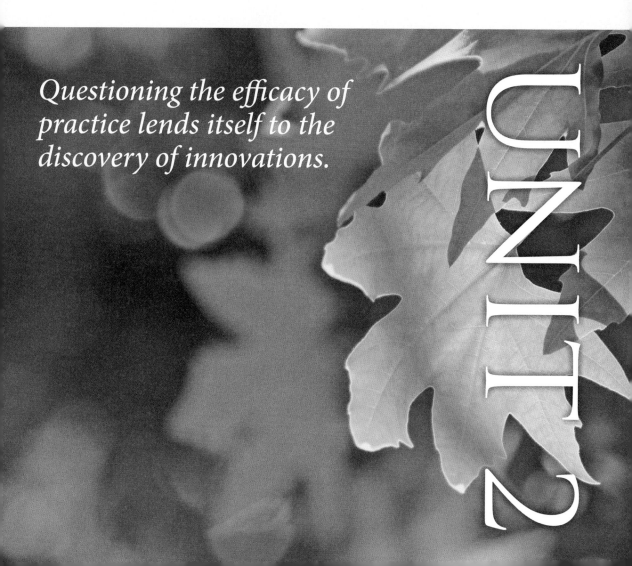

Questioning the efficacy of practice lends itself to the discovery of innovations.

UNIT 2

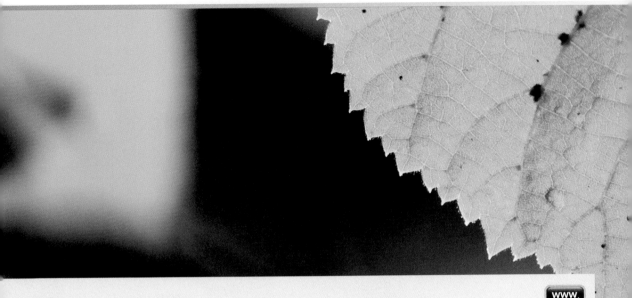

www

CHAPTER OBJECTIVES

At the end of this chapter, you will be able to:

< Discuss ways research problems are identified

< Describe relationships among the purpose statement, the research problems, and the research question

< Differentiate among associative, causal, simple, complex, directional, nondirectional, null, and research hypotheses

< Use criteria to appraise research questions

< Identify independent and dependent variables

< Compare the purposes of research questions and evidence-based practice questions

< Describe the PICO method

< Discuss ethical issues associated with the development of research and EBP questions

KEY TERMS

associative relationship
case studies
causal relationship
complex hypothesis
confounding variable
covary
dependent variable
directional hypothesis
empirical testing
extraneous variable

generalize
hypotheses
hypothesis testing
independent variable
nondirectional hypothesis
null hypothesis
PICO model
pilot
problem statement
purpose statement

replication
research hypothesis
research problem
research question
research topic
simple hypothesis
statistical hypothesis
systematic reviews

CHAPTER 3

Identifying Research Questions

Susie Adams

3.1 How Clinical Problems Guide Research Questions

At the end of this section you will be able to:

‹ Discuss ways research problems are identified

‹ Describe relationships among the purpose statement, the research problems, and the research question.

The primary goals for conducting nursing research are to generate new knowledge that has wide application to promote positive health outcomes for a particular patient population, enhance the overall quality and cost-effectiveness of care, improve the healthcare delivery system, and validate the credibility of the nursing profession through EBP. Determining what problems to study, framing research questions, and developing research hypotheses are often the most challenging aspects of the research process. Where does one begin?

Identifying Nursing Research Problems

There are an infinite number of nursing problems that merit investigation. The challenge is to narrow the focus of problems so they are clinically relevant and can be answered through empirical testing. **Figure 3-1** shows the logical flow for narrowing a nursing research problem. A *research problem* is an

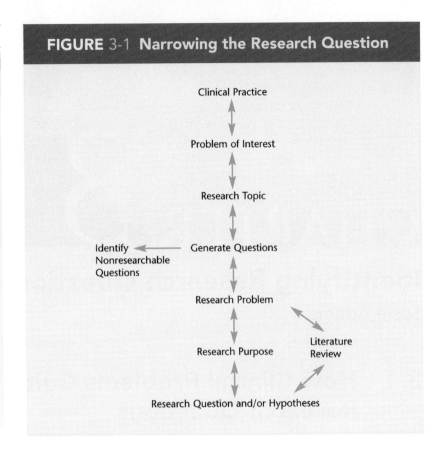

FIGURE 3-1 **Narrowing the Research Question**

area of concern when there is a gap in knowledge that requires a solution that can be described, explained, or predicted to improve nursing practice (Norwood, 2000). Research problems are identified through a variety of sources: personal clinical experience, professional literature, current nursing theories, previous research, and national initiatives. Nursing, like all healthcare professions, is constantly seeking ways to improve clinical outcomes and promote health across the lifespan.

Clinical Experience

Experience most often leads nurses to question whether there is a better approach to a clinical procedure or situation. Clinical curiosity and a desire to improve patient care can be the most important motivators to begin further inquiry that ultimately shapes research studies. Discussions with nursing colleagues regarding their clinical experiences and practice approaches can identify mutual clinical problems. Such discussions may stimulate shared interest for inquiry into best practice approaches for a specific clinical problem.

Professional Literature

Consulting the professional literature is another way to identify research problems. Journal clubs provide an approach to investigate clinical problems identified at the practice level. Internet search engines such Google Scholar (http://scholar.google.com/), PubMed (http://www.pubmedcentral.nih.gov/), and PsycINFO (http:// www.apa.org/ psycinfo/) provide access to scholarly literature across many disciplines and sources including books, abstracts, articles, and dissertations. Refinement of Internet search skills to extract relevant professional literature can be learned through online tutorials, formal classes, and assisted by public or university research librarians. Reading, sharing, and discussing clinical articles from professional journals typically lead to further inquiry into the clinical research literature.

Previous Research

Identifying and reading research articles on particular clinical problems helps nurses to understand the current knowledge about the topic. Reading research articles also reveals gaps about what is known or has not been tested or adequately evaluated. For example, there is a gap when nurses are not using a new clinical approach or intervention yielding better clinical results than the traditional intervention. A gap would also exist if there have been only one or two *case studies* reported in the literature. A gap may become apparent when the study design, method, measures, and outcomes apply to a small or limited sample. Traditionally, new interventions are tested with a small number of subjects in *pilot* studies before testing with larger samples. These types of studies begin to fill knowledge gaps. Testing whether this same intervention will result in a positive outcome in a more culturally diverse population, different age group, or different geographic sample merits investigation. This type of research is called *replication* studies. Finding that multiple studies have obtained similar positive results increases the extent to which one can *generalize* or apply findings to a wider population.

With the proliferation of professional journals across disciplines, it is no longer feasible to read all the published information on any given healthcare topic. A search of the literature about a narrowly focused clinical problem may yield dozens of relevant articles. Articles presenting a synthesis of several articles about a clinical topic, called *systematic reviews*, usually make gaps in the literature more apparent.

Current Nursing Theories

During the past 60 years, a variety of nursing theories have been developed to guide practice and predict nursing outcomes. Peplau's (1952) interpersonal

KEY TERMS

Case studies: A description of a single or novel event

Pilot: A small study to test a new intervention before testing with larger samples

Replication: Repeated studies to obtain similar results

Generalize: Applying findings from a sample to a wider population

Systematic reviews: A rigorous and systematic synthesis of research findings about a clinical problem relations theory, Orem's (2001) self-care deficit model, Roy's (1970) adaptation model, and Rogers's (1980) unitary man model are all examples of nursing theories that can generate nursing studies to test whether a given theory can predict outcomes. Developing studies that empirically test a specific nursing theory is challenging, and most nursing theories or models have few studies that validate major theoretical concepts. For example, Peplau's (1952) interpersonal relations theory has been widely cited in clinical papers; yet, only a few studies actually explore and test nurse–patient relationship factors derived from this theory (Forchuk, 1994; Forchuk, 1995; Forchuk & Reynolds, 2001). These types of studies are more likely to be initiated by experienced researchers who are well versed in theory construction and the measurement of concepts. However, beginning researchers may have opportunities to participate as a member of a research team engaged in testing a nursing theory. Novice researchers can gain valuable conceptual knowledge and pragmatic research skills and perhaps be equipped to develop their own programs of research to further test nursing theory.

National Initiatives

A number of U.S. government agencies routinely identify major health problems and establish national research priorities. These include the U.S. Surgeon General's Office (http://surgeongeneral.gov/) and the National Institutes of Health (NIH, http://www.nih.gov/) and their member institutes (http://www.nih.gov/icd/), such as the National Institute of Nursing Research (NINR, http://www.ninr.nih.gov/) and the National Institute of Mental Health (NIMH, http://www.nimh.nih.gov/). National research agendas identify areas of health concerns with significant implications for the general public, such as childhood obesity, oral health in children, health disparities in minority populations, cardiovascular disease in women, and disease prevention. These agencies identify areas with high priority for federal research funding to evaluate both prevention and intervention healthcare strategies. Nursing research studies derived from such national research agendas typically have greater opportunities for federal funding.

Narrowing the Problem of Interest

A clinical problem of interest is sometimes called the *research topic*. Because clinical problems tend to be quite broad in scope, it is essential to narrow the scope to design studies that are manageable. When narrowing clinical problems, it is important to consider several factors. Having a strong interest and passion for a clinical problem is vital because even a pilot study requires the investment of considerable time and effort. Sustained motivation is needed to see a study through to completion. The problem selected for study needs to be of clinical significance so it adds to the body of nursing knowledge. Consideration should be given to whether the problem affects a large number of people; if the outcomes will improve the care or quality of life for individuals, families, or groups; and if findings will be applicable in a practice environment. Additional considerations include feasibility in terms of time, research expertise, available resources, access to subjects, and ethical considerations for research subjects. When developing research questions about clinical problems, one must consider if the problem can be answered by the research process of empirical testing. Some questions are inherently philosophical in nature and cannot be answered by a research study. Questions that pose a moral choice are questions for philosophical inquiry and public policy deliberation. For example, stem cell research is a current clinical topic that may offer new solutions to a broad range of genetically linked disorders. The question, "Should stem cell research be limited to current strains, and should access to fetal stem cells be prohibited?" poses an ethical and philosophical question. However, reframing the question, "What are the attitudes of patients with Parkinson's disease and their family members toward research that could involve stem cells injected into brain tissue to generate myelinated neurons to reduce Parkinsonian tremors?" is empirically testable. Research questions must always be framed in a manner that can be empirically tested within ethical boundaries.

Even when questions can be framed for empirical testing, one must further consider if the question can be answered by existing knowledge or through basic problem-solving skills. For example, "Can stem cells be safely transplanted via injection into human bone marrow to treat leukemia?" is an EBP question that can be answered through consulting current literature (Laughlin & Lazarus, 2003). At an earlier time, this posed a researchable question, but that question has subsequently been answered. It is critical to investigate current literature because it would be a waste of resources to conduct research when knowledge already exists. Some questions may be answered through basic problem solving. For example, the question, "What is the best method to reduce fall risks among elderly clients served by a home healthcare agency?" could be addressed through a continuous quality improvement process. Initial and periodic fall risk assessments could be developed and compared with ongoing monitoring to track falls. Questions included in the fall risk assessment might be modified as data are obtained about client medications, cognitive function, and home conditions associated with falls and how to reduce these risks.

Problem Solving, Nursing Process, and Research Process

It is helpful to recognize the similarities and differences among the problem-solving process, nursing process, and research process. All three use abstract, critical thinking, and complex reasoning to identify new information, discover relationships, and make predictions about phenomena (Burns & Grove, 2001). All involve the scientific method of observation, data collection, problem identification, implementation of a solution, and evaluation of results. These processes are iterative, that is, continual refinement of knowledge occurs as the process is repeated.

Primary differences among the problem-solving process, nursing process, and research process are in their foci, purposes, and outcomes (Burns & Grove, 2001). The focus of the problem-solving process is on a specific goal in a particular setting for the purpose of generating the best solution to achieve the goal. The focus of the nursing process is on a specific patient care problem using assessment, nursing diagnosis, planning, implementation, and evaluation. The goal of the nursing process is to plan and direct care for a particular patient, family, or group of patients. The outcome is the improvement of health for a particular patient or family. In contrast, the research process has a broad focus drawing on knowledge from nursing and other disciplines. Rigorous application of scientific methods is used, and findings are disseminated through presentations and publications. The purpose of the research process is to generate new knowledge that has wide application to promote positive health outcomes for a particular patient population, enhance the overall quality and cost-effectiveness of care, and improve the healthcare delivery system.

Developing Problem Statements

Problem statements are derived from a research problem that has been identified as a situation that is unsatisfactory and requires further description, explanation, or a solution (Norwood, 2000). The *problem statement* formally identifies what problem is being addressed in the study. A problem statement must include the scope of the research problem, the specific population of interest, the independent and dependent variables, and the goal or question the study intends to answer (Gillis & Jackson, 2002). Additionally, the problem statement should implicitly or explicitly indicate that the proposed study is ethical, feasible, and of significant interest to nursing (Nieswiadomy, 2008). **Table 3-1** contains criteria nurses can use to evaluate problem statements. The research purpose and research questions logically flow from problem statements. The *purpose statement* is derived from the problem statement and indicates the aim of the study. The *research question* flows from the problem statement and study purpose, and often it is the interrogatory form of the problem statement. Examples illustrating the differences among the problem statement, the purpose of a study, and the research question are presented in **Box 3-1**.

TABLE 3-1 **Criteria for Evaluating Problem Statements**

1. Problem (or purpose) statement is clear and concise.
2. Problem statement is written as a declarative statement or a formal question (interrogatory).
3. Population of interest is clearly described.
4. Independent and dependent variables are identified.
5. Empirical data can be derived for the variables in the population of interest.
6. Indication that study is ethical.
7. Indication that study is feasible.
8. Indication that study is clinically significant and relevant to nursing practice.

Some researchers use the problem statement and research question interchangeably. The difference is the use of a declarative or an interrogatory sentence. The research problem when stated in the interrogative form is called the research question. Other researchers will frame the problem statement in a broader manner that generates several research questions, as in the example

BOX 3-1

Examples of Problem Statements, Purpose Statements, and Research Questions

Problem Statement: The use of alcohol by college freshmen contributes to alcohol-related injuries and emergency department visits at a state university.

Purpose Statement: To determine if brief screening and nursing intervention for alcohol use during freshmen orientation reduces self-reported alcohol use, alcohol-related injuries, and emergency department visits among college freshmen at a state university.

Research Question 1: Is there a difference in self-reported alcohol use between college freshmen who receive brief screening and nursing intervention for alcohol use during fall orientation and the previous class of freshmen students who did not receive brief screening and nursing intervention?

Research Question 2: Is there a difference in alcohol-related injuries and emergency department visits between college freshmen who receive brief screening and nursing intervention for alcohol use during fall orientation and the previous class of freshmen students who did not receive brief screening and nursing intervention?

TEST YOUR KNOWLEDGE 3-1

1. Researchable problems are identified through:
   a. current nursing theories
   b. personal clinical experiences
   c. philosophical questions
   d. national initiatives

2. A nurse is reading an article and reads the following statement: This study aims to examine the effect of guided imagery on postoperative pain in adults. This is an example of a:
   a. problem statement
   b. research question
   c. purpose statement
   d. hypothesis

How did you do? 1. a, b, d; 2. c

in Box 3-1. Not all research studies will include both a formal problem statement and a research question, but the research question can be implied from the problem statement.

3.2   Developing Hypotheses

At the end of this section, you will be able to:

‹ Differentiate among associative, causal, simple, complex, directional, nondirectional, null, and research hypotheses
‹ Use criteria to appraise research questions
‹ Identify independent and dependent variables

KEY TERM

Hypotheses: Formal statements of the expected or predicted relationship between two or more variables

Study *hypotheses* are formal statements regarding the expected or predicted relationship between two or more variables in a specific population. They are derived from either the problem statement or the research question. Some studies will not have formally stated hypotheses; yet, they can be implied from the research question. Hypotheses include independent and dependent variables that are directly linked to the problem statement and research question;

TABLE 3-2 **Criteria for Evaluating Hypotheses and Research Questions**

1. Does the study have an explicit hypothesis (or hypotheses)? Or does the study present a research question(s)?

2. Hypotheses are written in concise, present tense, declarative statements that are directly linked to the study problem.

3. For studies with an identified theoretical framework, each hypothesis is derived from the framework.

4. Each hypothesis clearly identifies the population and at least two variables that can be measured and empirically tested.

5. Each hypothesis will state one directional relationship between two variables, or a rationale will be stated for a nondirectional hypothesis.

6. For studies that present research questions (rather than hypotheses), the research questions are concise, clear, and specific.

7. Studies with research questions meet similar criteria to studies testing hypotheses with a clearly identified population, measurable variables, and theoretical framework.

predict the relationship between the independent and dependent variables in a specific population; and define the variables in a manner that empirical data can be gathered to test the predicted relationship between variables. Additionally, hypotheses need to be ethical, feasible, and relevant to nursing research practice. Criteria to evaluate hypotheses are outlined in **Table 3-2**.

Types of Hypotheses

Hypotheses can be categorized in four broad ways: 1) associative versus causal, 2) simple versus complex, 3) nondirectional versus nondirectional, and 4) null versus research. Hypotheses can fit into more than one category. For example, a researcher can state a simple, directional research hypothesis. Sometimes multiple independent and dependent variables can be included in a hypothesis.

Associative Versus Causal Hypotheses

Relationships identified in hypotheses are either associative or causal. Variables that have an *associative relationship* (**Figure 3-2A**) occur or exist together in the real world such that when one variable changes, the other variable changes. In an associative relationship, the two variables may change, or *covary*. When two variables covary in the same direction, a positive (Figure 3-2B) correlation results. For example, as people age, measures of blood pressure increase

KEY TERMS

Associative relationship: When one variable changes, the other variable changes

Covary: When change in one variable is associated with change in another variable

FIGURE 3-2 Associative and Causal Relationships

normally. There is a positive correlation between age and blood pressure. When variables vary in opposite directions, they are known as negative or inverse relationships (Figure 3-2C). The degree to which variables change may or may not be equal or proportional. This is different from a *causal relationship* in which one variable, the independent variable, is thought to cause or determine the presence of the other variable, the dependent variable (Figure 3-2D). One must be cautious not to misinterpret an associative relationship as one that is causal because association does not equal causation.

Simple Versus Complex Hypotheses

A *simple hypothesis* states or describes the relationship, associative or causal, between two variables. A simple associative hypothesis would state that variable X is related to variable Y (Figure 3-2A). A simple causal hypothesis would state that one independent variable is causally related to one dependent variable (Figure 3-2D). A *complex hypothesis* predicts the relationships, either associative or causal, among three or more variables. For example, multiple independent variables may act in a causal relationship to produce one or more dependent variables (Figure 3-2E). One independent variable may act in a causal fashion to produce multiple dependent variables (Figure 3-2F). Similar statements and illustrations could be made for associative relationships among three or more variables.

Nondirectional Versus Directional Hypotheses

Sometimes researchers have hunches about the direction that variables may take. Other times they may not. A *nondirectional hypothesis* is one that states that a relationship exists between two variables, but it does not predict the direction or nature of the relationship (Figure 3-2A). When no clear direction between the variables has been identified in clinical practice, natural observation of phenomena, relevant nursing theories, or in existing clinical or research literature, then no clear prediction can be hypothesized. Nondirectional hypotheses are commonly used in exploratory and descriptive studies. Common nondirectional descriptors include terms such as associated, correlated, or related. When a nondirectional hypothesis is used, a rationale is included in the problem statement explaining why a directional relationship cannot be predicted between the variables. By contrast, a *directional hypothesis* states the nature or direction of the relationship between two or more variables (Figure 3-2B-F). This type of hypothesis is based on nursing theories, observed phenomena, clinical experience, and existing clinical and research literature. Directional hypotheses are used to predict relationships between two or more variables. Common directional descriptors include terms such as increase, decrease, less, more, smaller, and greater. Directional hypotheses can also be categorized as associative or causal, simple or complex.

Null Hypotheses Versus Research Hypotheses

The fourth category of hypothesis includes the *null hypothesis* (H_0), which is also commonly called the *statistical hypothesis*. The null hypothesis states that there is no relationship between two variables, and statistical testing is used to either accept or reject this statement. Conversely, the *research hypothesis* (H_1) states that there is a relationship that exists between two or more vari-

KEY TERMS

Nondirectional hypothesis: Statement of the relationship between two variables that does not predict the direction of the relationship

Directional hypothesis: Describes the direction of a relationship between two or more variables

Null hypothesis: A hypothesis stating that there is no relationship between the variables

Statistical hypothesis: No relationship among the variables; null hypothesis

Research hypothesis: Indicates that a relationship between two or more variables exists

---

CRITICAL THINKING EXERCISE 3-1

A common problem in the newborn nursery is that infants undergoing circumcision show decreases in body temperatures following the procedure. A nurse researcher is interested in studying the effect of a warming tray on the body temperature of infants undergoing circumcisions. Write a research question, associative hypothesis, directional hypothesis, and null hypothesis that would be appropriate for this study.

TABLE 3-3 **Examples of Hypotheses for the Research Question: What is the relationship between self-esteem and adherence to a diabetic diet in adolescents with Type I diabetes?**

Type of Hypothesis	Hypothesis Statement
Associative	There is a relationship between the amount of self-esteem and adherence to a diabetic diet in adolescents with Type I diabetes.
Causal	Increased amounts of self-esteem increase adherence to a diabetic diet in adolescents with Type I diabetes.
Simple	Increased amounts of self-esteem increase adherence to a diabetic diet in adolescents with Type I diabetes.
Complex	Increased amounts of self-esteem increase adherence to diabetic diet and insulin administration in adolescents with Type I diabetes.
Directional	Increased amounts of self-esteem increase adherence to a diabetic diet in adolescents with Type I diabetes.
Nondirectional	There is an association between the amount of self-esteem and adherence to a diabetic diet in adolescents with Type I diabetes.
Null	There is no relationship between the amount of self-esteem and adherence to a diabetic diet in adolescents with Type I diabetes.
Research	Increased amounts of self-esteem increase adherence to a diabetic diet in adolescents with Type I diabetes.

KEY TERM

Hypothesis or empirical testing: Objectively measurable data gathered through the five senses to confirm or refute a hypothesis

ables. These relationships can be described and categorized as associative or causal, simple or complex, nondirectional or directional. *Hypothesis testing* or *empirical testing* involves the collection of objectively measurable data that are gathered through the five senses to confirm or refute a hypothesis. **Table 3-3** offers examples of how hypotheses can be worded.

What Is a Variable?

To understand hypothesis testing, it is important to understand the nature of variables. Variables may be phenomena that can be directly measured, such as pulse rate, blood pressure, respiratory rate, red blood cell count, antibody titer, thyroid stimulating hormone, or salivary cortisol level. Variables may

TEST YOUR KNOWLEDGE 3-2

Indicate which of the following terms best describes hypotheses 1–3 below:

a. associative

b. causal

c. simple

d. complex

e. directional

f. nondirectional

g. null

h. research

i. research question

1. Age, number of medical diagnoses, and number of medications affect the incidence of falls in older adults.

2. There is no relationship between seatbelt use and head injury in auto accidents.

3. Does consuming one glass of red wine daily reduce the incidence of heart disease in middle-aged men?

4. In the following hypothesis, scores on the Beck Depression Inventory will be lower in women who take yoga classes than in women who do not, the independent variable is:

a. score on Beck Depression Inventory

b. yoga ability

c. women

d. type of participation in yoga

How did you do? 1. a, d, f, h; 2. c, g; 3. i; 4. d

also be qualities, properties, or characteristics of people, groups, or objects, for example, socio-demographic characteristics, intelligence, social support, and self-esteem. Because these qualities, properties, and characteristics are not directly observable, they are measured indirectly using questionnaires and scales. Variables may also be derived from abstract concepts such as depression, anxiety, grieving, and quality of life, which require some indirect type of measurement. There is an entire body of research dedicated to the development and testing of variables used to measure such abstract concepts. The Beck

KEY TERMS

Independent variable: Variable that influences the dependent variable or outcome

Dependent variable: Influenced by the independent variable

Confounding or extraneous variable: Factors that interfere with the relationship between the independent and dependent variables

Depression Inventory (Beck, Ward, Mendelson, Mock, & Erbaugh, 1961), the Hamilton Anxiety Scale (Hamilton, 1959), and the Holmes and Rahe Social Readjustment Rating Scale (Holmes & Rahe, 1967) are several examples of ways to measure variables associated with abstract concepts.

Regardless of whether a variable is one that can be directly measured or requires some form of indirect measurement, variables are also categorized as independent, dependent, and confounding variables. The *independent variable*, commonly labeled the X variable, is the variable that influences the dependent variable or outcome. In experimental studies it is the intervention or treatment that is manipulated by the researcher. The *dependent variable*, commonly labeled the Y variable, is the variable or outcome that is influenced by the independent variable.

Confounding variables, or *extraneous variables*, commonly labeled Z, are factors that interfere with the relationship between the independent and dependent variables. Sometimes a confounding factor is known before a study begins; other times the confounding factor is identified while the study is being conducted or after the study is completed. If the confounding variable is known in advance, the researcher may try to use strategies to minimize or eliminate the effect of these variables. Another way to control for confounding variables is to use specific statistical tests. For example, in a study examining birth outcomes between women who receive prenatal care from midwives to women receiving care from a physician, the number of cigarettes smoked per day during pregnancy is an example of a confounding variable. Because smoking during pregnancy is known to reduce infant birth weights, either excluding mothers who smoke from the study or using statistical tests to control for this confounding variable would be needed.

3.3   Formulating EBP Questions

At the end of this section, you will be able to:

‹ Compare the purposes of research questions and EBP questions
‹ Describe the PICO method

While research and EBP both involve questions, their purposes are quite different. The primary purpose of nursing research is to generate new knowledge, and the purpose of EBP is to make decisions about patient care based on the best current evidence gathered from a systematic problem-solving approach. EBP incorporates a systematic search for evidence and a critical appraisal of the findings with clinical expertise and the patient's and family's values and preferences to provide the best patient care (Melnyk & Fineout-Overholt, 2005). Clinical curiosity motivates nurses and other healthcare providers to identify choices available for a particular patient to determine the best course of treatment. Given the burgeoning amount of new healthcare products, drugs, procedures, alternative medicine approaches, and the emerging information on risks, benefits, and efficacy of these products, procedures, and interventions, healthcare providers will be continually required to judiciously find the right evidence to make informed treatment care decisions in a time-efficient manner. In EBP, questions are generated in a manner slightly different from research questions. One widely used model in EBP is the *PICO model*. Clinical questions for specific patient problems are identified so that healthcare providers can find clinically relevant information using Internet search engines and databases (Higgins & Green, 2009). The acronym, PICO, stands for the following four components:

P = Patient population or patient condition of interest
I = Intervention of interest
C = Comparison of interest
O = Outcome of interest

The patient population or patient condition needs to be carefully delineated so that the search for evidence yields relevant information and prevents retrieval of too broad or off-target information. When retrieving information, it is important to keep in mind that findings may not be generalizable to a specific patient. For example, a teaching strategy that is successful with children may not be successful with adolescents.

In the PICO model, the intervention of interest requires similar delineation to yield focused, relevant information. When conducting a literature search, consider the main intervention or treatment, diagnostic test, procedure, or exposure. Also consider any factors that may influence the prognosis such as age, gender, ethnicity, coexisting conditions, and exposures to risk factors such as cigarette smoke, asbestos, or other toxins.

The comparison of interest can be a comparison with another intervention or treatment. The intervention of interest can also be compared to the standard of care. It is best to select the main alternative to the proposed intervention. For example, is the issue about trying to decide whether to implement a new treatment for sacral decubital ulcers in immobile elderly nursing home patients? An

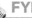
FYI

Nurses must consider patient preferences when making practice decisions, as well as take limited resources into consideration by selecting questions that are broad in scope and that can be completed. Priority should be given to studies that have the potential to generate significant contributions to patient outcomes.

KEY TERM

PICO model:
Patient population, intervention of interest, comparison of interest, and outcome of interest used to formulate EBP

BOX 3-2

Resource for Developing EBP Questions Using PICO Model

The University of Wisconsin-Madison Ebling Library for the Health Sciences website provides a resource for developing a PICO question (http://ebling.library.wisc.edu/portals/ebhc/pico.cfm). Be sure to check out the link to the PICO and Search Query Worksheet.

FYI

The primary purpose of nursing research is to generate new knowledge, and the purpose of EBP is to make decisions about patient care based on the best current evidence gathered from a systematic problem-solving approach.

approach to answer this question would be to compare the patient outcomes with the new treatment and the usual standard of care.

The outcome of interest is the desired accomplishment, measurement, or improvement as a result of the selected intervention or treatment approach. It is important to identify clear outcome measures to evaluate the efficacy of the intervention with the identified comparison. In the previous example, the outcome of decubital healing could be determined by measuring diameter and depth of ulcer, type and amount of drainage, formation of new tissue, and ulcer closure. Specifying the desired outcome measures further refines the literature search. Once the components of the PICO question have been identified, a statement can be written. **Box 3-2** includes a resource for developing EBP questions using the PICO model.

TEST YOUR KNOWLEDGE 3-3

True/False

1. There are no differences between research questions and EBP questions.

2. The PICO model is useful when considering EBP questions.

3. The standard of care or alternate interventions can be used as comparisons of interest in the PICO model.

How did you do? 1. F; 2. T; 3. T

CRITICAL THINKING EXERCISE 3-2

Consider how you would describe a group of patients similar to your specific patient. Include important patient characteristics, primary problem or disease, and any coexisting conditions. If age, gender, race, ethnicity, or other characteristics are relevant to the diagnosis or treatment, then those factors also need to be included.

3.4   Keeping It Ethical

At the end of this section, you will be able to:

< Discuss ethical issues associated with the development of research and EBP questions

Although there are not very many ethical issues involved with the development of research and EBP questions, the issues that exist are important. First and foremost, nurses must be certain that research questions posed can be answered while respecting the rights of human subjects. For example, it would be unethical to leave wounds untreated to determine how much time it takes for a stage four ulcer to develop because the intervention is less than the standard of

TEST YOUR KNOWLEDGE 3-4

1. Ethical issues associated with the development of research questions include:
    a. limited resources
    b. respecting human rights
    c. interests of the researcher
    d. patient preferences

How did you do? 1. a, b, c, d

care. Nurses must also keep in mind that EBP is not based solely on evidence. Regardless of answers that are found to questions, nurses must consider patient preferences when making practice decisions.

Researchers must also be aware that resources are limited. Problems that are broad in scope should be selected. Priority should be given to studies that have the potential to generate significant contributions to patient outcomes. It is also important to address questions that can be seen through to completion. Selecting problems that are of interest makes it easier for one to invest the time, energy, and resources necessary to finish a study.

Nurses need to recognize the difference between ethical questions and researchable questions. Although ethical questions do not lend themselves to research methods, discussion about them can make important contributions to nursing knowledge.

 ## *RAPID* **REVIEW**

 Identifying clinical practice and research questions is a critical skill for nurses and healthcare providers.

 A research problem is an area of concern when there is a gap in knowledge. These are identified through personal clinical experience, professional literature, current practice theories, previous research, and national initiatives.

 To narrow the problem of interest, it is best to select a problem that is of interest, can be answered by empirical testing, has not already been answered, or cannot be answered through basic problem-solving skills.

 Problem statements identify what the study is about, while purpose statements indicate why the study is being conducted.

 Research questions are interrogatory statements that flow from the problem statement.

 Hypotheses are formal statements regarding the expected or predicted relationships between two or more variables in a specific population. Hypotheses can be associative, causal, simple, complex, nondirectional, directional, null, and research.

 Variables can be measured directly or indirectly.

APPLY WHAT YOU HAVE LEARNED

So that you can better understand EBP, throughout the remainder of the book you will be guided through a series of exercises designed to involve you in the EBP process. The clinical problem used in this exercise is medication errors. You will find a variety of evidence on the companion website for your convenience. As you progress through the process, you will critique the evidence and decide what best practice to recommend. You will also design a policy and evaluate outcomes. By actively engaging in this exercise, you will be well prepared to be a leader who successfully moves evidence to the point of care.

Imagine you are assigned to a committee in your facility. The committee has been charged with determining best practices for reducing medication errors. To become familiar with the magnitude of this problem, visit the report brief, "Preventing Medical Errors," published by the Institute of Medicine (2006, see http://www.iom.edu/~/media/Files/Report%20Files/2006/Preventing-Medication-Errors-Quality-Chasm-Series/medicationerrorsnew.ashx). After reading the report, formulate possible PICO questions for the committee.

The independent variable, X, influences the dependent variable, Y, or outcome. In experimental studies, the intervention is the independent variable.

The dependent variable is the outcome that is influenced by the independent variable.

Confounding or extraneous variables, Z, are factors that interfere with relationships between independent and dependent variables.

The purpose of research questions is to generate new knowledge, while the purpose of EBP questions is to make decisions about patient care.

The PICO model is commonly used to formulate EBP questions. PICO stands for patient population, intervention of interest, comparison of interest, and outcome of interest.

Ethical considerations associated with research questions involve formulating questions that are answered by studies that respect the rights of human subjects, are feasible, and address questions of interest.

REFERENCES

Beck, A. T., Ward, C. H., Mendelson, M., Mock, J., & Erbaugh, J. (1961). An inventory for measuring depression. *Archives of General Psychiatry, 4,* 461–571.

Burns, N., & Grove, S. K. (2001). *The practice of nursing research: Conduct, critique, and utilization* (4th ed.). Philadelphia: Saunders.

Forchuk, C. (1994). The orientation phase of the nurse-client relationship: Testing Peplau's theory. *Journal of Advanced Nursing, 20*(3), 532–537.

Forchuk, C. (1995). Development of nurse-client relationships: What helps. *Journal of American Psychiatric Nurses Association, 1*(5), 146–151.

Forchuk, C., & Reynolds, W. (2001). Clients' reflections on relationships with nurses: Comparisons from Canada and Scotland. *Journal of Psychiatric and Mental Health Nursing, 8*(1), 45–51.

Gillis, A., & Jackson, W. (2002). *Research for nurses: Methods and interpretation.* Philadelphia: Davis.

Hamilton, M. (1959). The assessment of anxiety states by rating. *British Journal of Medical Psychology, 32*(1), 50–55.

Higgins, J. P. T., & Green, S. (editors). *Cochrane Handbook for Systematic Reviews of Interventions* Version 5.0.2 [updated September 2009]. The Cochrane Collaboration, 2009. Retrieved from www.cochrane-handbook.org

Holmes, T. H., & Rahe, R. H. (1967). Holmes-Rahe social readjustment rating scale. *Journal of Psychometric Research, 11,* 213–218.

Institute of Medicine. (2006). *Preventing medical errors.* Retrieved September 9, 2010, from http://www.iom.edu/~/media/Files/Report%20Files/2006/Preventing-Medication-Errors-Quality-Chasm-Series/medicationerrorsnew.ashx

Laughlin, M. J., & Lazarus, H. M. (2003). *Allogeneic stem cell transplantation: Clinical research and practice, Current clinical oncology.* Totowa, NJ: Humana Press.

McGillis Hall, L., Doran, D., & Pink, G. H. (2004). Nurse staffing models, nursing hours, and patient safety outcomes. *JONA, 34,* 41–45.

Melnyk, B. M., & Fineout-Overholt, E. (2005). *Evidence-based practice in nursing and healthcare: A guide to best practice.* Philadelphia: Lippincott Williams & Wilkins.

Nieswiadomy, R. M. (2008). *Foundations of nursing research* (5th ed.). Upper Saddle River, NJ: Prentice Hall.

Norwood, S. L. (2000). *Research strategies for advanced practice nurses.* Upper Saddle River, NJ: Prentice Hall.

Orem, D. E. (2001). *Nursing: Concepts of practice* (6th ed.). St. Louis, MO: Mosby.

Peplau, H. E. (1952). *Interpersonal relations in nursing.* New York: Putnam

Rogers, M. (1980). Nursing: A science of unitary man. In J. P. Riehl & C. Roy (Eds.), *Conceptual models for nursing practice* (2nd ed., pp. 329–337). New York: Appleton-Century-Crofts.

Roy, C. (1970). Adaptation: A conceptual framework for nursing. *Nursing Outlook, 18,* 42–45.

At the end of this chapter, you will be able to:

< Explain why performing a quality literature review is an essential skill for nursing students, researchers, and nurses

< Differentiate between searching for evidence and literature in lay and professional sources

< Explain the scientific literature publication cycle

< Differentiate between primary and secondary sources

< Identify different types of articles found in the literature

< Characterize the four major types of reviews

< Identify and use a variety of sources, both within and outside of the field of nursing, as appropriate

< Understand how the sources are structured

< Distinguish between the different sources' content, in both topic or subject matter and in format

< Perform various types of searches using basic and advanced source tools and search techniques

< List four databases where scholarly literature of disciplines is indexed

< Consider the ethical presentation and application of evidence

Boolean operators
call number
CINAHL
citation chasing
controlled vocabularies
electronic indexes
exploding
grey literature
indexes
integrative review
interlibrary loan
journal
keyword
magazine

meta-analyses
narrative reviews
nesting
peer review
periodical
plagiarism
popular literature
positional operators
precision
primary sources
print index
qualification
recall
record

scholarly literature
scientific literature
  publication cycle
search field
secondary sources
stopwords
subject headings
subject searching
systematic reviews
trade literature
truncation
wildcards

CHAPTER 4

Finding Sources of Evidence

Patricia Mileham

4.1 Purpose of Finding Evidence

At the end of this section, you will be able to:

‹ Explain why performing a quality literature review is an essential skill for nursing students, researchers, and nurses
‹ Differentiate between searching for evidence and literature in lay and professional sources

Most often, your first introduction to the literature review is tied to writing an academic paper. As undergraduate students, the focus of your papers is usually one of gathering information on a topic and perhaps sharing a resulting opinion about the findings. The literature review provides a consideration of what has been studied previously. For researchers, the literature review identifies gaps in the current research, highlights areas of needed change, increases awareness about practice, and helps sharpen and focus a research question. Because of the increasing emphasis on evidence-based practice (EBP), nurses must develop abilities to perform literature reviews to increase knowledge about a specific topic and provide the basis for an informed, professional opinion to champion EBP in clinical settings.

Knowing how to search for, access, and evaluate information is as key to your successful practice tomorrow as it is to earning a good grade in an academic paper today. In an insightful editorial directed to nursing faculty, Lander (2005) details the ties between research and EBP by delineating competencies nursing students should possess to complete this connection themselves:

Research questions and practice considerations must be based on informed, ethical opinions resulting from consideration of evidence that is currently available. This requires a detailed review of the literature.

They need to know what sources of information are reliable and credible and how to gain access to them. They need some specific skills that enable them to comprehend designs and specific design issues. They need to know how to differentiate poor quality from good quality reports of studies, systematic reviews, and clinical guidelines. They need an approach for assessing the value of an intervention for clinical practice. Above all, they need access to computers and technical resources. (p. 300)

These are competencies needed to perform quality literature reviews, not just an academic exercise left behind when your diploma is in hand.

Whether you are performing a literature review for the 1st, 15th, or 50th time, consider it a part of your practice worth doing well every time. Just as patients are assessed before treatment recommendations are made, literature reviews are assessments of topics before the research or practice continues. Whether the purpose of the literature review is an EBP proposal in your workplace, a research question in your graduate studies, or part of an academic paper as an undergraduate, the process is the same. Depending on the situation, search complexity and access to resources may be different; however, the procedural steps and attention to quality work will remain the same. This is because the desired outcome stays the same: Research questions or practice considerations must be based on informed, ethical opinions resulting from consideration of evidence that is currently available.

With staggering amounts of information available via the Internet and the proliferation of journal and monograph materials, skilled literature review practices have never been more necessary. While it is well known that anyone can publish anything on the Internet, today's more sophisticated tools, such as wikis and blogs, increase the challenge of evaluating the validity of information. Information of all types travels rapidly from source to source. This results in mixing hoaxes, urban legends, and other types of misinformation along with accurate and reliable information. Nurses not only face this situation as information consumers, but they must also consider it within their roles as patient advocates. Patients are bombarded with information as well. Their desire to be knowledgeable about their illnesses and health care often makes them even more vulnerable to misinformation. Most patients do not have the knowledge base possessed by nurses to evaluate information and make informed decisions. Books such as *Internet Resource Guide for Nurses and Health Care Professionals* (Hedba, Czar, & Mascara, 2005) and *The Nurses' Guide to Consumer Health Web Sites* (Fitzpatrick, Romano, & Chasek, 2001) provide nurses with an insightful understanding of the structure and use of healthcare resources available on the Internet. Resources such as these position nurses to assist patients with obtaining accurate information.

Nurses have an ethical responsibility to skillfully use all tools and resources available. Not everything is, or will ever be, available electronically. Nurses should be aware of and use print materials that are still current and viable. Conversely, because not all electronic resources that are based on print resources are comprehensive or contain older or archival information, research questions can take reviewers back to older print journals or *indexes*.

There are many reputable government, organizational, and educational resources available on the Internet (sites that are free and accessible to all), such as the University of Washington's HealthLinks EBP site http://health-links.washington.edu/ebp. There are also many restricted resources, such as literature databases (often paid for by a school or hospital) or resources within organizational sites available only to members. These restricted resources usually contain professional literature that has been compiled, sorted, indexed, and made available. Content in these resources is written for professional colleagues, not for the lay person or the consumer. It is not unreasonable to expect nurses to be well versed in both the professional and lay perspectives, using professional resources to keep current about practice while also helping patients as consumers of health care.

KEY TERM

Indexes: A listing of electronic or print resources

TEST YOUR KNOWLEDGE 4-1

1. Learning to perform a quality literature review is essential for which of the following reasons?
   a. Lays the foundation for writing quality undergraduate academic papers
   b. Identifies gaps in current research
   c. Provides basis for making best practice decisions
   d. Develops skills necessary for lifelong learning

True/False

2. All sources retrieved from the internet are applicable to EBP.

3. Access to computers and technical resources is critical to link research to EBP.

4. Librarians are searching and system experts.

5. All useful resources on the web are free and accessible to all.

How did you do? 1. a, b, c, d; 2. F; 3. T; 4. T; 5. F

Access to academic, health sciences, or hospital library resources is vital to quality literature review. Because each library and database has its own best practice procedures, initial time spent orienting with an expert about these systems is worthwhile. Just as nursing faculty are subject content experts, librarians are searching and system experts.

4.2   Types of Evidence

At the end of this section, you will be able to:

[www]

< Explain the scientific literature publication cycle
< Differentiate between primary and secondary sources
< Identify different types of articles found in the literature
< Characterize the four major types of reviews

Not all information is created equal, nor is it presented in the same manner. Being able to identify various types of information and sources is fundamental to starting a successful literature review search.

Scientific Literature Publication Cycle

It is helpful to first consider the *scientific literature publication cycle* to make searching easier (University of Washington Libraries, 1999). As shown in **Figure 4-1**, the cycle generally begins with the idea and the research itself, which is available only informally through raw data reports, grant proposals, and perhaps as-yet-unpublished conference papers. At the next point, when researchers are confident in the findings and their presentations, information is prepared for dissemination as a professional, scholarly paper. Papers judged to be of high quality about studies using sound research methods are accepted by editors of scholarly journals and indexed in literature indexes and databases so that others may find them when conducting literature searches. After this point, papers, or information contained within them, move into a more generalized publication format where they may be summarized or compiled with other like-topic papers. They are typically published in reviews or magazines directed toward a wider, less professionally focused audience. Finally, if findings are considered noteworthy, they may be cited in textbooks or reference materials, such as encyclopedias or bibliographies.

KEY TERM

Scientific literature publication cycle: A model describing how research becomes disseminated in publications

Keeping the scientific literature publication cycle in mind, you might now realize that when looking for the most current, authoritative information on a topic, you should be checking the published, scholarly literature. If the goal is to

FIGURE 4-1 The Scientific Publication Cycle

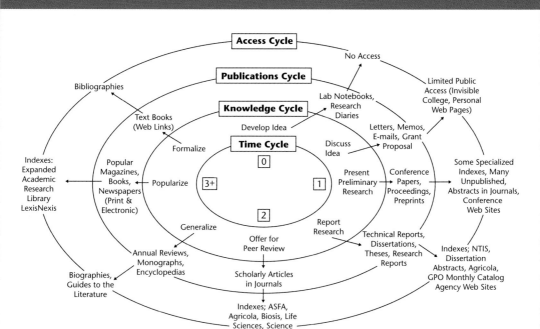

Source: University of Washington Libraries (1999).

compare evidence, systematic reviews are a useful way to locate similar topics quickly. By keeping in mind the publication dates of the studies contained in the systematic review, the search can be completed by searching for evidence published during time spans not covered by the systematic review.

Making Sense of Types of Evidence in the Literature

Evidence in the literature can be categorized in a variety of ways. Nurses find that understanding the terms associated with these categories is helpful when making decisions about evidence. Evidence can be categorized as: 1) primary or secondary, 2) peer reviewed or not peer reviewed, and 3) scholarly, trade, or popular.

Primary and Secondary Sources

Primary sources present original information by the person or people responsible for creating it. Paintings, speeches, diary entries, autobiographies, and

KEY TERM

Primary sources:
Original information presented by the person or people responsible for creating it

interviews are some common examples. In the world of research, however, primary sources are the journal articles, book chapters, dissertations, or conference proceedings written by the people involved in the original research. Primary sources always provide full references to others' work cited within the paper. *Secondary sources* are the resulting commentaries, summaries, reviews, or interpretations of primary sources. Always written after primary sources are presented, and often written by those not involved in the original work, secondary sources can provide new insights or historical perspectives not previously available. Some common secondary sources are textbooks, systematic reviews, biographies, and general magazines. Secondary sources often do not cite the work of others.

For example, an original research paper on Internet use by patients with diabetes is published in the scholarly journal, *Nursing Research*. This publication is considered to be a primary source. Several weeks later, *Newsweek* published a more general article about the effect of the Internet on patient education. In the article, results from the original paper published in *Nursing Research* are mentioned along with a short quote. This article constitutes a secondary source about the original research conducted. Sometimes it is important to eliminate secondary sources because of the bias inherent when someone other than the original researcher provides the information. When creating EBP, nurses should always read primary sources and draw their own conclusions.

Peer Reviewed and Refereed Sources

Research and empirical papers, published as primary sources in scholarly literature, undergo rigorous evaluation by experts and editors, which is known as *peer review* or refereed judging. Subject significance, methods, and conclusions are judged by peer reviewers. When papers meet established criteria, they are accepted for publication. This process is designed to ensure high quality of published works and allows readers who are noted experts to have confidence in what is being presented.

Scholarly, Trade, and Popular Literature Categories

Distinguishing between different types of information categories can help determine the type of information contained within them. There are generally three broad categories: *scholarly*, *trade*, and *popular literature*. Scholarly works are written and edited by professionals in the discipline for other colleagues. They are the vehicles for publication of original research, focus on narrow topics within the discipline, and are often filled with discipline-specific vocabulary. For example, the *Journal of Nursing Scholarship*, published by Sigma Theta Tau International, is a scholarly journal. Trade publications are also written for professionals within a discipline but are written with a more casual tone. They contain information related to professional development, products, practices, or trends in the discipline. *American Journal of Nursing* and *RN Magazine* are examples of trade publications. Popular literature is written to inform or entertain the general public. The writing level is very basic, and graphics often get as much space as the text. For example, *Prevention* is a source of information about health written for the general public.

Periodicals, Journals, and Magazines

Few terms used in libraries cause more confusion than these three: periodicals, journals, and magazines. While some people use these terms as synonyms, it is best to understand the differences between these terms and to use them correctly. *Periodical* is the broadest term of the three and indicates a resource that is published periodically, usually on a set schedule. In many libraries, periodical is the term used to designate these types of publications as a collection. Both journals and magazines are designated as periodicals. *Journal* is the term used to indicate resources of a scholarly or professional nature. *Magazine* indicates a resource targeted for the general reading audience, most often in the popular works category. When having difficulty distinguishing between these three types of resources, a quick consultation with a librarian or a search of a library website for information about this topic can be helpful.

Understanding Types of Reviews

Before the electronic information age, researchers developed ways to keep up to date by creating early forms of reviews to summarize information. Because of the increased volume of information being made available as a result of information technology, there is some cause for concern. Evans and Kowanko (2000) state:

> As the volume of research literature increases, reliance on these summaries will also increase. This reliance will see literature reviews forming the basis of many health care decisions rather than the original primary research. It is therefore important that they are conducted with similar rigour to the studies they summarize. (p. 37)

Consider the implications of a poorly conducted summary when contrasting the academic and clinical settings. When literature reviews conducted for academic papers lack precision and quality searching, the results often lead to a lower grade. Likewise, when considering decisions about EBP, a poorly conducted literature review may negatively impact patient care.

Reviews can be conducted in a variety of ways. Whittemore (2005) details differences among the major types of reviews. Echoing Evans's and Kowanko's (2000) concerns, Whittemore also notes that the "literature search stage is a critical element to conducting a quality research review because incomplete and biased searches result in an inadequate database for the review and the potential for faulty conclusions" (p. 58). To make good decisions about best practice, nurses should familiarize themselves with the major types of reviews: narrative, integrative, meta-analysis, and systematic.

Narrative Reviews

Narrative reviews are the most traditional type of review, thus the most familiar. These kinds of reviews are frequently found in trade publications. Because writers judge which works to include and exclude, narrative reviews are subjective. Often based on only the very common or uncommon elements of the various works, writers are not particularly concerned with widely varying research methods, designs, or settings. For example, the review of literature section in most published articles is a traditional narrative review.

Integrative Reviews

Jackson (1980) defined an *integrative review* as "generalizations about substantive issues from a set of studies directly bearing on those issues" (p. 438). Integrative reviews are scholarly papers that synthesize published studies and articles to answer questions about phenomena of interest. They are typically found in peer-reviewed professional publications. Ganong (1987) is credited with clarifying the steps of conducting integrative reviews in nursing. Ganong's article provides a grid layout that many find useful as a tool to track and compile data from various research papers. Components of the grid include methods, theories, and empirical findings of the reviewed papers. These grids are often included in published integrative reviews. Whittemore (2005) notes that an advantage to integrative reviews "is the ability to combine data from different types of research designs and include theoretical, as well as, empirical literature" (p. 57). In other words, integrative reviews do not need to include works that use the same designs or research methods.

Meta-Analyses

Meta-analyses combine results of studies into a measurable format and statistically estimate the effects of proposed interventions. Unlike in an integrative review, meta-analyses include works that are similar or identical so that statistical comparisons can be made. Another difference between these two types of reviews is that meta-analyses include both published and unpublished works. Evans and Kowanko (2000) surmise that meta-analysis reviews grew from narrative reviews when the increasing amounts of numerical data grew too cumbersome. According to Whittemore (2005), meta-analyses are especially useful as sources of evidence when large randomized trials are not feasible.

Systematic Reviews

Systematic reviews combine elements of the three previously discussed methods. These are "scientific tools which are used to summarize and communicate the results and implications of otherwise unmanageable quantities of research" (Evans & Kowanko, 2000, p. 35). Articles included in systematic reviews all address the same clinical problem. "A well-specified clinical question, use of the best available evidence, explicit methods, and an exhaustive search for

KEY TERM

Systematic reviews: A rigorous, methodical synthesis of research findings about a clinical problem

TEST YOUR KNOWLEDGE 4-2

1. Put the following points of the scientific literature publication cycle in order:
   a. finding cited in textbook
   b. paper accepted for publication in scholarly journal
   c. idea for research identified
   d. article cited in indexes in databases
   e. findings included in magazine article

2. Which of the following are primary sources?
   a. biography
   b. systematic review
   c. research article
   d. dissertation

3. Which of the following journals are considered scholarly journals?
   a. *Nursing Research*
   b. *RN Magazine*
   c. *American Journal of Nursing*
   d. *Journal of Nursing Scholarship*

4. A review that synthesizes only published articles to answer questions about phenomena of interest is known as:
   a. narrative review
   b. integrative review
   c. meta-analysis
   d. systematic review

How did you do? 1. c, b, d, e, a; 2. c, d; 3. a, d; 4. b

relevant primary studies are hallmarks of this method" (Whittemore, 2005, p. 58). Systematic reviews, combined with other types of guidelines, are sources that can be helpful in situations when evidence is needed quickly. Systematic reviews can be found online at the Joanna Briggs Institute and the Cochrane Center and in some professional publications.

4.3   How Sources Are Organized

At the end of this section, you will be able to:

‹ Identify and use a variety of sources, both within and outside of the field of nursing, as appropriate
‹ Understand how the sources are structured
‹ Distinguish between the different sources' content, in both topic or subject matter and in format

Consider your first clinical experience with a patient. Before that experience, you were educated about various aspects of patient care and equipment. No one just handed you a stethoscope and a blood pressure cuff and wished you luck. Most likely, you first read about the various procedures, learned what to expect in typical situations, and then practiced in a laboratory setting. Learning to search for information can be approached in a similar way. Gaining insight about how information resources are structured, what their contents contain, and what search techniques work best will increase your skill and efficiency.

Many factors come into play when conducting a search of the literature. What interests you about the topic should determine the depth and breadth of the search, which sources to search, and the dates of publication to include. Immediate access to sources being sought is not always possible. Sometimes it may take several weeks to acquire sources, while other sources may be unobtainable. Knowing this encourages implementing strategies to ensure that you are able to meet deadlines.

After the research question is developed, the researcher is ready to proceed through the steps of the literature review process. Using selected search words and terms based on the topic, databases are searched, search results are organized, full content of the materials are located, and the evidence is evaluated for its usefulness. Being aware of these steps focuses attention on the process and results.

When information applicable to the subject has been gathered, it is important to keep in mind that the process might not be finished. It is not usual

FYI

To create an EBP, nurses must be aware of information retrieval options. Librarians are an excellent resource for becoming an effective researcher.

for individuals to quit at this point, satisfied that the information they have gathered will somehow work within their needs. Carefully reviewing obtained materials to ensure that they are appropriate can save time and money. Reexamine the original focus and search strategy to ensure that the information obtained is indeed useful. If it is not, determine where the search was flawed and decide whether a new search is necessary.

Finally, make sure that the information gathered is scholarly. Information should be written by knowledgeable authors, published by respected sources, and appropriately current. The content of information should always be evaluated, appraising it on criteria such as intended audience, depth of coverage, objectivity, and related reviews. When you are unsure of the credibility of information, nursing faculty or librarians can provide guidance.

Consult With an Expert

Working with a librarian is guaranteed to save you time. "In addition, there is evidence that library services can lead to time savings for health-care professionals and, thus, to cost savings and health-care benefits" (Weightman & Williamson, 2005, p. 5). Few others on a campus or in a healthcare institution know as much about information structure, storage, retrieval, and evaluation as librarians. Most academic libraries have subject-specialty librarians for specific disciplines, and at health sciences libraries, specialties become even more specific. While reference desk inquiries are appropriate for general questions, an appointment with a subject-specialty librarian is the best way to obtain specific information in a shorter amount of time.

To create an EBP, nurses must be aware of information retrieval options. Hospitals often support library resources and a librarian. Academic or health sciences libraries, especially at state-funded institutions, may allow community members access to their holdings. Academic libraries are especially useful because they have strong collections in the scholarly literature, while public libraries have more consumer-oriented materials.

Looking at the Structure of Sources

When information sources are organized using basic principles of consistent record formatting and field labels, searchers can rely on finding similar information each time they perform the same search, even if new information has been added to the system. For example, if the keyword "anxiety" is entered into a database, the searcher would expect the search to yield information such as author, title of article, year of publication, and the abstract each time the keyword is entered. Each time "anxiety" is entered, the same sources should be seen. If any new sources have been added to the database since the previous search, these should also appear. Considering familiar organizational structures of sources will help in understanding more complex systems. Perhaps the first organizational system you ever learned was the alphabet. Children in kindergarten learn to line up in alphabetical order according to their last names. They do not line up according to height or hair color because those system labels are not as straightforward and consistent as the alphabet. The phone book is another example of a structure for organizing information. The white pages are arranged in alphabetical order. This is a very effective way to organize information when one knows the name of the business one is seeking. The yellow pages offer another organizational structure for searching. Subject listings in the yellow pages were created so that if one knows the type of business, but not its name, the information can be found. The key to using the yellow pages, though, is to know exactly what terms the creators used for the subject areas. For example, if you need a haircut, would you use "hair," "barber," or "beauty shop" as a keyword? While this example might seem very elementary right now, understanding how the phone book is organized will be beneficial when considering the most common types of electronic searches.

Structures can also be designed to organize physical objects. For example, in bookstores, books are organized in subject areas around the store, and within each area, they are perhaps grouped into subcategories and shelved by the author's last name. Libraries are arranged in the same manner, but, because there are many more books to organize, a consistent number or letter/number combination system is used. Most public and school libraries use the Dewey decimal system, while most academic libraries in the United States use the Library of Congress system. Many health sciences libraries use the National Library of Medicine system. Here too, when the books are in their general subject areas, they are then categorized into smaller subcategories and then shelved according to the author's last name. In the library system, every item has its own unique *call number* according to its subject area and author's last name. No other item will have that same number. Familiarity with the system and knowing which system the library uses makes searching for sources more efficient.

Knowing general call numbers of a subject can also expedite searches for items in a library collection. For example, in academic libraries using the Library of Congress method, medical books are located within the R area shelves and nursing books are on the RT shelves. Further knowledge of what subjects the numbers connote can lead to more detailed browsing, such as knowing that the nursing research texts' section is RT 81.5, while writings about nursing history are in the RT 31 shelves. Call numbers for specific books are easily found through searching the library's catalog.

KEY TERM

Call number: Unique number assigned to items in a library by subject and author name

While the structure used in libraries is quite efficient for locating sources, confusion can occur when sources can be classified in more than one way. Information on a specific topic might be scattered throughout the collection. For example, when searching for sources on the topic of ethical practices and how they relate to health care, it is helpful to browse multiple areas, such as nursing ethics, medical philosophy, medical ethics, law of the United States, and medical legislation.

There are other structures that aid in finding information. For example, the table of contents in a book helps readers find information located within the text without having to read every single page. The table of contents narrows the search from hundreds of pages to perhaps 20 or 30 pages. The search can be narrowed even further by using the index that provides a very detailed listing of words contained in the book. By using the index, the search can be narrowed to a few pages.

The concept of indexes has proved to be a very useful structure to assist researchers with finding scholarly articles and reports. Prior to the electronic age, printed indexes of professional literature covering only the information in one particular discipline provided listings of all information produced in that discipline in a particular time span. For nursing, the most recognized and used *print index* started in the 1940s and was known as the *Cumulative Index to Nursing and Allied Health Literature*. Today, nurses use the electronic version known as *CINAHL*. *Electronic indexes* are most commonly referred to as databases.

In the print indexes, information is organized three ways: author listings, title listings, and subject listings. In early print indexes, subject listings offered a new organizational structure. Publishers of the indexes began to choose keywords that would always represent the subject regardless of the words used by authors. For example, the term *heart attack* is always listed as "myocardial infarction." The consistent use of keywords provided a solid foundation for the electronic searching conducted today.

With the advent of electronic resources and the Internet, another type of searching became possible. Searching does not need to be limited to keywords because entire bodies of text can be searched. This is known as *keyword* searching. This type of searching in electronic databases allows searching for the author's words, not the subject terms assigned by the database publisher. Keyword searching is not without its challenges. For example, the word "diet" as it is used by the general public usually is defined as a meal plan to lose weight. Healthcare professionals typically use the word "diet" to refer to meal plans that are therapeutic for patients. When conducting a keyword search, entering "diet" will achieve different results depending on the source. Keyword

KEY TERMS

Print index: Printed listing of electronic or print resources

CINAHL: *Cumulative Index to Nursing and Allied Health Literature; database for nursing and health-related literature*

Electronic indexes: Electronic listing of electronic or print resources

Keyword: A significant word from a title or document used as an index to content searches will also provide results that are exactly what the searcher intends, or not, depending on how the word is used in the text. The source searched does not know the searcher's intent; it only knows what term has been entered.

The Internet, while an accessible source of abundant information, has a very unorganized and inconsistent structure. Tools are being developed to support Internet searching that are comparable to those used in electronic databases. Google Scholar and the advanced search options for Google and Yahoo! browsers give users specific search options, such as searching for phrases, broad subject areas, and document types. As with all organizational structures, knowing how to use the tool results in more productive searches.

Being aware of these simple facts can facilitate searching in indexes and databases. As mentioned earlier, not all electronic resources that were once in print format are comprehensive in their coverage. They may go back only 20 to 25 years in the literature. Foundational or key studies could be missed if they were conducted prior to the date the electronic database began. Keep in mind the frequency with which the database is updated. For example, a database updated monthly will not yield a new search on a daily basis. Searches can be programmed to be performed regularly so that new literature is identified when it is added to the database. Practicing this as a student prepares you to find evidence for implementing best practice.

Databases: The Same but Different

There are variations in databases just as there are variations in the human body. In healthy people there are variations in height, weight, age, and appearance, but overall their organ systems perform in the same manner. Databases also vary in appearance (color, graphics, results display) even though content is the same or very similar. Understanding how a search strategy works in one database can be helpful in understanding how to use another database. When using databases to search for information, if the results of the search are unsatisfactory, the help feature can offer guidance. The fact that not all databases are provided by the same information vendor can be a source of confusion. Consider the many different fast food restaurants that offer variations of the hamburger. Each company touts a special bun, sauce, or grade of hamburger. In the same way, vendors who provide access to the same databases do so in various manners. Companies such as EBSCOhost, Ovid, SilverPlatter, Elsevier, and Thomson Gale purchase database content from the original creator and sell the content with their own design, search options, and date ranges. For example, suppose you are using CINAHL in the EBSCOhost system and a friend at another institution is using it through the Ovid system. While the content and search strategies the two of you use will be similar, your resulting searches and appearance of the screens will be very different. Another cause of confusion for users and librarians alike is that content may change in a database. These changes are due to interactions among vendors and journal publishers who provide the articles. Sources available in full text one day may be found in a citation-only option the next. When this happens, it may not be the result of errors made while searching. Talking to a librarian may resolve the situation and result in obtaining the information desired.

Topic and Subject Matter

Information about scholarly literature of disciplines is collected and indexed in subject-specific databases, such as CINAHL. There is not much, if any, popular-content works contained in them. Additionally, information about works yet to be published, called *grey literature*, includes unpublished reports, conference papers, and grant proposals. Grey literature is often indicative of upcoming hot topics in the field. Databases can also cite professional information, such as organizational guidelines, editorial essays, and letters to the editor. For example, commentaries to authors' work that has generated controversy can be useful sources.

General content databases offer a mix of scholarly, trade, and popular works. Professional journals, popular magazines, newspapers, and industry bulletins may all be part of the search results (unless you limit the search accordingly). These databases are helpful when gathering information on current news events, government reports, and health care from the consumer point of view.

Databases also contain citations useful to patient education. In the healthcare literature, there are distinctions made between consumer health materials and patient education materials. Consumer health materials are general articles about topics such as maintaining a healthy lifestyle. Patient education materials are items that are designed to assist patients in making informed decisions regarding their medical care. Nurses are often asked to decipher what patients hear in the news and refer them to additional, reliable information sources.

Format

In print and electronic information sources, the basic building block is called a *record*. Each piece of information contained in the record has been entered into what is referred to as a *search field*, which makes electronic searching possible. Each record minimally consists of a citation of information and a record number. Citations provide author name, title, publication date, and depending on the type of item, publisher information and page numbers. Citations are the

KEY TERMS

Grey literature: Unpublished reports, conference papers, and grant proposals

Record: Basic building block of print and electronic information sources

Search field: Where each piece of information contained in the record is entered minimal amount of information needed to locate items, and they contain information required for a reference list. Record numbers, similar to call numbers for books, are numbers assigned by the information source and are unique to each record. Depending on the information source, other fields of information may be available about the citation. Subject terms and *subject headings* are often listed. An abstract may be included and is helpful to quickly determine the item's content. Sometimes references cited in the item are also included in the format. Reference information can be helpful for locating other relevant information. Other fields might be added to the record, such as text language, type of publication, or designating an item as research that is evidence based or peer reviewed. While all databases offer citations, these come in three formats: citation only, citation with full content, or a mix of both. Because print indexes are citation only, it always requires an additional step to obtain the full content. Most electronic information sources are mixed. Very few databases provide only full content records, and they are the exception rather than the rule. Because librarians understand the need to have full content available as easily as possible, systems have been created to meet that need. These systems basically tie citations in one database to full content available in other databases or to print resources within the library. If a hyperlink in the record is available to link to full content, no additional step is needed.

When items are not available in full content within any database or within library print holdings, a copy of the item can be retrieved through the *interlibrary loan* system. For your convenience, most records provide a hyperlink to interlibrary loan request forms so that requests can be made immediately when you determine that an item is not available locally. Most of the time, this service is subsidized by the library and is available at no cost. Because it usually takes 7 to 10 days after making a request to receive materials, it is prudent to begin

TEST YOUR KNOWLEDGE 4-3

True/False

1. All libraries use the same system for organizing their collections.

2. Table of contents and indexes can be useful to narrow searches for evidence.

3. Knowing key terms used in an index can facilitate effective searches.

How did you do? 1. F; 2. T; 3. T

searches well before deadlines. Journal articles are usually copied and sent to the requester to keep. Books, videos, and other such items are sent on loan and must be returned to the lending library. Because each library's procedure is slightly different, it is important to understand how to request materials prior to needing this service. You might not receive everything requested because copyright issues, limited numbers of available copies, and other restrictions can impact requests.

4.4   How to Search for Evidence

At the end of this section, you will be able to:

< Perform various types of searches using basic and advanced source tools and search techniques
< List four databases where scholarly literature of disciplines is indexed

Access to Content: Tools and Techniques

There are three types of access to information: free access, access paid by an institution, and access paid by an individual. Most electronic sources provided by the U.S. government are free access. Most libraries grant free access to their holdings to those physically present. If the item is available for borrowing, a library card is needed to check out the item. Although these services are provided to patrons for free, the library is paying the costs. Nurses can often access resources for free at their places of work. Like libraries, the healthcare organization is charged to provide the services. Regardless, access to electronic sources is being paid for by someone. For example, if there were a nurse who was self employed, that nurse may have to subscribe as an individual to access CINAHL.

General Search Strategies

Searching for evidence does take time, but knowing the organization of the system and doing a search correctly can improve efficiency. Novice searchers often begin by searching for a specific type of document, such as a nursing research article reporting outcomes of an experimental study. While it is good to have an idea of the evidence that you would like to find, do not discount other evidence uncovered during the search. Sometimes a continuing education article that mentions a particular study or a literature review in an article on a related topic may provide sources not found through other methods of searching. Another helpful strategy to locate evidence is to build searches both backward

FYI

Knowing a variety of search techniques—such as keywords, Boolean operators, and truncation—is essential to effective research, while accessing the most reliable databases ensure EBP.

and forward in time. This is sometimes called *citation chasing*. For example, a nurse locates a single article about community preparations for bioterrorism. The nurse examines the references listed to determine if there are other sources on this topic that seem to stand out as foundational or noteworthy. If so, the nurse obtains these sources and proceeds to appraise their reference lists as well. This strategy is an effective way to search previous literature and often identify the articles that were first published about the topic. Forward searching strategies are made possible by electronic databases. For example, the nurse enters information for a single article and uses a hyperlink option "times cited in this database." This link connects to other documents that have cited that article since its publication.

Hints for Searching Print Indexes

Because of the convenience of electronic resources, most individuals are unfamiliar with print indexes. Typically, print indexes are used to search for older literature that has not been indexed in electronic databases. Therefore, perhaps the best strategy when using print indexes is to ask a librarian for help. Librarians are familiar with the sources and know which sources will be most useful. Because older print resources are primarily organized by time, usually in spans of a year or two, knowing the years to search can help immensely. Keeping in mind that search terms change over time is also important when using print indexes. For example, while "patient education" is the correct subject term today, if searching records created before 1988, the correct term is "health education, information services."

Hints for Searching Electronic Databases

Parameters of recall and precision provide conceptual baselines for refining search strategies in electronic databases. The successful integration of these parameters results in retrieved records that more closely match the desired focus and number of sources that are desired.

Recall describes the broad "catch" of retrieved records. Those records, usually high in number, will display a wide range of what has been classified as related records. Recall is a strategy best used when the information being sought is uniquely detailed, a new topic or procedure, or has not been widely written about in the literature. By gathering a large number of records, there can be some assurance that the information needed is somewhere within them, even though many of the records retrieved will not be relevant.

Precision is a search strategy that narrows the parameters of the search. When a search term displays a precise retrieval, the records are usually smaller in number but more closely matched to the entered search terms. This search strategy is best when the information being sought has been written about in a number of authoritative sources by a number of knowledgeable people. The search can be narrowed without undue concern about the loss of some relevant records because it is likely that the search contained needed information in the retrieved records.

An effective technique, especially for novices whose skills are not yet finely tuned, is to combine these search strategies. Beginning with a recall strategy will retrieve many records. Following with precision search strategies will narrow the field of the originally recalled records.

Basic Searches: Using Keywords

There are two basic types of search queries when searching electronic databases: keyword and controlled vocabulary. Each has its own benefits and constraints, but the key to successful searching is knowing which type of query is being used. Because the Internet is easy to use, bad search habits have resulted. Internet search engines are eager to please and therefore usually produce results for the entered search term. However, the results often include unrelated items. The definition of terms may not match, the websites identified may be of dubious quality, or perhaps a misspelled search term retrieves matches from others who have misspelled words the same way. Electronic databases hold searchers to a higher level of use. For example, correct spelling really counts. When words are misspelled, databases reply with "zero results retrieved." By practicing good search habits, databases can offer consistency in searching, reliability of information found, and access to information not available on the open Internet. Keyword searching allows you to enter a search term that best describes it as it is used in information source records. While this search strategy will retrieve related records, searches will also need to include synonyms and variations of the search term to ensure that all relevant records were retrieved. For example, when searching for information about newborns and their mothers, a keyword search using the terms "bonding" and "attachment" would be necessary. Keyword searches are often best for searching full text or citation records. In most databases, keyword searching also considers words in the title, content notes, and author fields of each item's record.

Search tools are used to refine keyword searches. While the underlying concepts of these tools remain constant across various applications and resources, some electronic databases do not support all of them, or their symbols may be slightly different. To make the best use of powerful search strategies, it is essential to check the database's help files to make sure the tools are available and that the chosen symbols are entered correctly.

Search operators, also known as *Boolean operators*, are words that specify the relationship between two or more search terms. Search terms can be linked in a number of ways using the terms *and, or,* or *not*.

Using "and" narrows a search. Both of the search terms entered must be found somewhere in the record, though not necessarily in the same place. For example, terms may be a part of an author's name and part of a title. In most databases, the Boolean operation of "and" is automatically used when two or more keywords are entered. For example, a nurse is searching for information about eating disorders. Entering the keywords "anorexia" and "bulimia" will return only records containing both terms.

Using the Boolean operation of "or" broadens a search. When using this approach, either search term must be found somewhere in the record. This is especially helpful when searching synonyms or words with various forms. Unlike electronic databases, most Internet search engines default to the "or" operation when two or more keywords are entered. This explains why a search can retrieve so many irrelevant records. For example, a search strategy of "anorexia or bulimia" will return records that contain either one or both terms.

Searches can be narrowed by using the Boolean operation of "not." Using this operation, a record can be retrieved only if the first search term is present and the second search term is not present. In the example of eating disorders, entering keywords "anorexia not bulimia" will return results that contain only anorexia.

Search operators can also be used with Internet search engines. It is essential to check the help files of the search engine. Some search engines require that the search operators be typed in all capital letters, some accept two of the three operators and not the other, and some require the combination "and not" for the "not" operator.

Another helpful strategy when conducting basic searches is *truncation*, which is the ability to retrieve records of search terms that share a common root. In each database, a symbol of some sort is placed at the end of the group of letters forming the root search term. The symbol is usually an asterisk, but sometimes a colon, a question mark, a dollar sign, or a pound sign might be used. Check the help files to see which symbol is used in the database being used. Using the longest root possible increases the accuracy of the search. For example, instead of entering all of the terms "nurse," "nurses," and "nursing" in a search, truncation would replace all three with "nurs*." The challenge with truncation, however, is that it is often surprising to find how many words share common roots. In this example, records that include nursery and nursing home will also be retrieved.

The use of *wildcards* is another strategy that involves substituting symbols for one or more letters in a search term. Many databases use the question mark as a wildcard. The help section provides information about how wildcards are used. For example, instead of entering both "woman" and "women" as search terms, use the wildcard entry "wom?n" instead.

Nesting, or grouping, is a strategy best used when a search contains two or more Boolean operators. Parentheses, and sometimes quotation marks, are used to indicate which search terms are grouped together. Just as in elementary algebra problems, the information within the parentheses will be processed first and then applied to the information outside the parentheses. Another way to use nesting is to place the parentheses around a phrase or proper noun to instruct the database to search for the terms exactly as entered. For example, if searching for information about the use of herbal remedies, entering "(herbal remedies)" would generate records about this topic. Nesting is becoming a useful option with many Internet search tools and databases.

In most databases, the first screen allows searchers to apply limits to fields being searched within records, thereby filtering searches from the very start. Limits can be set for fields such as search term, language, publication type, and publication date. Limiting a set after an initial search will create a new list of records, drawn from the original set of records that is narrower in scope. In some databases, it is possible to apply consecutive limits, which further narrows each subset.

Stopwords are words that are so commonly used in records that they are a hindrance to accurate record retrieval. These words are usually articles of speech, conjunctions, and pronouns. Although database searching has been programmed to ignore stopwords, some databases still show "failed search" when stopwords are used. While stopwords can vary among databases, the most common ones to avoid are *a, an, and, for, in, of, the, this,* and *to.*

Advanced Searches: Controlled Vocabulary

Controlled vocabularies are standardized, hierarchical lists that have been designated to represent major subject concepts and conditions contained within a database. Vocabularies usually change from database to database. The hierarchical nature of the lists benefits search strategies by allowing broad concepts to be narrowed in a manner that stays consistent within that framework. CINAHL's list is called CINAHL Headings. MEDLINE and The Cochrane Library use Medical Subject Headings (MeSH). Before items are added to a database, subject matter is determined. Specific terms that apply to the determined subjects will be chosen from the standardized list, regardless of the terminology used by authors. This approach provides a consistent method for retrieving the

KEY TERMS

Wildcards: Symbols substituted for one or more letters in a search term

Nesting: A strategy best used when a search contains two or more Boolean operators

Stopwords: Words, such as a, the, and in, that are so commonly used that they can hinder accurate record retrieval

Controlled vocabularies: Standardized hierarchical lists that represent major subjects within a database

Subject searching: Searching databases using controlled vocabulary

Exploding: Technique for searching subject headings that identifies all records indexed to that term

Qualification: Limiting fields of search, commonly using limits such as author, title, or subject

Positional operators: Specify the number of words that can appear between search terms

records even when different terminology is used in the text. For example, the term *heart attack* is always listed as "myocardial infarction" within a controlled vocabulary structure. Using controlled vocabulary searching is called *subject searching*. Unless otherwise noted, only records that match exactly to the terms as they were entered will be displayed. The challenge is to determine what term is being used to represent the subject matter that is being sought. It is possible to find standardized lists used in databases to determine the best terms to use. In most databases, terms are hyperlinked for ease of use. Do not assume that a keyword in one database will be the same one to use in another database. For example, a search conducted in the PsycINFO database may use a different subject term than a search conducted in the MEDLINE database, even though both are science-related databases. When this happens, the search "fails" and the searcher is mistakenly led to believe that the second database contains no information on the topic. *Exploding* is one of the most powerful techniques for searching subject headings. When a subject term is exploded, the database is instructed to search all the records indexed to that term as well as any terms that are in a related, narrower category. For example, exploding the search term "headache" in a CINAHL search would result in a search that includes the terms "rebound headache" and "vascular headache." Exploding can dramatically increase the number of records generated by the search. Most health sciences databases support this technique. One of the benefits of knowing both keyword and subject searching is that they can be combined to increase the effectiveness and efficiency of the search. Qualification and positional operators are more advanced keyword techniques that can be very powerful when used in combination with subject searching. *Qualification* designates which fields are to be searched in the record. The most common ways to limit searches are by author (au), title (ti), subject (su), publisher, and publication date. Placement of the punctuation can be important when using limiting search terms. These options may be available only using the advanced search methods in databases.

The proximity of search terms to one another can be specified using *positional operators*. The most commonly used are "adj" (adjacent), "near," and "same." Usually, "adj" and "near" can be grouped with a number to specify the number of words that can appear between search terms. "Same" designates that the search terms are found in the same field of the record such as the title or the abstract. Because order is not designated with "same," search terms will not necessarily be next to one another. When using this technique, it is best to check the help section for instructions.

Best Sources for EBP

Both print and electronic resources contain useful information to answer EBP questions. Many useful encyclopedias, handbooks, guides, and care plan manuals are available in print-only format. Asking a librarian for details on the collection can provide valuable insight. Electronic sources offer a mix of scholarly, trade, and popular works. Professional journals, popular magazines, newspapers, and industry bulletins may all be part of the search results. The three most commonly found general databases are Academic Search Premier, Expanded Academic ASAP, and LexisNexis Academic. The first two databases contain very similar content and have a higher percentage of scholarly work than LexisNexis Academic. LexisNexis Academic is all full content and offers a wider range of news, business, and legal sources than do the other two databases. In subject-specific databases, scholarly literature of professions and disciplines is indexed. Because most electronic sources are international in their collection scopes, a separate distinction has been made for those resources produced by the U.S. government. **Table 4-1** provides categorization and general information about subject-specific databases that are extremely useful when creating EBP. The URL is provided for access to additional information, but if the database is proprietary, it will not provide access to the content. Ac-

TABLE 4-1 Subject-Specific Databases

CINAHL	*http://www.ebscohost.com/cinahl/*	CINAHL is the premier database covering the areas of nursing and allied health. Online coverage is usually comprehensive back to 1982 with monthly updates. After beginning with the indexing of 5 journals in the 1940s, there are currently more than 2,800 journals indexed, resulting in more than 1,000,000 records.
MEDLINE via PubMed	*http://www.ncbi.nlm.nih.gov/pubmed/18335860*	Providing coverage of MEDLINE and other medical sciences and biomedical literature back to the 1950s, PubMed is a service of the U.S. National Library of Medicine, providing free access on the Internet to more than 17,000,000 citations. While this link is to the free version available on the Internet, your library might provide access to other vendor-created versions that might provide a familiar search environment and then also link directly to library resources (and it will be called MEDLINE, not PubMed).

PubMed Clinical Queries	*http://www.ncbi. nlm.nih.gov/sites/ pubmedutils/clinical*	The Clinical Queries search supports specialized PubMed queries for clinicians in areas of clinical studies, systematic reviews, and medical genetics.
Evidence-Based Nursing/EBN Online	*http://ebn.bmj.com/*	EBN Online seeks to help practicing nurses keep up with the evidence-based literature in a manageable manner. Each study presented on the website begins with a brief but detailed abstract followed by expert commentary on the potential for clinical application of the study.
Joanna Briggs Institute	*http://www. joannabriggs.edu. au/about/home.php*	Based in the Royal Adelaide Hospital and the University of Adelaide (Australia), the institute was established in 1996 to offer collaboration in EBP with healthcare professionals and researchers across the professional continuum in more than 40 countries.
The Cochrane Collaboration and Library	*http://www. cochrane.org*	An international not-for-profit organization, the collaboration seeks to provide timely, up-to-date research evidence. Not a physical entity, the Cochrane Library is a database collection, providing access to systematic reviews, controlled trials, methodology registry, technology assessment, and more. DARE (Database of Abstracts of Reviews of Effects) is also part of the library.
Centre for Evidence-Based Research	*http://www.cebm. net/?o=1013*	Established in Oxford, England, the centre's mission is to provide free and open access to support and resources in the field of evidence-based health care to anyone who wants to make use of them.
The TRIP Database	*http://www. tripdatabase.com*	In support of EBP, the TRIP database aims simply to provide healthcare professionals with easy access to high-quality material on the web. Its contents are evaluated by the Centre for Evidence-Based Medicine. After 4 years of being a subscription-only service, it resumed as an open access service in September 2006.

Virginia Henderson International Nursing Library	*http://www. nursinglibrary.org/ portal/main.aspx*	With a primary goal of becoming a comprehensive nursing resource, the library, and its Registry of Nursing Research database, offers nurses access to reliable, easy-to-use information.
Agency for Healthcare Research and Quality (AHRQ): Evidence-based Practice	*http://www.ahrq. gov/clinic/epcix.htm*	This site provides open internet access to categorized EBP resources, reports, and related issues. There are links to other parts of the AHRQ site as well, in clinical practice guidelines, outcomes and effectiveness, technology assessments, and preventive services.
National Guideline Clearinghouse	*http://www. guideline.gov*	An initiative of the AHRQ, the clearinghouse serves as an open-access, public resource for evidence-based clinical practice guidelines.
National Quality Measures Clearinghouse	*http://www. qualitymeasures. ahrq.gov*	Another resource sponsored by AHRQ, this site serves as a public repository for evidence-based quality measures and measure sets.
National Institute of Nursing Research	*http://www.nih.gov/ ninr*	NINR is a foundational resource in supporting and improving health across the spectrum. Among other initiatives, the institute supports and conducts its own clinical research and provides training on health and illness issues.
BMJ Clinical Evidence	*http://www. clinicalevidence. com/ceweb/index. jsp*	Owned by the British Medical Journal Publishing Group Ltd., this internet site adds the fluidity of web-based updates to an already respected, authoritative peer-reviewed journal that provides access to systematic reviews of clinical conditions.
EMBASE	*http://www.embase. com*	With more than 18,000,000 records, EMBASE provides comprehensive online access to recent literature in pharmacological and biomedical literature. It includes MEDLINE records in those topic areas from 1966–present.

ClinicalTrials.gov	*http://clinicaltrials. gov/ct/gui*	A collaboration between the National Library of Medicine and the Food and Drug Administration, Clinical Trials.gov offers access to more than 36,000 clinical studies sponsored by various federal agencies and private industry. The website offers up-to-date information on the various federal and private clinical trials. All 50 states and over 130 countries have trials listed within the collection.
American FactFinder	*http://factfinder. census.gov/home/ saff/main .html?_lang=en*	The definitive source for population, housing, economic, and geographic data as provided by the U.S. Census.
PsycINFO	*http://www.apa.org/ pubs/databases/ psycinfo/index.aspx*	Dating back to 1887 in its electronic coverage, PsycINFO is the definitive source of psychology literature, claiming that more than 97% of its content material is peer-reviewed.
ERIC	*http://www.eric. ed.gov*	The Educational Resources Information Center (ERIC) is the definitive source of education literature. While this link is to the free version available on the internet, your library might provide access to other vendor-created versions that might provide a familiar search environment and then also link directly to library resources.
Sociological Abstracts	*http://www.csa.com/ factsheets/socioabs-set-c.php*	Sociological Abstracts provides access to international literature in sociology and in the related social sciences and behavioral disciplines.
Social Services Abstracts	*http://www.csa. com/factsheets/ssa-set-c.php*	Social Services Abstracts provides access to current research in social work, human services, social welfare, social policy, and community development.
ABI Inform	*http://proquest. com/products_pq/ descriptions/abi_ inform.shtml*	Serving here as an example of an excellent business literature source, ABI Inform is the comprehensive business database, covering all areas of business conditions and related topics. While some business-related materials are within CINAHL, searching the business literature for issues of human resources, staffing, customer service, and so on, can be helpful.

Dissertation Abstracts Online	http://www.proquest.com/en-US/products/dissertations/	Coverage includes dissertations and theses from the United States, Canada, Britain, and other European countries. Searching dissertation topics is a great way to learn what is new in the disciplines as well as gain access to comprehensive reference lists.
Google Scholar	http://scholar.google.com/	Google Scholar allows you to use the familiarity of Google to search the Internet in an interdisciplinary way. Citation results are scholarly in nature and will direct you to full content if it is available on the Internet. Google Scholar also partners with libraries to set up linking with their full content resources. Your librarian can tell you if this is possible in your system.

cess may be available through local libraries or places of employment. After evidence has been gathered, materials must be appraised for their integrity and applicability. Sources chosen by your library, a respected professional organization, or a reputable government agency have already been through an evaluation process. Most individuals struggle with evaluating other Internet sources. A couple of general guidelines will serve you well:

< If you have any doubts at all about the information, do not use it. Or, minimally, verify it elsewhere in a reputable source.
< Ask your nursing faculty or librarian for insight on the situation. Chances are your discussion with them will clarify your concerns, and as often happens in a discussion of this type, your decision will become apparent.

CRITICAL THINKING EXERCISE 4-1

Which of the following two articles would you recommend to your unit supervisor for changing practice? Explain why you would make this recommendation. One article contains general referrals to the foremost authorities on the topic, and five research studies are cited. The second article contains a summative review of research conducted by authorities in the field, various application scenarios for different institutions, and a comprehensive reference list.

TEST YOUR KNOWLEDGE 4-4

Match the following:

1. Boolean operator
2. Wildcard
3. Stopwords
4. Qualification
5. Positional operator

a. ?
b. Near, same, or adj
c. Or, and, or not
d. au, ti, or su
e. for, this, or to

How did you do? 1. c; 2. a; 3. e; 4. d; 5. b

There are many guides and resources available in local libraries that help evaluate Internet materials. Evaluating sources is not as simple as just using a checklist. LoBiondo-Wood (2002) notes that we all have "choices . . . when using information from any source. Certainly any source of information can be misinterpreted but you are less likely to misuse information or obtain poor information if you think through both the validity and the reliability of the information" (p. 11). In other words, if you discover a piece of evidence that is not confirmed in any other sources and is never mentioned as new, foundational, or groundbreaking, the information is questionable.

4.5   Keeping It Ethical

At the end of this section, you will be able to:

‹ Consider the ethical presentation and application of evidence

The phrase, "give credit where credit is due" is familiar to most individuals. There are few places that more stringently apply the concept of attribution than the university setting. For those new to academic writing, the reference list and citing of sources within papers is confusing and is often considered a purposeless task imposed by the professor. Often, the citation of references is the last thing done when deadlines are approaching. Consequently, not much thought is given to the importance of attributing information to appropriate sources.

Citations of sources provide acknowledgments of others' ideas and contributions to the subject. Ideas are owned by those individuals who first wrote about them. For example, when you submit a paper to a professor, you have created a piece of original work. No one else has written about the topic in quite the same way, used the same sources in the same way, or drawn conclusions in the same way.

To a degree, there are cultural differences regarding the formal acknowledgment of the work of others. In Western academic culture, it is considered *plagiarism* to use another's work without giving proper credit. A simple rule to avoid plagiarism is if you have read it, heard it, or viewed it and want to include it, cite it. If the thought, wording, or graphic is not your original work, cite the source. Because plagiarism is considered to be a serious violation of ethical standards, penalties can be severe. Plagiarism is easy to avoid by providing proper citations.

Things get a little less clear when it comes to paraphrasing the work of others. This is when unintentional plagiarism can occur, even by the most conscientious students. There are examples of both direct quotes and paraphrasing in this chapter. Paraphrasing can be identified by noting the citation for the author names and publication dates. Depending on the sentence construction, paraphrasing either precedes or follows those indicators. Paraphrasing can be very challenging. If you have difficulty with this technique, use direct quotes or seek assistance from your school's writing center.

Using the common knowledge test can help determine if a citation is required. Like paraphrasing, over time you will become more comfortable with this. As you become more knowledgeable about accepted facts in nursing, you will be able to recognize common knowledge situations. Another simple rule is if you have to look it up, cite it. For example, it is common knowledge that antibiotics are used to treat infections. But if information is presented about a new antibiotic that is not well known, a citation would be required. It is better to err on the side of caution and write a paper with too many citations than to accidentally plagiarize.

Your authority as a writer in the discipline is increased when proper credit is given to the work of others. Practiced professionals often skim a reference list to see if foundational studies are included, and if not, they may disregard the paper. By placing your original thoughts within the context of others who are already known and respected, you are continuing the scholarly conversation from your perspective. Given the increase in undergraduate research, your contributions could provide a new insight that results in being cited by others.

KEY TERM

Plagiarism: The use of another's work without giving proper credit

 FYI

Keeping the review of the literature ethical requires giving full credit to sources, which entails keeping accurate citations.

TEST YOUR KNOWLEDGE 4-5

1. Plagiarism is avoided by:
   a. using quotations with proper citations
   b. paraphrasing the work of others
   c. erring on the side of caution
   d. cutting and pasting from websites

How did you do? 1. a, b, c

Citation formatting is not just busywork to add stress to the completion of a paper. Just as the proper information in search fields provides consistency and reliability to searching, providing citation information that is correct and in the right format increases the reliability and ease of locating those sources if desired. Providing the correct citation information allows your work to serve as a conduit for those who are citation chasing.

 RAPID **REVIEW**

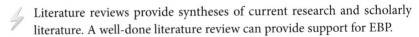

Today's work environment requires that nurses be adept at gathering and appraising evidence for clinical practice and assisting patients with health-care information needs.

Literature reviews provide syntheses of current research and scholarly literature. A well-done literature review can provide support for EBP.

An understanding of the scientific literature publication cycle provides a basis for making decisions about the most current information on a topic.

Primary sources are original sources of information presented by the people who created them. Secondary sources are resulting commentaries, summaries, reviews, or interpretations of primary sources.

Many research journals involve peer review.

There are many ways to categorize sources. Scholarly, trade, and popular literature is one way. Another categorizing system involves periodicals, journals, and magazines.

APPLY WHAT YOU HAVE LEARNED

The EBP Committee has agreed upon the following PICO question: Are other strategies more successful for reducing medication errors involving hospitalized adults than the current way that meds are administered? The next step for the committee is to find pertinent literature.

1. What keywords would you use to conduct a search of CINAHL to retrieve sources of evidence?

2. The Internet is another source of evidence. What websites in Table 4-1 might provide additional information? On the companion website, you'll find items of evidence that were obtained through a search of CINAHL and websites. The next task for committee members is to read and analyze each piece of evidence. The committee has decided to use a grid to organize and summarize the evidence so that the information is presented in a consistent and succinct format. This is helpful because trends can be easily identified and gaps in the knowledge base are made apparent. Organizing the review with a grid is a positive strategy to overcome the barrier of lack of time because it reduces the need to repeatedly sort through articles during future discussions. Also on the companion website, you will find a grid to use for this exercise. Two articles (Cohen & Shastay, 2008; Rothschild et al., 2005) are summarized as an example.

3. Read the following articles: Fowler, Sohler, and Zarillo (2009) and Kliger, Blegen, Gootee, and O'Neil (2009). Enter information about these articles into the first two columns. In column one use APA format, like in the example, because this is the most commonly used style for nursing publications.

There are four types of review: narrative, integrative, meta-analysis, and systematic.

Understanding how sources are structured can simplify a search of the literature.

Sources can be identified through both print indexes and electronic databases. Topics, subject matter, and format may vary but all include citation information.

Helpful strategies to use when conducting a search include: citation chasing, measurements of recall and precision, keyword and controlled vocabulary searches, Boolean operators, truncation, wildcards, nesting, limits, stopwords, exploding, qualification, and positional operators.

Databases can be either general content sources or subject-specific content sources. CINAHL is nursing's premier subject-specific database.

 By interacting with professional literature through writing, creating literature reviews, and conducting research, nurses are part of the scholarly conversation taking place within their discipline. Correct attribution to sources of others' original work, as well as proper construction of citations, demonstrates the ethical sense of responsibility and professionalism.

REFERENCES

Cohen, H., & Shastay, D. (2008). Getting to the root of medication errors: *Nursing 2008, 38*(12), 39–49.

Evans, D., & Kowanko, I. (2000). Literature reviews: Evolution of a research methodology. *The Australian Journal of Advanced Nursing, 18*(2), 33–38.

Fitzpatrick, J. J., Romano, C. A., & Chasek, R. (2001). *The nurses' guide to consumer health web sites.* New York: Springer.

Fowler, S. B., Sohler, P., & Zarillo, D. F. (2009). Bar-code technology for medication administration: Medication errors and nurse satisfaction. *MEDSURG Nursing, 18,* 103–109.

Ganong, L. H. (1987). Integrative reviews of nursing research. *Research in Nursing & Health, 10*(1), 1–11.

Hedba, T., Czar, P., & Mascara, C. (2005). *Internet resource guide for nurses and health care professionals* (3rd ed.). Upper Saddle River, NJ: Pearson Prentice Hall.

Jackson, G. B. (1980). Methods for integrative reviews. *Review of Educational Research, 50,* 438–460.

Kliger, J., Blegen, M. A., Gootee, D., O'Neil, E. (2009). Empowering frontline nurse: A structured intervention enables nurses to improve medication administration accuracy. *The Joint Commission Journal on Quality and Patient Safety, 35,* 604–612.

Lander, J. (2005). Finding, evaluating, and using research for best practice. *Clinical Nursing Research, 14,* 299–302.

LoBiondo-Wood, G. (2002). Evaluating the validity of internet resources. *Inside Case Management, 8*(11), 1, 3–4, 11.

Rothschild, J. M., Keohane, C. A., Cook, E. F., Orav, E. J., Burdick, E., Thompson, S., . . . Bates, D. W. (2005). A controlled trial of smart infusion pumps to improve medication safety in critically ill patients. *Critical Care Medicine, 33,* 533–540.

University of Washington Health Sciences Libraries. (2007). *Evidence-based practice.* Retrieved August 15, 2010, from http://healthlinks.washington.edu/ebp

University of Washington Libraries. (1999). *Scientific publication cycle.* Retrieved August 15, 2010, from http://www.lib.washington.edu/subject/ environment/imt220/pubcycle.jpg

Weightman, A. L., & Williamson, J. (2005). The value and impact of information provided through library services for patient care: A systematic review. *Health Information and Libraries Journal, 22*(1), 4–25.

Whittemore, R. (2005). Combining evidence in nursing research. *Nursing Research, 54*, 56–62.

www

CHAPTER OBJECTIVES

At the end of this chapter, you will be able to:

< Define the terms *theory* and *research* as they relate to the practice of nursing

< Distinguish between conceptual and empirical definitions

< Describe how theory and research influence each other in a professional discipline

< Apply the language of the discipline in describing the relevance of linking theory, research, and practice in nursing

< Discuss how honoring prior work ethically builds nursing knowledge

KEY TERMS

concepts
conceptual definitions
construct
empirical indicators

metaparadigm
model
operational definitions
proposition

theoretical frameworks
theory

CHAPTER 5

Linking Theory, Research, and Practice

Elsabeth Jensen

5.1 How Are Theory, Research, and Practice Related?

At the end of this section, you will be able to:

< Define the terms *theory* and *research* as they relate to the practice of nursing
< Distinguish between conceptual and empirical definitions
< Describe how theory and research influence each other in a professional discipline
< Apply the language of the discipline in describing the relevance of linking theory, research, and practice in nursing.

"The bringing together or nexus of nursing theory, practice and research creates a true integration of knowledge designed to support the service to clients and the health of society" (Butcher, 2006, p. 112). In the profession of nursing, theories and research provide an essential foundation for practice and exist to serve the goals of practice. At the same time, practice is the source of the questions to be addressed by research. The relationships among theory, research, and practice are reciprocal in that each informs the other in the development of disciplinary knowledge. Practice is also the testing ground for theory, where only those theories found helpful to practice survive and evolve. Practice is also a source for new theories. In the same way, the disciplinary knowledge that is nursing knowledge is also dynamic and evolving. As

FYI

Knowledge
is not static,
but rather
it develops
out of asking
questions and
seeking answers.
Learning to ask
good questions
is as essential
as learning how
to find good
answers.

students prepare for practice as nurses, it is easy to believe that what is being learned is sound and should never be questioned. Learning to ask good questions and developing a critical mind is essential. Knowledge is not static, but rather it develops out of asking questions and seeking answers. Learning to ask good questions is as essential as learning how to find good answers.

Understanding Theory, Research, and Practice From a Practice Perspective

There are terms applicable when discussing theory, research, and practice. Understanding these terms allows nurses to communicate ideas effectively with other members of the healthcare team to develop an evidence-based practice.

The Special Language of Theory

A *theory* is a set of concepts linked through propositions to provide an explanation of a phenomenon. Nursing theories are belief systems that guide practice (Parse, 2006). Theory provides the lens through which nurses view clients. In any discipline there is usually one model that defines it at any point in time (Butcher, 2006). Currently in nursing, the concepts of person, environment, health, and nursing are the focus of the development of disciplinary knowledge (Fawcett, 1984; Graham, 2003). These four concepts have been present from the time of Nightingale (1969). Nurses have many formal nursing theories available from which to choose. While it is beyond the scope of this chapter to describe them, it is important for students and nurses to study them because they represent the many ways that nursing practice can be approached. Using theory in practice provides a framework to nurses as they assess and provide care. The study of theory introduces a new language that is specific to nursing. Fawcett and Downs (1992) are considered to be authorities on the study of theory and research. As mentioned earlier, the concepts that are core to nursing are person, environment, health, and nursing. These are known as the *metaparadigm* of nursing. The concepts are very broad, and each nursing theory provides definitions for how they are used in that model. *Concepts* are the words or phrases that convey a unique idea or mental image that is relevant to the theory. For example, Hildegard Peplau (1952) defined health as the forward movement of personality, while Martha Rogers (1970) defined health as being what the person says it is, that is to say, individuals define health for themselves, and nurses need to know what that definition is for each person. As another example, Nightingale (1969) defined environment as everything outside the person, while Rogers (1970) defined environment as being integral with the person. These are different views and lead to some differences in the focus of practice of nurses guided by each of these theories.

KEY TERMS

Theory: A set of
concepts linked
through propositions
to explain a
phenomenon

Metaparadigm: Four
broad concepts core
to nursing: person,
environment, health,
and nursing

Concepts: Words or
phrases that convey
a unique idea that is
relevant to a theory

CRITICAL THINKING EXERCISE 5-1

In your nursing program, how are the concepts of the metaparadigm defined? Is there a model or theory that is used?

Concepts are individual building blocks joined together in statements to create propositions. A *proposition* is a statement about the relationship between two or more concepts. For example, Nightingale (1969) linked a concept from the environment, sunlight, to the concept of health when she wrote:

> It is the unqualified result of all my experience with the sick, that second only to their need of fresh air is their need of light . . . not only light, but direct sunlight they want . . . People think the effect is upon the spirits only . . . we must admit that light has quite as real and tangible effects upon the human body. (p. 84)

Nightingale's proposition is that exposure to sunlight promotes healing and recovery in the person. Knowing this, nurses will expose people to sunlight to promote health.

Another important word in the language of theory is *construct*. A construct is a property that is neither directly nor indirectly observed. It is a word or phrase to communicate a specific, key idea to others. One example of a construct is social support. Social support cannot actually be seen, but it can be inferred through assessment of other observable attributes. To assess social support, nurses could count the number of people in a patient's circle of family and friends or could assess the quality of social support by asking patients about their perceptions of the support they receive.

The Importance of Testing Theory

Nurses look to research to develop and test ideas that may be useful and also look to researchers to address practice questions for which there are no answers. Nursing researchers are responsible for developing and testing knowledge to guide nursing practice (Butcher, 2006). There are important distinctions to note in order to understand what is and what is not nursing research. Nursing research is research that provides results that are relevant for practice, either at the level of basic research or at the level of applied research. Some researchers claim their work is nursing research because the researcher is a nurse or because the researcher studied nurses. But it is the focus on nursing practice

KEY TERMS

Proposition: A statement about the relationship between two or more concepts

Construct: A word or phrase used to communicate a specific key idea to others

 FYI

Nursing research provides results that are relevant to and expand or enhance practice. For research to be considered *nursing* research, the focus is on nursing practice, rather than research that happens to be conducted by a nurse.

CASE EXAMPLE 5-1

Early Methods of Resuscitation: An Example of Practice Based on Untested Theory

Throughout the past century, nursing students have been taught how to resuscitate patients who stop breathing. As early as 1912, students were taught a variety of methods for providing artificial respiration. It was theorized that moving air in and out of the lungs would be effective. One of these techniques was designed for resuscitating infants. Byrd's Method of Infant Resuscitation (Goodnow, 1919) directed the nurse to hold the infant's legs in one hand, and the head and back in the other. The nurse would then double the child up by pressing the head and the knees against the chest. Then the nurse would extend the knees to undouble the child. This would be repeated but "not too rapidly" (Goodnow, 1919, p. 305). At intervals, the nurse would dip the child into a mustard bath, in the hope that this would also stimulate respiration. The nurse would continue this until help arrived.

Other methods of artificial respiration taught included Sylvester's method for adults (Goodnow, 1919). The patient was placed flat on his back. The nurse would grasp his elbows, and press them close to his sides, pushing in the ribs to expel air from the chest. The arms would then be slowly pulled over the head allowing the chest to expand. The arms would be lowered to put pressure on the chest, and the cycle was then repeated. This was to be done at the rate of 18 to 20 cycles per minute.

By 1939, postmortem examinations after unsuccessful resuscitations showed veins to be engorged while the arteries were empty (Harmer & Henderson, 1942). Although this evidence indicated other factors needed to be considered, resuscitation techniques continued to focus only on the respiratory system. The same methods of resuscitation that were in use in 1919 were still being taught in 1942. Although students were still being taught the Sylvester method, they were also learning the new "Schäfer method" (Harmer & Henderson, 1942, p. 941). This method involved placing the patient in a prone position. The nurse would straddle the thighs, facing the patient's head, and alternatively apply and remove pressure to the thorax.

Eventually, it was noted that what was believed to be best practice was not effective. Results of postmortem examinations indicated that something was missing in the techniques, and therefore research was begun to determine best practice. Today, nursing students are taught cardiopulmonary resuscitation techniques based on updated research and theories.

that defines nursing research. The mere fact that the research was conducted by a nurse or that nurses were studied does not necessarily qualify the research as nursing. Historically, and even today, approaches to practice are often based on "professional opinion" when research is absent. The preceeding historical Case Example 5-1 provides such an illustration. It also demonstrates the value of systematically studying the effects of interventions.

This case example clearly illustrates how knowledge changes over time and ineffective practices are replaced with innovations. What is considered to be state-of-the-art practice at one time is replaced when new knowledge based on evidence emerges. Understanding the cycle of science compels nurses to continue learning throughout their careers to avoid becoming laggards. This case also underscores the importance of ordinary observations in the field of practice. In this case example, postmortem observations pointed to the need for another sounder approach to resuscitation. This case also illustrates how slowly innovations are adopted, even with evidence that a current practice is unsound.

The Special Language of Research

It is important to understand the special language associated with research (Fawcett & Downs, 1992). Research can be either deductive or inductive. It can be quantitative, qualitative, or a combination of both approaches. Regardless of the approach used, theory provides a framework for the design. Deductive research typically involves quantitative designs and begins by deriving testable ideas from theories (Case Example 5-2). Reports of deductive research describe the theoretical assumptions used to guide the study in the introduction section. Reports also include a critical review of previous research that both supports and refutes aspects of the theory. Because theories are abstract in nature, there is a language of research that corresponds to the language of theory. Unlike terms associated with theory, the language of research refers to the empirical or that which can be observed. Researchers cannot measure concepts; however, they can measure variables. A variable is an observation that can be measured by assigning a number to each dimension. For example, a researcher may choose to study the abstract concept of health by measuring the empirical variable of number of acquired upper respiratory infections per year. A hypothesis is a special type of proposition that can be tested empirically. There should be a theoretical basis for hypotheses. For example, a nurse may wish to test the relationship between exposure to sunlight and number of acquired upper respiratory infections per year in people receiving nursing care to test Nightingale's (1969) observations. The stated hypothesis could be that there is a relationship between exposure to sunlight and the number of acquired upper respiratory infections per year. The researcher would statistically test the null hypothesis that exposure to sunlight does not affect the acquisition of upper respiratory infections. Statistical methods are such that a hypothesis, and by extension, a theory, is never proved. It can only be supported. A theory holds only until evidence comes forward to refute it (Johnson, 1983). This is a hard concept for students to grasp because the logic of building knowledge by rejecting opposite ideas seems backwards. This is one reason why research can be slow and painstaking. Using deduction, researchers formulate hypotheses based on clear definitions of concepts and variables. Often, formulating hypotheses coincides with stating definitions. There are two kinds of definitions: conceptual and operational. *Conceptual definitions* are the definitions of concepts contained in the theory that is being used. These definitions sound like those found in dictionaries. *Operational definitions* are definitions that explicitly state how the variable will be measured or operationalized. For example, using Nightingale's theory (1969), the conceptual definition of health would be the absence of disease. A researcher could operationalize health as the number of self-reported upper respiratory infections per year. Environment was defined as everything outside the person (Nightingale, 1969); this would be the conceptual definition. The number of hours a person is in the light of the sun is an operational definition of environment. Defining concepts and variables allows researchers to collect quantitative data and apply statistics to learn about the phenomenon of interest.

Operational definitions can vary across studies because there are many different ways to measure any given concept. In the example, exposure to sunlight

CASE EXAMPLE 5-2

Nightingale's Work to Reduce Death Rates During War: An Example of Theory and Deductive Research

Nightingale theorized that five factors were essential for promoting health: pure or fresh air, pure water, efficient drainage, cleanliness, and light—especially direct sunlight (Nightingale, 1969). Through the application of her theory about what was required for the sick to recover, the death rate at Barrack Hospital during the Crimean War dropped from 42% to 2.2% in the first 6 months after her arrival. Nightingale was able to document this through the use of statistics (Strachey, 1918). Through careful collection and tracking of data, she was able to confirm that nursing interventions based on her theory were effective. Nightingale remains the first known quantitative researcher in nursing. Her work is an excellent example of theory applied to practice and supported and validated by deductive research.

could also be measured using an instrument that would provide a value for the intensity of sunlight over a period of time. The researcher would need to decide if exposure to sunlight through a glass window is appropriate or if exposure needs to be unobstructed by glass. The instruments used to measure the amount of time exposed to sunlight and the method of recording the number of self-reported acquired upper respiratory infections would be considered the *empirical indicators* of the variables being studied.

When researchers formulate their plans of research, they use theories to create *theoretical frameworks*. A theoretical framework provides the structure for the study by linking the abstract to the empirical. Sometimes researchers depict their frameworks using a *model*, which is essentially a pictorial representation of the concepts and their interrelationships.

Inductive research is used to develop theory and is usually qualitative. Researchers typically begin data collection before reading the literature to avoid biasing the data collection process. When reporting inductive research, authors use quotes to highlight key points of the theory that has emerged. An example of how a theory can be developed inductively using one particular qualitative method follows (Case Example 5-3).

There are also researchers who use both qualitative and quantitative methods in the same study. Studies can also have both deductive and inductive elements. The development of the transitional discharge model in mental health is an

KEY TERMS

Empirical indicators: Measures of the variables being studied

Theoretical framework: The structure of a study that links the theory concepts to the study variables

Model: Pictorial representation of concepts and their interrelationships

CASE EXAMPLE 5-3

Understanding and Helping Depressed Women: An Example of Theory and Inductive Research

Schreiber, a clinical nurse specialist, noticed that twice as many women as men suffered from depression. She found little in the way of nursing research that could help her care for these women. In order to better understand the recovery process for these women, she used a grounded theory approach (Glaser & Strauss, 1969), to guide her work (Schreiber, 1996). A sample of 21 women who had recovered from depression was interviewed for the study. Schreiber identified that women need to tell their story, and "seek understanding," in order to proceed to the stage of "cluing in," which is a stage of recovery. By identifying stages of recovery and formulating a theory about the process of recovery, specific nursing interventions were able to be identified. For example, implications for nursing practice include recognizing the importance of facilitating women telling their stories.

CASE EXAMPLE 5-4

A Transitional Discharge Model for Mental Health: An Example of Theory and Research Using Mixed Methods

As an advanced practice nurse in a tertiary care mental health setting, Forchuk noted that more clients left the unit due to death than by discharge. Those that had been discharged were often re-admitted within a month of leaving the hospital. Her challenge was to find a way to help discharged clients return to the community and successfully remain there. She worked systematically with staff, clients, family members, and former clients in the community to discover what interventions might be helpful. From these efforts, it became clear that patients were discharged to an environment where all of their relationships were within a community in which they felt alone and isolated. This conclusion was reached inductively. Because no nursing theory could be found to effectively explain the observations, Forchuk began developing a model to explain successful discharge of mental health clients. The model combined continuing staff support from professionals who had established therapeutic relationships with clients and with peer support from former users of mental health services who successfully transitioned to the community. Professionals continued interactions with clients until they established a working relationship with the community. The model was piloted and the results were impressive (Forchuk & Brown, 1989). All nine clients discharged during the study year were successful in their return to the community, reducing the cost of their care (Forchuk et al., 1998a; Forchuk, Jewell, Schofield, Sircelj, & Valledor, 1998b; Schofield et al., 1997). Both quantitative and qualitative measures were used to collect data. As a result of the pilot, funding for a large clinical trial to test the model in an experimental study was obtained (Forchuk, Martin, Chen, & Jensen, 2005).

example of this mixing of methods and approaches (Forchuk & Brown, 1989; Forchuk, et al., 1998a; Forchuk et al., 1998b; Forchuk, dt al., 2005).

Case Example 5-4 illustrates how researchers may use multiple approaches when addressing clinical questions. It also demonstrates that it takes more than one study to build knowledge. Work replicated in Scotland with similar positive results (Reynolds et al., 2004) lends further support to the transitional discharge model for mental health.

Theory in Practice

The American Nurses Association (ANA) has defined the practice of nursing as the "protection, promotion, and optimization of health and abilities, prevention of illness, injury, alleviation of suffering through the diagnosis and treatment of human response, and advocacy in the care of individuals, families,

CRITICAL THINKING EXERCISE 5-2

A nurse on a surgical floor observes that there are several new approaches being used to dress wounds. She observes that some methods appear to promote healing faster than others. While reviewing the research literature, she is unable to locate any research about the dressings she is using. How might she go about testing her theory that some methods are better than others? Can this be done deductively, inductively, or using mixed methods? Are there any theories presently available to her related to wound healing, and if so, where might she locate these? What concepts might be important in forming the question?

communities, and populations" (ANA, 2003, p. 6). From the early days of the profession, students have been taught that a scientific attitude and method of work combined with "experience, trained senses, a mind trained to think, and the necessary characteristics of patience, accuracy, open-mindedness, truthfulness, persistence, and industry" (Harmer, 1933, p. 47) are essential components of good practice. Harmer goes on to say, "Each time this habit of looking, listening, feeling, or thinking is repeated it is strengthened until the habit of observation is firmly established" (p. 47). This still holds true today. Benner (1984) studied nurses in practice and concluded that to become an expert nurse one has to practice nursing a minimum of 5 years. There are no shortcuts to becoming an expert in one's field. The development of knowledge and skill takes time and work. As nurses encounter new situations, learning takes place. Nursing knowledge develops and is refined as nurses practice (Waterman, Webb, & Williams, 1995). In this way, nurses adapt theories to fit their practices. Unfortunately, much that is learned about theory during practice remains with the nurse because nurses rarely share their practice expertise through conference presentations and publications. The discipline will be enriched when nurses engage more formally in disseminating their knowledge about theory in practice.

The Relationships Among Theory, Research, and Practice

Practice relies on research and theory and also provides the questions that require more work by theorists and researchers. Each informs and supports the other in the application and development of nursing knowledge. When the relationships among theory, research, and practice are in harmony, the discipline

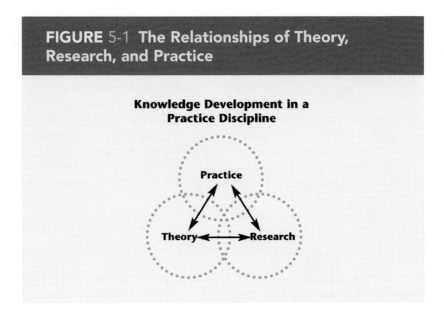

FIGURE 5-1 **The Relationships of Theory, Research, and Practice**

is best served, ultimately resulting in better patient outcomes (Maas, 2006). The relationships are dynamic and flow in all directions. Practice informs and is informed by theory development as well as research. Research and theory development inform and are informed by each other (see **Figure 5-1**).

The literature reflects that in the nursing profession there is tension about the relationships among theory, research, and practice. Too often theorists, researchers, and nurses work in isolation from each other. Some see research as serving to develop theory that should then drive practice (Mitchell, 1997), while others see theory as driving research that should then drive practice (Billings & Kowalski, 2006). Still others see practice as informing and being informed by research and theory (Schmelzer, 2006). As Butcher (2006) points out, practicing nurses focus on unique individuals, researchers focus on systematically collecting knowledge about samples and populations, and theorists focus on abstract and general concepts and their interrelationships. Understanding the different perspectives of each of these activities in knowledge building shows them to be complementary.

At a micro level, each nurse engages in research and theory development. For example, each patient encounter can be considered to be a study with one subject. Assessment can serve as data collection involving both quantitative and qualitative data, and the plan of care emerges from the analysis. The result is a theory of what will work for this person. The theory is tested as care

CRITICAL THINKING EXERCISE 5-3

Reflect on your most recent patient encounter. When you assessed your patient, what theoretical assumptions guided your data collection? Were there questions you had about nursing needs or health circumstance that puzzled you? How did you go about addressing these questions? How might you go about that in the future? Who might you involve in addressing questions? What did you do that worked when providing care for this patient? Would you use the approach with another patient? Why or why not?

is delivered, and if positive outcomes are achieved, the theory is validated. If outcomes are not positive, the theory is refuted and a new theory is created, resulting in a revised plan of care. Learning from each patient encounter is applied to new encounters. Case by case, the nurse learns about both the unique and universal characteristics of individuals.

Researchers engage in a similar process but from a different perspective. Nursing researchers systematically study individuals in groups to uncover knowledge about universal characteristics of individuals as they apply to their health. Knowledge from research assists nurses to choose interventions that have a known probability of success. Although research findings help nurses predict what will be successful for the majority of individuals, outcomes cannot be predicted for an individual. When an individual does not respond like the majority of people, a nurse will rely more on clinical judgment and patient preferences.

Like researchers, theorists also work at a macro level building knowledge that can be universally applied. Theory provides understanding and guidance to the practice of nursing. It also provides language for describing nursing's work.

It is clear from the debate in the literature that nurses, researchers, and theorists can work more closely together and that such partnerships will be very fruitful for the development of nursing knowledge. Schmelzer (2006) encourages nurses to collaborate with researchers to find answers for practice problems. Waterman et al. (1995) also supports closer working relationships among nurses, researchers, and theorists. It is quite reasonable for nurses to be members of formal research teams as content experts. Another way to increase collaboration is for more researchers and theorists to engage in practice.

TEST YOUR KNOWLEDGE 5-1

Fill in the blanks:

1. A concept at the abstract level is comparable to a _____ at the operational level.

2. A _____ at the abstract level is comparable to a hypothesis at the operational level.

3. Quantitative research typically _____ theory, while qualitative research typically _____ theory.

True/False

4. Theory, research, and practice should be developed in isolation.

5. Nurses are encouraged to collaborate with researchers and theorists to expand nursing knowledge.

6. Concepts of the metaparadigm of nursing include: nursing, health, disease, social interaction, and persons.

How did you do? 1. variable; 2. proposition; 3. tests, builds; 4. F; 5. T; 6. F

5.2   Keeping It Ethical

At the end of this section, you will be able to:

‹ Discuss how honoring prior work ethically builds nursing knowledge

FYI

Credit must be given for ideas built on earlier work as well as for new ideas generated by challenging old ideas.

Students of any discipline are taught the body of knowledge that has been built over time, including the origins of the ideas that comprise that body of knowledge. As individuals contribute to the body of knowledge, credit should be given to those on whose work they are building.

Knowledge in a discipline is built in small steps that in time mark a long and fruitful journey of discovery. When reading the works of nurses, researchers, and theorists, students of the discipline should be able to trace the evolution of ideas. Credit must be given for ideas built on earlier work as well as for new ideas generated by challenging old ideas. This trail can be followed by examining references and reading the work of those who made

TEST YOUR KNOWLEDGE 5-2

True/False

1. In the discipline of nursing, it is easy to follow how knowledge has developed because theorists have carefully provided citations for their ideas.

2. Giving credit to those who provide the basis for ideas is ethical practice.

How did you do? 1. F; 2. T

earlier contributions. Sadly, nurses have been poor at leaving such a trail. Few theorists cite the nurses who influenced their thinking. For example, Peplau (1952) gives credit to Adler, a psychologist, for influencing her thinking, but she makes no mention of nurses who may have influenced her despite the fact that she published for nurses practicing in mental health areas. Likewise, Rogers (1970) does not credit the sources of her nursing knowledge even though she published a model for nurses in all settings. In other cases, an author may state that an idea came from another individual but does not provide a reference, or an author may use a secondary source for a quote when a primary source is available. Failure to honor the work of others creates problems for nurses trying to understand the evolution of nursing knowledge and practice.

When studying the writings of nurses who are contributors to disciplinary knowledge, it is important to look for the foundation of their ideas. Where information about these ideas is lacking, nurses should critically appraise claims that the work is a legitimate part of the disciplinary knowledge of nursing. To write as a contributor to the disciplinary body of knowledge without giving credit to those who provided the basis for the ideas is not just poor practice; it is unethical, and is, in fact, plagiarism.

 FYI

To write as a contributor to the disciplinary body of knowledge without giving credit to those who provided the basis for the ideas is not just poor practice; it is unethical, and is, in fact, plagiarism.

 RAPID **REVIEW**

 Theories are sets of concepts linked by propositions that explain phenomena. They provide a belief system to guide practice.

 Concepts are words or phrases conveying unique ideas or mental images. They are the building blocks of theories.

The metaparadigm of nursing has four concepts: person, health, environment, and nursing.

 Propositions are statements describing relationships between two or more concepts.

 Constructs are properties that are inferred because they cannot be directly observed.

 Variables describe how concepts will be measured at the empirical level, and hypotheses are propositions that can be tested empirically.

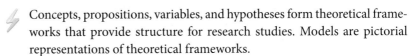 Concepts, propositions, variables, and hypotheses form theoretical frameworks that provide structure for research studies. Models are pictorial representations of theoretical frameworks.

 Conceptual definitions are like definitions found in dictionaries and are abstract in nature. Operational definitions specify how variables will be measured. Empirical indicators are the instruments used to measure variables.

 Deductive quantitative research is typically used to test theory, while inductive qualitative research can be used to build theory. Mixed methods can also contribute to the development of theory.

APPLY WHAT YOU HAVE LEARNED

WWW

A committee member tells you she has found two articles (Mark, Salyer, & Wan, 2003; Rich, 2005) that use a theoretical framework. She is excited about these and would like the committee to consider how these models might be useful to its work. As the chairperson, you are responsible for facilitating discussion. To prepare, you read the articles and consider the following questions.

1. The article by Mark and colleagues (2003) describes a study that uses a structural contingency theory. How does this framework influence the study?

2. In the article by Rich (2005), the corkscrew model of error reduction is discussed. How might this model be used as a framework for designing interventions that reduce medication errors?

3. Enter information about these two articles into the first and second columns of your grid on the companion website.

⚡ In practice, nursing knowledge is developed and refined through patient encounters.

⚡ The relationships of theory, research, and practice are dynamic and complementary.

⚡ In practice, nurses learn about unique and universal characteristics of individuals. Researchers use systematic study to discover knowledge about universal characteristics of people. Theorists build knowledge that can be universally applied.

⚡ The ethical practice of honoring the work of others creates a trail whereby nurses can follow the building of nursing knowledge.

REFERENCES

American Nurses Association. (2003). *Nursing's social policy statement* (2nd ed.).Washington, DC: Author.

Benner, P. (1984). *From novice to expert: Excellence and power in clinical nursing practice*. Menlo Park, CA: Addison-Wesley.

Billings, D. M., & Kowalski, K. (2006). Bridging the theory-practice gap with evidence-based practice. *The Journal of Continuing Education in Nursing, 37*, 248–249.

Butcher, H. (2006). Integrating nursing theory, nursing research, and nursing practice. In P. S. Cowen & S. Moorhead (Eds.), *Current issues in nursing* (pp. 112–122). St. Louis, MO: Mosby.

Fawcett, J. (1984). The metaparadigm of nursing: Current status and future refinements. *Image: Journal of Nursing Scholarship, 16*, 84–87.

Fawcett, J., & Downs, F. S. (1992). *The relationship of theory and research* (2nd ed.). Philadelphia: Davis.

Forchuk, C., & Brown, B. (1989). Establishing a nurse-client relationship. *Journal of Psychosocial Nursing, 27*(2), 30–34.

Forchuk, C., Chan, L., Schofield, R., Sircelj, M., Woodcox, V., Jewell, J., … Overby, B. (1998a). Bridging the discharge process. *Canadian Nurse, 94*(3), 22–26.

Forchuk, C., Jewell, J., Schofield, R., Sircelj, M., & Valledor, T. (1998b). From hospital to community: Bridging therapeutic relationships. *Journal of Psychiatric and Mental Health Nursing, 5*, 197–202.

Forchuk, C., Martin, M. L., Chan, Y. L., & Jensen, E. (2005). Therapeutic relationships: From psychiatric hospital to community. *Journal of Psychiatric and Mental Health Nursing, 12*, 556–564.

Glaser, B., & Strauss, A. (1969). *The discovery of grounded theory*. Chicago: Aldine.

Goodnow, M. (1919). *First-year nursing* (2nd ed.). Philadelphia: Saunders.

Graham, I. W. (2003). The relationship of nursing theory to practice and research within the British context: Identifying a way forward. *Nursing Science Quarterly, 16*, 346–350.

Harmer, B. (1933). *Textbook of the principles and practice of nursing* (2nd ed.). New York: Macmillan.

Harmer, B., & Henderson, V. (1942). *Textbook of the principles and practice of nursing* (4th ed.). New York: Macmillan.

Johnson, M. (1983). Some aspects of the relation between theory and research in nursing. *Journal of Advanced Nursing, 8*(1), 21–28.

Maas, M. L. (2006). What is nursing, and why do we ask? In P. S. Cowen & S. Moorhead (Eds.), *Current issues in nursing* (pp. 5–10). St. Louis, MO: Mosby.

Mark, B. A., Salyer, J., & Wan, T. T. H. (2003). Professional nursing practice: Impact on organizational and patient outcomes, *JONA, 33*, 224–234.

Mitchell, G. J. (1997). Questioning evidence-based practice for nursing. *Nursing Science Quarterly, 10*, 154–155.

Nightingale, F. (1969). *Notes on nursing: What it is, and what it is not*. New York: Dover.

Parse, R. R. (2006). Research findings evince benefits of nursing theory-guided practice. *Nursing Science Quarterly, 19*, 87.

Peplau, H. E. (1952). *Interpersonal relations in nursing: A conceptual frame of reference for psychodynamic nursing*. New York: Putnam.

Reynolds, W., Lauder, W., Sharkey, S., MacIver, S., Veitch, T., & Cameron, D. (2004). The effect of transitional discharge model for psychiatric patients. *Journal of Psychiatric and Mental Health Nursing, 11*, 82–88.

Rich, V. L. (2005). How we think about medication errors: A model and a charge for nurses. *AJN, 105*(3) (Suppl.), 10–11.

Rogers, M. E. (1970). *An introduction to the theoretical basis of nursing*. Philadelphia: Davis.

Schmelzer, M. (2006). Personal reflections about the theory-research-practice connection. *Gastroenterology Nursing, 29*, 489–491.

Schofield, R., Valledor, T., Sircelj, M., Forchuk, C., Jewell, J., & Woodcox, V. (1997). Evaluation of bridging institution and housing—A joint consumer care provider initiative. *Journal of Psychosocial Nursing, 35*, 9–14.

Schreiber, R. (1996). Understanding and helping depressed women. *Archives of Psychiatric Nursing, 10*, 165–175.

Strachey, L. (1918). *Eminent Victorians.* New York: Garden City.

Waterman, H., Webb, C., & Williams, A. (1995). Parallels and contradictions in the theory and practice of action research and nursing. *Journal of Advanced Nursing, 22,* 779–784.

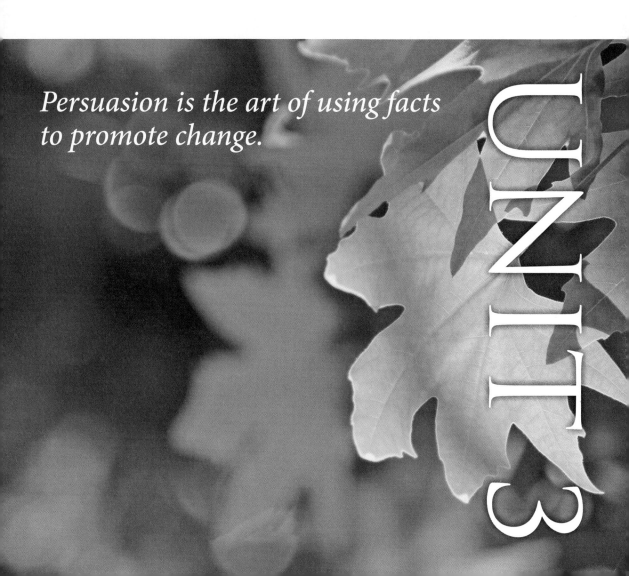

Persuasion

Persuasion is the art of using facts to promote change.

UNIT 3

CHAPTER OBJECTIVES

At the end of this chapter, you will be able to:

< Explain the relationships among the study purpose, literature review, research questions or hypotheses, study framework, and the study design

< Define key concepts relevant to quantitative research designs including experimental, nonexperimental, causality, probability, control, manipulation, bias, randomization, between-subjects, within-subjects, and study validity

< List elements to be considered when appraising quantitative designs

< Define the four types of validity

< Describe seven threats to internal validity

< Describe six threats to external validity

< Identify strategies used to reduce threats to internal and external validity

< Differentiate the time dimension of data collection across retrospective, cross-sectional, and longitudinal and prospective designs

< Discuss ethical issues related to internal and external validity

KEY TERMS

attrition rate
between-groups design
bias
case-control
causality
cohort comparison
construct validity
control
crossover
cross-sectional
double-blind experimental
    designs
effects of selection
ex post facto
external validity
extraneous variables

follow-up
Hawthorne effect
history
instrumentation
interaction of treatment
    and history
interaction of treatment
    and setting
interaction of treatment
    with selection of
    subjects
internal validity
longitudinal design
manipulation
maturation
mortality

panel design
probability
prospective design
random assignment
random sampling
randomization
reactivity
retrospective design
selection bias
statistical conclusion
    validity
study validity
testing
trend
type II error
within-groups design

CHAPTER 6

Key Principles of Quantitative Designs

Rosalind M. Peters

6.1 Chart the Course: Selecting the Best Design

At the end of the section, you will be able to:

< Explain the relationships among the study purpose, literature review, research questions or hypotheses, study framework, and the study design

< Define key concepts relevant to quantitative research designs including experimental, nonexperimental, causality, probability, control, manipulation, bias, randomization, between-subjects, within-subjects, and study validity

< List elements to be considered when appraising quantitative designs

Introduction to Design

You will see the term *research design* used two different ways. Many people use the term broadly to encompass multiple aspects of the research process including the sampling plan, data collection procedures, implementation strategies, and data analysis. In this context, the broad use of the term implies the overall method of the research study. Another way the term can be used is to refer to the specific plan or blueprint that will be used to meet the stated purpose of the study. When evaluating the appropriateness of the research design, it is important to realize that the design is not developed in a vacuum. Instead, it should reflect an integration of the theoretical and empirical literature that was presented in the review of the literature section of the study. This section usually ends by identifying a gap in current knowledge about the phenomenon of interest. The purpose of the proposed study should be to fill some portion of that gap in knowledge with the research questions or hypotheses determining what specific new knowledge will be generated. The research design should flow from the stated purpose and provide a plan that can answer the research questions and test the stated hypotheses.

Quantitative designs used to examine relationships among variables are categorized as experimental or nonexperimental. These designs can be used to meet four key purposes. Experimental designs are used for the purpose of examining causality. Nonexperimental designs can be used for the purposes of describing a phenomenon in detail, explaining relationships and differences among variables, and predicting relationships and differences among variables. The major difference between nonexperimental and experimental designs is the role of the researcher. In experimental designs, researchers actively manipulate the independent variable (IV), sometimes known as the causal variable, to determine its effect on the dependent variable (DV) or outcome variable. In nonexperimental designs, researchers are observers noting the occurrence of the variables of interest and trying to determine relationships and differences. Other quantitative designs are used for the purpose of addressing methodological issues such as instrument development, or in the case of a meta-analysis to examine outcomes across a number of studies.

As you appraise an article for the quality of the study presented, you should find that there is a logical flow of information from the literature reviewed and study framework. This information leads you to agree that the study is needed, that the purpose is appropriate given the literature presented, and that the planned design will be able to generate quantitative information to address the stated research questions and hypotheses.

Understanding Key Concepts in Quantitative Designs

Best practice means that nurses must have confidence in the evidence that they are applying to patient care. Having confidence in findings requires that nurses be able to critically appraise quantitative studies before applying findings to practice. Therefore, understanding key concepts and principles related to the design of quantitative studies is necessary.

Causality and Probability

Causality refers to the relationship that exists between a cause and its effect. The cause has the ability or power to produce a specific effect. The assumption is made that the cause precedes the effect. Being able to determine causality requires that the variables of interest are studied in chronological order: the causal variable, or IV, has to occur prior to the occurrence of the DV, or the effect. From a research perspective, causality is the belief that researchers, using stringent controls, can manipulate a cause to produce the effect or result that can be repeated. Experimental designs are used to examine causality, with researchers manipulating the IV while observing its effect on the DV. When working with people, nurse researchers recognize that there are multiple factors that can contribute to an outcome. Rarely do nurses deal with problems that have only one cause and one effect. When outcomes have many causes, it is known as multicausality. Therefore, it is important to consider multicausality when evaluating research designs. Because it is possible that there are multiple, interrelated factors causing an outcome, it is important for researchers to try to identify and control for as many of those factors as possible. When appraising research studies, nurses need to familiarize themselves with the variables included in the study and evaluate the discussion section of the study report to determine if researchers identified other possible causes for the results. **Table 6-1** outlines points that should be considered when appraising quantitative designs.

KEY TERM

Causality: The relationship between a cause and its effect

TABLE 6-1 Elements to Consider When Appraising Quantitative Designs

What type of quantitative design is being used?
Can causality be inferred?
Did researchers use the highest level of design possible to answer the research questions?
What strategies did the researcher use to control for the effects of extraneous variables?
What threats to internal and external validity might be present, and were any strategies used to reduce them?
Were there any ethical concerns about the design?

Closely related to the idea of multicausality is the idea of *probability*. Again, because nursing is a human science rather than a basic science, such as biology or chemistry, nurse researchers are unlikely to be able to assert with absolute certainty that the IV caused the effect in the DV. Instead, research related to human health and functioning results in assertions of probability or how likely it is that the change of the DV was caused by the IV. Probability assertions leave open the possibility that there are other causes and factors affecting the result seen in the DV.

Control, Manipulation, and Bias

Control refers to the ability to manipulate, regulate, or statistically adjust for the multitude of factors that can influence the DV. Control is necessary to make assertions about cause and effect. *Manipulation* is an important aspect of control in experimental designs and refers to the ability of researchers to control the IV. It is considered to be the intervention, or treatment, that is being tested in an experimental study. The intervention may be physiological, psychological, behavioral, educational, or a combination of these.

For example, a researcher hypothesizes that educational interventions will result in increased condom use among sexually active teens and wants to test a newly developed computer-based intervention. The researcher manipulates the IV, the educational intervention, by determining what content will be included, how it will be delivered, in what environment it will be delivered, and who will receive it. The researcher in this example would then compare preintervention condom usage with postintervention usage. The researcher also could compare the difference in condom usage between the intervention group and a control group. In health-related experimental designs, the control group of subjects usually receives the standard of care but does not get the intervention. The control group of teens, in this example, would participate in the traditional sex education classes offered in their school but would not be able to access the computer-based program. However, because factors other than education can affect condom use, the researcher also needs to control for these extraneous or confounding factors.

Extraneous variables are those that confound, or confuse, the effect of the IV on the DV. Researchers can control for extraneous variables through careful selection of participants, use of consistent data collection procedures, randomization, or by using certain statistical tests. Examples of confounding variables in the example might be the age of the teen, religious beliefs, self-efficacy for resisting peer pressure, cost of condoms, ease of purchasing them, and whether or not the teen has a current sexual partner. Without careful control of extraneous variables, bias can be introduced into the study.

Bias results when extraneous variables influence and distort the relationship between the IV and the DV so that the findings are not really reflecting the true relationship. For example, if the study included students without a current sexual partner, it would be highly likely that the intervention would result in no significant difference in condom use. This lack of difference might be attributed to the intervention being ineffective when it is actually due to the fact that the teen is not currently engaging in sexual activity requiring a condom. Researchers control for this type of bias by clearly specifying criteria required for subjects to be included in a study. After subjects are enrolled in a study, it is important for researchers to control how the study is actually conducted. This includes controlling the environment in which the study is conducted, providing consistency in how interventions are delivered, and collecting data in a careful and consistent manner. For example, asking students to report their condom use during an interview where others might hear their responses could bias the results because students may not feel comfortable responding truthfully. A better way to obtain this information may be to have students complete a self-report of their condom use on an anonymous questionnaire.

Randomization

Randomization is an effective way to control extraneous variables. Randomization can occur either with random sampling of the subjects to be studied or by random assignment of subjects to intervention or control groups. *Random sampling* means that all people in the population of interest have the same probability of being selected to be included in the study. This occurs infrequently in health-related research because researchers usually do not have the time or money to randomly sample from all people who could potentially participate. For example, it would be very difficult to randomly sample sexually active teens from around the country. Instead, in this example the researcher would most likely use a convenience sample of students from high schools within their area. They would then randomly assign the students into the intervention and the control groups. *Random assignment* means that all subjects in the sample (not the population) have an equal chance of being assigned to either the treatment or the control group. Random assignment increases the likelihood that extraneous variables that may affect the DV will be equally distributed between the two groups. Using random assignment allows researchers to be more confident that it was the IV rather than the extraneous variables that caused the effect on the DV. Although researchers may be very careful about selecting representative samples and using random assignment to groups to control for extraneous variables, these techniques do not guarantee that extraneous variables will be equally distributed between the two groups.

KEY TERMS

Bias: When extraneous variables influence the relationship between the independent and dependent variables

Randomization: The selection, assignment, or arrangement of elements by chance

Random sampling: Technique for selecting elements whereby each has the same chance of being selected

Random assignment: Subjects have an equal chance of being in either the treatment or the control group

Between-groups design: Study design where two groups of subjects can be compared

When groups are different, researchers will need to apply certain statistical tests to control for the effect of extraneous variables on the DV.

Between-Groups and Within-Groups

Quantitative studies often are designed for the purpose of making comparisons either by comparing different groups of subjects or by comparing the same subject at different points in time. Studies developed to compare two different groups of subjects use a *between-groups design*. For example, a researcher who is studying condom use among adolescents may wish to know the practices of

TEST YOUR KNOWLEDGE 6-1

1. When designing a study, which of the following should the researcher consider:
   a. research question
   b. review of the literature
   c. theoretical framework
   d. study purpose

2. Which of the following is *not* a purpose of nonexperimental designs:
   a. describe phenomenon
   b. explain relationships
   c. predict relationships
   d. examine causality

3. The researcher's ability to manipulate or regulate extraneous variables is known as:
   a. control
   b. manipulation
   c. bias
   d. probability

4. When a researcher assigns subjects to groups by tossing a coin, the researcher is using:
   a. random selection
   b. random assignment
   c. bias
   d. within-groups design

How did you do? 1. a, b, c, d; 2.d; 3. a; 4. b

high school juniors and seniors as well as college freshmen and sophomores. The researcher could make comparisons among these four groups about the frequency of condom use.

While comparisons among diverse subjects are important, there may be other situations when researchers are more interested in making comparisons within the same subject. For example, a researcher is interested in the effect of music therapy on patients' levels of pain. Using a *within-groups design*, the researcher would measure the subjects' levels of pain before the intervention, conduct the intervention, and then measure pain levels after the intervention. By comparing the subjects' pain scores before and after the intervention, the researcher is able to determine the effectiveness of music therapy as a pain relief measure.

Researchers can combine between-groups and within-groups designs within the same study to compare the effectiveness of more than one intervention. In the pain example, the researcher might offer music therapy as an intervention to one group of subjects and relaxation therapy as another intervention to a different group of subjects. The researcher could analyze the within-groups results to determine the level to which each intervention reduced pain, and the researcher could compare between-groups to determine if there was a difference in the amount of pain relief provided by the music and relaxation.

6.2   What Is Validity?

At the end of this section, you will be able to:

< Define the four types of validity
< Describe seven threats to internal validity
< Describe six threats to external validity
< Identify strategies used to reduce threats to internal and external validity

Exerting control over extraneous variables affecting the DV is one important factor to ensure valid results. *Study validity* refers to the ability to accept results as logical, reasonable, and justifiable based on the evidence presented. Validity is sometimes described as the truth or accuracy of the results. Evaluating the quality of quantitative evidence requires nurses to identify potential threats to validity, evaluate the seriousness of those threats, and determine if results are valid for application to patient care. Threats are forces that can change the results of studies. Campbell and Stanley (1966) identified two major types of

FIGURE 6-1 **Relationships Among Types of Validity**

> *External Validity:* The degree to which the results of this study can be generalized to other subjects, settings, and time.
>
> > *Construct Validity:* The degree to which the instrument or empirical indicator actually measures the theoretical concept of interest.
> >
> > > *Internal Validity:* The degree to which we can conclude that it was the independent variable, not the extraneous variables, that produced the change in the dependent variable.
> > >
> > > > *Statistical Conclusion Validity:* The confidence we have that the results from the statistical analysis accurately reflect the true relationship between the independent and dependent variables

validity: internal and external (see **Figure 6-1**). Internal and external validity were originally developed to evaluate cause and effect relationships, making them most relevant for experimental designs. However, validity should be considered with all quantitative designs. It is important when appraising research articles to identify threats and consider how these threats may have influenced the DV.

Internal Validity

Internal validity is the degree to which one can conclude that it was the IV, not extraneous variables, that produced the change in the DV (Cook & Campbell, 1979). To establish internal validity, researchers must demonstrate that results obtained were caused by the IV. Common threats to internal validity include selection bias, history, maturation, testing, instrumentation, mortality, and statistical conclusion validity.

Selection Bias

Selection bias occurs when the change in the DV is a result of differences in the characteristics of subjects before they entered a study, rather than as a result of the IV. Suppose a researcher wants to compare the effectiveness of group teaching to one-on-one teaching. At the hospital where the study is being conducted, patients are allowed to choose the kind of teaching they want.

It is possible that people who select group teaching will be different on some characteristics from those who select one-on-one teaching. Selection bias can be minimized somewhat by the use of random assignment to groups.

History

The threat of *history* occurs when the DV may have been influenced by some event, other than the IV, that occurred during the course of the study. In the example of condom use, it might be difficult to attribute increased use of condoms to the computer intervention if during the same time as the study was being conducted MTV or VH1 aired public service announcements encouraging safe sex practices. In such a situation, it is difficult for the researcher to know if it was the IV or the increased awareness from television that produced the change in the DV. The threat of history could have been decreased by having a control group that would have been exposed to the television ads but did not receive the computer intervention.

Maturation

Over the course of a study, subjects may change either by growing or becoming more mature. This is known as the threat of *maturation*. Changes such as these are more likely to influence the DV when a study continues over time. For example, if subjects during the study on condom use came of age to obtain a driver's license and get a job, it would be difficult to determine if an increase in condom use was a result of the IV or to the subjects' increased ease of purchasing condoms for use. A control group may help limit this threat to internal validity.

Testing

The threat of *testing* occurs when a pretest influences the way subjects respond on a posttest. Repeated testing can cause familiarity with the test itself, and answers may reflect subjects' abilities to remember how questions were answered previously rather than reflecting current knowledge and beliefs.

Instrumentation

When there are changes made in the way variables are measured, the threat of *instrumentation* can occur. For example, in a study measuring blood pressure, if the original measurement is taken using an aneroid sphygmomanometer but later measurements are taken using an automated device, it makes it difficult to determine if any change in blood pressure readings is a result of the IV or the change in devices. Another potential instrumentation threat arises when data are collected by observation or interview using different data collectors.

KEY TERMS

History: A threat to internal validity when the dependent variable is influenced by an event that occurred during the study

Maturation: A threat to internal validity when subjects change by growing or maturing

Testing: A threat to internal validity when a pretest influences the way subjects respond on a posttest

Instrumentation: Threat to internal validity when there are inconsistencies in data collection

To control for this threat, researchers need to ensure comprehensive training of all data collectors. Researchers also evaluate interrater reliability to determine the degree of consistency among individuals collecting data.

Mortality

Mortality refers to the loss of subjects before the study is completed. Loss of subjects may be a threat to internal validity if there is a difference in the characteristics of the subjects who dropped out compared to those who completed the study. Internal validity is also threatened when there is a difference in the loss of subjects between the experimental and control groups. Mortality tends to increase the longer a study lasts. In health-related research, emotional states such as depression and anxiety, as well as physical states such as fatigue, may influence dropout rates. When appraising a study for the threat of mortality, it is important to compare the number of subjects who entered the study with the number of subjects in the final sample. In a research article, the term *attrition rate* refers to the dropout rate. If the attrition rate is high, the author of the article should provide an analysis and explanation for the dropout rate.

Statistical Conclusion Validity

Statistical conclusion validity refers to the confidence one has that the results of the statistical analysis accurately reflect the true relationship between the IV and DV. This does not happen when researchers make a *type II error*. Type II errors occur when researchers inaccurately conclude that there is no relationship between the IV and DV when an actual relationship does exist. A type II error is more likely to occur when the sample size is small. Often large samples are needed in order to detect the effect of the IV on the DV. Low reliability of the measures is another factor that can interfere with researchers' abilities to draw accurate conclusions about relationships among the IV and DV. When appraising research articles for threats to statistical conclusion validity, it is important to consider the information presented in the methods section that details the reliability of instruments. Researchers can control for low reliability of the measures by using well-established and well-designed instruments.

CRITICAL THINKING EXERCISE 6-1

A researcher is interested in studying the effect of hearing loss on self-esteem in adolescents attending grades 6–12. What threats to internal validity should the researcher address? What controls could the researcher use to minimize these threats?

External Validity

External validity refers to the degree to which the results of the study can be generalized to other subjects, settings, and times (Cook & Campbell, 1979). One kind of threat, construct validity, is concerned about whether the instrument is really measuring the theoretical concept under investigation. Other threats to external validity are ones that occur because of interactions between the IV and the subjects, setting, or history.

Construct Validity

Construct validity is an important consideration when evaluating external validity. Assessing construct validity allows researchers to determine if instruments are actually measuring the theoretical concepts that are intended to be measured. A threat of construct validity can lead to unintentional confounding of the results. For example, a researcher is studying the effect of anger on blood pressure; however, the instrument used to measure anger contains some items that might also reflect depression. The relationship between anger and blood pressure is confounded because the instrument measures two theoretical concepts. Therefore, the researcher would be unable to determine if changes in blood pressure were a result of anger or depression. When appraising an article for threats to construct validity, it is important to consider information presented in the methods section of the article. This section should contain information on the reliability of the instrument used and details as to how the validity of the instrument was established.

Reactivity

Sometimes subjects are influenced by participating in a study. Changes noted in the DV can be a result of subject *reactivity* and not a result of the IV. This is known as the *Hawthorne effect*. The Hawthorne effect was first recognized in studies done at the Western Electric Corporation's Hawthorne plant. One of the studies attempted to determine if changing the amount of lighting in the work environment changed productivity. In this study, productivity increased regardless of changes made to lighting. One explanation for this result was that the increased productivity occurred because the employees knew they were

KEY TERMS

External validity: The degree to which the results of the study can be generalized

Construct validity: A threat to external validity when the instrument does not accurately measure the theoretical concepts

Reactivity: The influence of participating in a study on the responses of subjects

Hawthorne effect: Subjects' behaviors affected by personal values or desires to please the experimenter

CRITICAL THINKING EXERCISE 6-2

Have you ever participated in a research study? Do you think your behaviors were different because you knew you were being studied?

being studied. Therefore, the behaviors of subjects in a study may be affected by their personal values, their desires to please the experimenter or provide the results the experimenter wants, and whether the study is congruent with their personal interests and goals.

Experimenter expectancy is another type of reactivity that threatens external validity. When researchers have desired outcomes in mind, they may inadvertently affect how interventions are conducted and how they interact with subjects. For example, a researcher may be friendlier to subjects in the experimental group than to subjects in the control group. As a result, subjects in the experimental group may perceive involvement in the study more positively than subjects in the control group.

Double-blind experimental designs have been used in health research to control for threats of reactivity. In double-blind studies, neither subjects nor individuals administering the treatments know if subjects are receiving experimental interventions or standard of care. This design is fairly common in drug studies where a placebo pill can be manufactured to appear exactly like the drug being studied.

Effects of Selection

Because researchers most often study samples, rather than an entire population, representativeness of the sample is essential. If the sample does not represent the population, *effects of selection* limit the ability to generalize to the population. For example, a researcher is interviewing mothers. Because interviews are being conducted only during the day and no child care is provided, individuals who work during the day or have small children are less likely to participate in this study. Consequently, researchers would not be able to generalize to all mothers but only to mothers who do not work during the day and mothers without young children.

Interaction of Treatment and Selection of Subjects

Because external validity is concerned with generalizing to other individuals, it is only natural to ask, "Will this IV affect other people in the same way?" The *interaction of treatment with selection of subjects* must be considered (Cook & Campbell, 1979). This requires consideration of the difference between the accessible population and the target population of interest (Kempthorne, 1961). In the condom use example, the target population is all sexually active teens. The accessible population is the group of teens from which the researcher is actually able to obtain a sample of subjects. So, if the computer-based intervention is found to be effective in increasing condom use in a sample of students from a Midwestern suburban high school, how generalizable are those findings to teens living in urban centers in the west or rural areas of the south?

Interaction of Treatment and Setting

Sometimes an *interaction of treatment and setting* can affect external validity. This interaction is concerned with whether results from an intervention conducted in one setting can be generalized to another setting where the same intervention is used. If the study on condom use was conducted with teens waiting to be seen in a family planning clinic, can the findings from that study be generalized to teens in a high school setting?

KEY TERM

Interaction of treatment and setting: A threat to external validity when an intervention conducted in one setting cannot be generalized using the same intervention

TEST YOUR KNOWLEDGE 6-2

1. The degree to which the results of studies can be generalized to other individuals, settings, or time is:

    a. external validity

    b. construct validity

    c. internal validity

    d. statistical conclusion validity

2. During a study examining nurses' job satisfaction, the union decides to hold a strike. This is what type of threat to internal validity:

    a. selection bias

    b. mortality

    c. history

    d. testing

3. A researcher plans to observe children in a kindergarten class. Students have always been told to be on their best behavior when guests are present in the classroom. What is the greatest threat to external validity:

    a. construct validity

    b. Hawthorne effect

    c. selection

    d. interaction of treatment setting

How did you do? 1. a; 2. c; 3. b

Interaction of Treatment and History

Interactions of treatment and history can also occur. This threat is concerned with how the effects from the intervention might be changed by events occurring in the past or in the future. For example, if the researcher found that the computer-based intervention increased condom use, would those results be generalizable to the future if a cure for HIV were to be discovered?

6.3   Categorizing Designs According to Time

At the end of this section, you will be able to:

‹ Differentiate the time dimension of data collection across retrospective, cross-sectional, and longitudinal and prospective designs

KEY TERMS

Interaction of treatment and history: A threat to external validity when historical events affect the intervention

Retrospective design: Research design when researchers look back in time to determine possible causative factors

Ex post facto: Retrospective research design

Case-control: Retrospective study where research begins with people who already had the disease

Evaluating the strength of the evidence obtained with quantitative designs includes evaluating the timing of data collection. The time dimension of a study may be classified as retrospective, cross-sectional, and longitudinal or prospective.

Retrospective Designs

Retrospective designs may also be referred to as *ex post facto*, which means after the fact. When designing retrospective studies, researchers start with the DV and look back in time to determine possible causative factors. Retrospective designs are considered to be after the fact because the DV has already occurred, which means that the IV cannot be manipulated and subjects cannot be randomly assigned. Thus, retrospective designs are never experimental in nature. Retrospective designs are often used in epidemiological studies. For example, causes of AIDS were discovered by researchers who started noticing an unusual increase in the number of cases of Kaposi's sarcoma occurring in young men. By taking careful histories, researchers were able to look back in time to determine behaviors and risk factors common to men who developed AIDS. Behaviors were compared with behaviors of men who did not have the disease. This type of retrospective study is called a *case-control* study because researchers started with a group of people who already had the disease. Identifying smoking as a cause of lung cancer also resulted from examining retrospective data. In both of these examples, retrospective designs were appropriate because it would have been unethical for researchers to deliberately expose subjects to either the HIV virus or to tobacco smoke. When conducting quality control studies, researchers often use retrospective designs. In these types of studies, researchers may want to gather information about an organization's status related to a patient problem such as falls. Chart audits can be done to determine the number of falls that occurred in the past 6 months. Information can be gathered on patients who have fallen to identify potential causative factors such as age, diagnoses, units where falls occurred, and staffing levels at the time of falls. Thus, retrospective studies can provide important data using nonexperimental designs. However, because retrospective designs are not experimental, a disadvantage is that researchers cannot say definitively that the IV caused the DV. Instead, researchers can conclude that there is an increased likelihood or probability that the IV caused the outcome in the DV.

Cross-Sectional Designs

Cross-sectional studies are nonexperimental designs that researchers use to gather data from a group of subjects at only one point in time. Cross-sectional designs provide a snapshot by collecting data about the IV and DV at the same time. Because data are collected at one time, it is difficult to establish cause and effect using cross-sectional designs. For example, a researcher is studying the effect of self-efficacy on condom use in adolescents. If a cross-sectional design is used, it would be difficult to determine if increased self-efficacy caused increased condom use or if increased condom use resulted in a sense of increased self-efficacy. Using a strong theoretical framework can guide the researcher when speculating about the relationships of the variables being studied with a cross-sectional design. It is important not to confuse cross-sectional studies with other designs. For example, a researcher who is interested in subjects' cardiovascular responses to stress may start by measuring blood pressures, exposing subjects to a stressful video clip, and then re-measuring blood pressures during and immediately after the video. Although data are collected in the immediate present, data about the IV and DV are not collected at the same point in time. Therefore, this is an example of an experimental design rather than a cross-sectional design. *Cohort comparison* studies are a specific type of nonexperimental cross-sectional design where more than one group of subjects is studied at the same point in time. Cohort comparison designs allow researchers to draw conclusions about variables over time even though data were collected at only one point in time. In the example of condom use, a cohort design could be used to study the factors associated with condom use among high school freshmen as well as high school sophomores, juniors, and seniors. The variables related to condom use in each group could be analyzed and compared to see if the same variables applied across the groups or to find out at what grade level the variables changed. Because following the same subjects

 FYI

as they progress through high school would take 4 years, gathering data from different subjects at each grade saves time. The advantages of cross-sectional designs are that they are easier to manage and are more economical. Because data are collected only one time from each subject, the threats of mortality, maturation, and testing are minimized. A limitation of cross-sectional designs is that it is difficult for researchers to make claims about cause and effect.

Longitudinal Designs

Longitudinal designs are used to gather data about subjects at more than one point in time. These may be either experimental or nonexperimental designs. Longitudinal designs are sometimes called *prospective designs*, which are studies that begin in the present and end in the future. Nonexperimental, prospective designs are commonly used in epidemiological studies where researchers begin by identifying presumed causes and then follow subjects into the future to determine if the hypothesized effects actually occur. In *panel designs*, the same subjects are used to provide data at multiple points in time. The observational study component of the well-known Women's Health Initiative (WHI) is an example of a prospective, nonexperimental, panel design (National Heart, Lung and Blood Institute [NHLBI], 2010). In the WHI, researchers funded by the NHLBI gathered data over an 8-year period from postmenopausal women between 50 and 79 years of age. The purpose of the study was to determine reliable estimates of the extent to which known risk factors predict heart disease, cancer, and fractures in older women. Women who joined the panel study were asked at different points in time to provide data about their health behaviors. They were not required to change any of their health habits—only to report them. *Trend* studies use nonexperimental designs to gather data about the variables of interest from different samples from the target population across time. An example of this is the Youth Risk Behavior Surveillance System (YRBSS) conducted by the Centers for Disease Control and Prevention (http://www.cdc.gov/HealthyYouth/yrbs/index.htm). Since 1992, the YRBSS has surveyed representative samples of students in grades 9–12. Repeated every 2 years, surveys provide data regarding the prevalence of risk behaviors among high school students. By using different samples of teens, researchers are able to determine if the rates of risky behaviors are increasing, decreasing, or staying the same over time. Another type of longitudinal design is the *follow-up* study. Researchers use this design to follow subjects into the future. These may be either experimental or nonexperimental designs. Nonexperimental follow-up studies differ from panel studies in that the samples are not drawn from the general population (e.g., not from all postmenopausal women or all teens in high school), but instead samples are selected because they have a specific characteristic or condition that researchers are interested in studying.

KEY TERMS

Longitudinal designs: Designs used to gather data about subjects at more than one point in time

Prospective designs: Studies over time with presumed causes that follow subjects to determine if the hypothesized effects actually occur

Panel design: Longitudinal design where the same subjects provide data at multiple points in time

Trend: A type of longitudinal design to gather data from different samples across time

Follow-up: A longitudinal design used to follow subjects into the future

An example of a nonexperimental follow-up design is a study involving the breastfeeding behaviors of new mothers. The researcher would select a sample of new mothers and follow them for a period of months to determine variables associated with their continuing or discontinuing breastfeeding.

Follow-up studies may also be experimental in design. A researcher may design a supportive educational intervention to increase new mothers' confidence in breastfeeding. The researcher would randomly assign mothers to either the new educational intervention group or the standard of care group. Mothers would be followed over the next few months to determine if the educational intervention made a difference in the length of time that mothers breastfed their infants. The hormone replacement component of the WHI Clinical Trial and Observational Study (http://www.nhlbi.nih.gov/whi/ctos.htm) is another example of an experimental follow-up study. In this study, women were randomly assigned to either a treatment or placebo group and then followed for 8 years to determine the effect of hormone replacement therapy on the prevention of coronary heart disease and osteoporotic fractures.

Crossover designs are a type of longitudinal study in which subjects receive more than one experimental treatment and are then followed over time. Subjects act as their own control group. Researchers manipulate the IV by randomizing the order in which the treatments are provided. An example of a crossover design is one in which the researcher is interested in determining whether relaxation techniques or exercise has a greater effect on reducing blood pressure. Some subjects would be randomly assigned to receive training in relaxation techniques first while others would be given instructions about exercise first. As subjects enter the study, baseline measures of blood pressure would be obtained. They would then do either the exercise or relaxation procedures for a set time period and would have their blood pressure measured at different points in time. Subjects would then be asked to stop the intervention and resume their normal habits while blood pressures are measured again. At a later time, subjects would receive instructions about the experimental treatment they had not done initially. Again, subjects would be followed for a set period of time with their blood pressures being measured. At the end of the study, the researcher would be able to determine which intervention produced the greatest reduction in blood pressures. One problem with crossover studies, however, is the possibility of a carryover effect. Even though subjects would be asked to stop performing the first intervention, sometimes they may continue to use it during the second phase of the study.

Gathering data at multiple points in time does not necessarily make a study longitudinal. Usually the term *longitudinal* is reserved for studies in which data are gathered over extended periods of time rather than in just a few hours or

KEY TERM

Crossover:
Experimental design using two or more treatments; subjects receive treatments in random order

TEST YOUR KNOWLEDGE 6-3

True/False

1. In retrospective designs, also known as ex post facto designs, the researcher manipulates the IV.

2. Cohort comparison studies can save time because more than one group of subjects is studied.

3. The threat of mortality is greater in cross-sectional designs than in longitudinal designs.

4. Any study that involves collecting data at multiple points in time is a longitudinal study.

How did you do? 1. F; 2. T; 3. F; 4. F

days. In some nursing situations, data may be repeatedly gathered but only for a relatively short period of time. For example, a researcher is studying the effects of music therapy on blood pressure of patients who are admitted to the intensive care unit. Although blood pressure is measured every hour for a 24-hour period, this study would not be described as a longitudinal study.

Longitudinal designs provide important information about the chronological relationships that exist between the IV and DV by determining changes over time. Another advantage is that this type of design can be used to test cause and effect. One disadvantage of longitudinal studies is their cost in following subjects over an extended period of time. The threat of mortality is increased; thus researchers need to make special plans to encourage subjects to complete the studies. Maturation is another threat inherent in longitudinal designs because changes of subjects are inevitable. Because longitudinal studies involve repeated measurements, the threat of testing is often increased.

6.4 Keeping It Ethical

At the end of this section, you will be able to:

< Discuss ethical issues related to internal and external validity

Researchers are obligated to conduct well-constructed studies. If a study does not have adequate controls in place, then the researcher has wasted valuable resources such as time, money, and subject volunteerism. Furthermore, failure to control jeopardizes the integrity of the findings. When findings are flawed, patient safety could be affected when practice is changed based on the evidence. Researchers should make every effort to implement strategies that enhance control and manipulation while reducing bias.

Implementation of strategies needs to be balanced with protecting the rights of human subjects. For example, when individuals are recruited for a study that involves two or more groups, they often express a desire to choose their group assignment. Allowing subjects to select their group assignment introduces the threat of selection bias. Most researchers would opt to randomly assign subjects to groups to reduce this threat. Therefore, it would be important for the researcher to inform subjects, during the recruitment process, that they will not be allowed to choose their own groups. Doing so allows individuals to make informed decisions about participating.

 FYI

Researchers are obligated to conduct well-constructed studies. If a study does not have adequate controls in place, then the researcher has wasted valuable resources such as time, money, and subject volunteerism.

 RAPID **REVIEW**

 Quantitative designs are used to describe phenomena, explain relationships, predict relationships, and explain causality.

 Nurses must consider elements of design when appraising quantitative studies.

- There are three major categories of quantitative designs: experimental, quasi-experimental, and nonexperimental.

- Causality refers to a relationship that exists between a cause and its effect. The IV must occur prior to the DV in order to claim a cause and effect relationship. Because outcomes can have multiple causes, probability assertions leave open the possibility for multicausality.

- In quantitative designs, researchers control, manipulate, and randomize to control for extraneous variables.

- Randomization is used in two ways to control for extraneous variables. Random sampling is the process of selecting a sample whereby each element in the population has an equal chance of being selected. Random assignment to groups means that all subjects in the sample have an equal chance of being assigned to either the intervention or control group.

- Researchers use within-groups designs to examine how subjects in the same group change over time. Between-groups designs involve comparisons of subjects of one group to subjects in another group.

APPLY WHAT YOU HAVE LEARNED

Consider the designs used in Fowler, Sohler, and Zarillo (2009), Kliger, Blegen, Gootee, and O'Neil et al. (2009), and Mark, Salyer, and Wan (2003). Identify any threats to internal and external validity of these studies. Discuss strategies that the researchers used to minimize these threats.

There are two major types of validity: internal and external. Internal validity is the degree to which one can conclude that it was the IV, not extraneous variables, that produced the change in the DV. External validity refers to the confidence one has that findings can be generalized across different types of people, settings, and times.

There are seven threats to internal validity: selection bias, history, maturation, testing, instrumentation, mortality, and statistical conclusion validity.

There are six threats to external validity: construct validity, reactivity, selection, interaction of treatment and selection of subjects, interaction of treatment and setting, and interaction of treatment and history.

Quantitative studies can be classified as follows according to the timing of data collection: retrospective, cross-sectional, longitudinal, and prospective.

REFERENCES

Campbell, D. T., & Stanley, J. C. (1966). *Experimental and quasi-experimental designs for research*. Chicago: Rand McNally.

Cook, T. D., & Campbell, D. T. (1979). *Quasi-experimentation: Design and analysis issues for field settings*. Boston: Houghton Mifflin.

Fowler, S. B., Sohler, P., & Zarillo, D. F. (2009). Bar-code technology for medication administration: Medication errors and nurse satisfaction. *MEDSURG Nursing, 18*, 103–109.

Kempthorne, O. (1961). The design and analysis of experiments with some reference to education research. In R. O. Collier & S. M. Elan (Eds.), *Research design and analysis* (pp. 97–126). Bloomington, IN: Phi Delta Kappa.

Kliger, J., Blegen, M. A., Gootee, D., & O'Neil, E. (2009). Empowering frontline nurses: A structured intervention enables nurses to improve medication administration accuracy. *The Joint Commission Journal on Quality and Patient Safety, 35*, 604–612.

Mark, B. A., Salyer, J., & Wan, T. T. H. (2003). Professional nursing practice: Impact on organizational and patient outcomes. *JONA, 33*, 224–234.

National Heart, Lung, and Blood Institute (2010, September 21). Women's health initiative. Retrieved from http://www.nhlbi.nih.gov/whi/index.html

CHAPTER OBJECTIVES

At the end of this chapter, you will be able to:

< Explain the three essential components of experimental designs

< Identify major experimental designs

< Discuss the advantages and disadvantages of various experimental designs

< Discuss the key difference between quasi-experimental and experimental designs

< Identify major quasi-experimental designs

< Discuss the advantages and disadvantages of various quasi-experimental designs

< Describe the purpose of nonexperimental designs

< Identify major nonexperimental designs

< Discuss the advantages and disadvantages of various nonexperimental designs

< Define translational research, community-based participatory action research, and health services research

< Discuss ethical issues related to quantitative designs

KEY TERMS

community-based participatory action research
comparative design
correlational design
covary
crossover design
descriptive correlational design
descriptive design
experimental design
exploratory design
factorial design
health services research

model-testing
multiple experimental groups design
nonequivalent control group pretest-posttest design
nonequivalent groups posttest only design
nonexperimental design
one group posttest only design
predictive correlational design

preexperimental
quasi-experimental design
Solomon four group design
survey design
time series design
translational research
two group posttest only design
two group pretest-posttest design

CHAPTER 7

Quantitative Designs: Using Numbers to Provide Evidence

Rosalind M. Peters

7.1   Experimental Designs

At the end of this section, you will be able to:

< Explain the three essential components of experimental designs
< Identify major experimental designs
< Discuss the advantages and disadvantages of various experimental designs

Quantitative designs can provide evidence that describe a phenomenon, explain relationships and differences among variables, predict relationships and differences among variables, or determine causality (Campbell & Stanley, 1966; Cook & Campbell, 1979). *Experimental designs* provide the best evidence for claiming that a cause and effect relationship exists. This type of design often includes the terms *pretest* and *posttest*. These terms refer to the point in time when data collection is taking place. Sometimes these are labeled "before" and "after" designs because pretest means data are collected prior to or before the intervention group receives the treatment, while posttest refers to data collected after the intervention is completed. Experimental designs look for differences between treated and untreated subjects. Therefore, there must be a minimum of two groups. To be considered a true experimental design, three features must be present: randomization, control, and manipulation.

CRITICAL THINKING EXERCISE 7-1

Remember an experiment you conducted in your chemistry class. Identify the three essential components of an experiment and tell how each was accounted for in your example.

KEY TERM

Experimental design: Design involving random assignment to groups and manipulation of the independent variable

Essential Components of Experimental Designs

Randomization in experimental designs is used in two ways. One way requires researchers to randomly select subjects from the target population. The other way is to randomly assign subjects to groups. Because random selection of the sample usually is not possible in nursing research, random assignment to groups is considered to be sufficient to meet the criteria of randomization for an experiment.

The second component of experimental designs is control, which is related to randomization. A control group, for comparison to the experimental group, is one strategy researchers use to control for extraneous variables. In addition to a control group, other ways researchers control for extraneous variables are by exerting the highest level of control over the selection of subjects, the definitions of the variables, and the environment in which the experiment is conducted.

Manipulation is the third essential component. Researchers must be able to manipulate the independent variable (IV) for a design to be considered experimental. This is accomplished by consistently administering the intervention.

True Experimental Designs

FYI

Experimental designs look for differences between treated and untreated subjects. The untreated group is the control group.

When creating an evidence-based practice (EBP), experimental designs are most valued. When appraising quantitative research studies, you may see the term *randomized controlled trial* (RCT), a term used to describe an experimental study that is conducted in healthcare settings. The RCT designation refers to the fact that the study is "clinical" in nature rather than a specific type of design. Regardless of the specific experimental design used, RCTs are characterized by the following considerations: 1) they involve a large number of subjects, often from diverse geographic areas, 2) there are strict guidelines for including subjects in a study, 3) subjects are randomly assigned to intervention and control groups, 4) groups must be comparable (equivalent) on key characteristics at baseline, 5) the intervention is consistently implemented to all subjects in the experimental group following a very rigidly defined protocol for implementation, and 6) all subjects in both groups are measured on the dependent variable (DV) using the same method of measurement at the same points in time.

There are six types of true experimental designs commonly reported in the scientific literature. These include: 1) two group pretest-posttest, 2) two group, posttest only, 3) Solomon four group, 4) multiple experimental groups, 5) factorial, and 6) crossover designs.

KEY TERM

Two group pretest-posttest design:
Subjects are randomly assigned to the experimental or control group, and measured before and after the intervention

Two Group Pretest-Posttest Designs

The *two group pretest-posttest design* is considered to be the "classic" experimental design. Subjects are randomized to either the experimental group receiving the intervention or the control group. They are measured before and after the intervention is implemented (see **Table 7-1**). This design allows researchers to examine within-subjects results as well as between-subjects results. For example, a researcher wants to test a new teaching strategy for diabetic patients. Patients in a diabetic clinic are randomly assigned to either the computerized learning module group or the standard of care group. Knowledge

TABLE 7-1 **Experimental Designs**

Two Group Pretest–Posttest (Classic)				
Experimental Group:	R	O_1	X	O_2
Control Group:	R	O_1		O_2
Two Group Posttest Only				
Experimental Group:	R		X	O_2
Control Group:	R			O_2
Solomon Four Group				
Experimental Group 1:	R	O_1	X	O_2
Experimental Group 2:	R		X	O_2
Control Group 1:	R	O_1		O_2
Control Group 2:	R			O_2
Crossover Design (randomization of treatment order)				
Experimental Group 1:	O_1 O_2 R X_1 O_3 O_4 $(-X)$ O_5 O_6 X_2 O_7 O_8			

Key: R = Randomization; O = Observation or Measurement; X = Treatment or Intervention; –X = Treatment Withdrawn

KEY TERMS

Two group posttest only design: An experimental design when subjects are randomly assigned to an experimental or control group and measured after the intervention

Solomon four group design: An experimental design with four groups—some receive the intervention, others serve as controls; some are measured before and after, others are measured only after the intervention

about diabetes is measured before and after teaching for all subjects. One way the researcher can determine the efficacy of the intervention is to compare the pretest and posttest scores of subjects in the intervention group to see if learning occurred. Another way to evaluate the intervention would be to compare posttest scores from the two groups to determine if one teaching method is better than another.

A potential disadvantage of the two group pretest-posttest design is that threats to internal validity are introduced from repeated testing. In the previous example, the threat of testing could be reduced by providing subjects with alternate forms of the diabetic knowledge test. Mortality is another threat because subjects are measured more than once. Also, when the intervention is burdensome, subjects may be more likely to withdraw from studies.

Two Group Posttest Only Designs

In experimental *two group posttest only designs*, researchers randomly assign subjects to either an intervention group or a control group. In nursing studies, the intervention is conducted with the experimental group (see Table 7-1), while the control group receives standard of care. After the intervention is completed, the DV is measured at the same point in time in both groups. This type of design is used when it is not possible or practical to measure the DV before the intervention is implemented. For example, a researcher is interested in examining the effect of music therapy on pain levels of patients undergoing invasive procedures. Because patients have no pain prior to invasive procedures, it would be impossible to determine if the intervention decreased levels of pain. Therefore, the only way a researcher can determine if music therapy effectively reduced pain would be to use a between-subjects design. Pain levels from subjects who used music therapy would be compared to the pain levels of subjects who did not. Because subjects are measured only once, threats of testing and mortality are minimized. A disadvantage of the two group posttest only design is that it is susceptible to the threats of selection bias. One cannot assume that the two groups are equivalent, because there was no measurement at baseline. Selection bias should be minimized because subjects are randomly assigned to groups. The characteristics of subjects that might affect the DV should be equally distributed between the two groups through the use of random assignment.

Solomon Four Group Designs

As the name implies, there are four groups of subjects involved in the *Solomon four group design*. Two groups of subjects receive the intervention, and two groups of subjects receive standard of care or a placebo. One experimental group and one control group are measured before and after the intervention, while the other experimental and control groups are measured only after the intervention (see Table 7-1). Researchers select this four group design over the two group pretest-posttest design to reduce the threat of testing. This design is also superior to the two group posttest only design because selection bias is minimized. Consider the diabetic teaching intervention example again. Suppose the researcher is concerned that subjects will learn information by taking the diabetic knowledge test. By adding two more groups that do not take the pretest, the researcher can compare posttest scores from subjects that took the pretest to scores of subjects that did not take the pretest. If testing is a threat, the researcher can expect that the pretest groups will have higher posttest scores than those who did not take the pretest.

While the Solomon four group design is a strong design, it has limitations. Because there are more groups, sample sizes must be large. This means that subjects must be available, recruitment of subjects will take longer, and costs will be increased.

Multiple Experimental Groups Designs

It is possible for researchers to use either the posttest alone or the pretest-posttest design with *multiple experimental groups designs*. To conduct this type of study, researchers would have multiple experimental groups and one control group. In the example of interventions to reduce pain during invasive procedures, the researcher might be interested in testing two different interventions. The researcher could randomly assign subjects to experimental group one, which would receive music therapy. Other subjects would be randomly assigned to experimental group two, where they would receive therapeutic touch. Other subjects would be randomly assigned to the control group for standard of care. The advantage of the multiple group design is that it allows researchers to compare the effect of different interventions on the DV. A major disadvantage of this design is that a large number of subjects is needed to detect differences across multiple groups.

Factorial Designs

In the previously discussed designs, only one intervention has been manipulated. Even in multiple group experiments, each experimental group receives only one intervention. *Factorial design* allow researchers to manipulate more than one intervention during the same experiment. Researchers may compare multiple interventions (e.g., music *and* therapeutic touch combined) or multiple levels of interventions (e.g., music with therapeutic touch for 10 minutes, 15 minutes, or 20 minutes). For example, a researcher is interested in increasing

KEY TERMS

Multiple experimental groups design: Experimental design using two or more experimental groups with one control group

Factorial design: Experimental design allowing researchers to manipulate more than one intervention

TABLE 7-2 Factorial Design

		Website InterventionWebsite Intervention	
		YES	NO
Home Visit Intervention	YES	Both home visit and website	Home visit alone
	NO	Website alone	No intervention control group

self-care behaviors of people with high blood pressure. The researcher hypothesizes that home visits and an interactive website will be effective in lowering blood pressures. Two experiments could be used to test each intervention separately, or a factorial design could be used to test both interventions separately, while testing the effects of a combined intervention for controlling high blood pressures. **Table 7-2** depicts the 2 × 2 factorial design for this example. Note that there are three intervention groups (home visit alone, website alone, and combined home visit and website) and one control group that receives neither the home visits nor the interactive website.

Because of its complex nature and sophisticated data analysis, more experienced researchers tend to use this type of design. Like Solomon four group designs, sample sizes need to be large because there will be a minimum of four

TEST YOUR KNOWLEDGE 7-1

True/False

1. All experiments must include a minimum of two groups of subjects.

2. The Solomon Four Group design is more effective at controlling for the threat of testing than is the two group pretest-posttest design.

3. In a factorial design, only one group of subjects is required because they act as their own control.

4. Patients who are not in the intervention group must receive the standard of care.

How did you do? 1. T; 2. T; 3. F; 4. T

groups. However, time and effort are saved by not having to conduct multiple studies.

Crossover Designs

In the discussion of longitudinal designs, *crossover designs* were mentioned. Although only one group of subjects is used, crossover designs include the three essential components of an experiment (see Table 7-1). Independent variables are manipulated by the researcher, and the order in which the interventions are administered to subjects is randomized. Because subjects serve as their own control group, the criterion of control is met because it is assumed that each subject will remain stable on the extraneous variables during the study.

Smaller sample sizes will be needed because only one group of subjects is required, and subjects serve as their own controls. A disadvantage is that subjects may continue to engage in the first intervention after moving to the second.

KEY TERM

Crossover design: Experimental design using two or more treatments and subjects receive both treatments in a random order

7.2   **Quasi-Experimental Designs**

At the end of this section, you will be able to:

< Discuss the key difference between quasi-experimental and experimental designs
< Identify major quasi-experimental designs
< Discuss the advantages and disadvantages of various quasi-experimental designs

Quasi-experimental designs are like experimental designs; they involve manipulation of the IV but do not meet one of the other essential components of experimental designs (Campbell & Stanley, 1966; Cook & Campbell, 1979). They either lack randomization or a control group, which makes claims of cause and effect weaker than in experimental designs. Because of this, studies using quasi-experimental designs are ranked lower as sources of evidence than studies using experimental designs. However, there are many situations involving the study of human health when it is not feasible or ethical to conduct an experiment. Therefore, quasi-experimental designs serve an important function in providing beginning evidence of causality. There are three commonly used quasi-experimental designs: 1) nonequivalent control group pretest-posttest, 2) time series designs, and 3) preexperimental designs (see **Table 7-3**).

KEY TERM

Quasi-experimental design: Research designs involving the manipulation of the independent variable but lacking either random assignment to groups or a control group

TABLE 7-3 **Quasi-Experimental Designs**

One Group Pretest-Posttest (no randomization)					
Group 1:			O_1	X	O_2
Nonequivalent Control Group Pretest-Posttest (no randomization)					
Experimental Group:			O_1	X	O_2
Comparison Group:			O_1		O_2
One Group Time Series (no randomization)					
Group 1:	O_1	O_2	O_3	X	O_4	O_5
One Group Posttest Only Design (no randomization, no pretest)					
Group 1:				X	O_2
Nonequivalent Control Group Posttest Only (no randomization, no pretest)					
Experimental Group:				X	O_1
Comparison Group:					O_1

Key: R = Randomization; O = Observation or Measurement; X = Treatment or Intervention;
    –X = Treatment Withdrawn

Nonequivalent Control Group Pretest-Posttest Designs

The *nonequivalent control group pretest-posttest design* differs from the classic experimental design in that researchers are unable to randomly assign subjects to groups. Because researchers are unable to randomize in these designs, the nonintervention group is referred to as a comparison group rather than a control group. Researchers are able to measure both groups on the DV prior to and after the intervention (see Table 7-3). For example, the faculty of a nursing college is considering changing a nursing research course offered to junior students. In one semester, a professor administers a pretest measuring knowledge about nursing research. The professor then teaches the course content in the usual lecture style. At the end of the semester, the final exam is used as a posttest to measure students' knowledge of research. The next semester, another group of students enter the research course. They are given the same pretest, but the instruction is online with no class lectures. At the end of the semester, the same comprehensive final exam is administered. The faculty would then be able to compare students' knowledge pre- and postintervention and make

KEY TERM

Nonequivalent control group pretest-posttest design: A quasiexperimental design is where two groups are measured before and after an intervention a determination regarding the effect of the different teaching methods on students' knowledge about research. Because students were unable to be randomly assigned to a teaching method, this is not an experimental design. Without randomization, it is possible that the students are not equivalent on important factors that may affect how they learned the course materials. This contributes to selection bias and weakens the design. Threats to internal validity as a result of testing, maturation, and mortality can exist.

Time Series Designs

The second most commonly seen quasi-experimental design is the *time series design*. This type of design may be used when neither randomization nor a comparison group is possible. Researchers may opt to study one group over a prolonged period of time prior to administering the intervention and then make multiple observations after the intervention is conducted. For example, the faculty decides to change the pass rate on exams from 75% to 80%. They could compare the number of student nurses passing at 75% for four semesters to the number who pass at 80% over four semesters. Although there are many factors that contribute to pass rates among student nurses, following the data for an extended period of time helps faculty to determine the effect of a policy change.

Preexperimental Designs

One group posttest only and *nonequivalent groups posttest only designs* are often referred to as *preexperimental* rather than quasi-experimental. The difference between pre- and quasi-experimental designs is that quasi-experimental designs, while lacking some elements of an experiment, use other strategies to control for extraneous variables. Many threats to internal validity can be found in these posttest only designs. An example of a one group posttest only study is when a researcher implements an educational intervention to teach new mothers the benefits of breastfeeding. After the intervention, the mothers' knowledge of breastfeeding was tested. Without a pretest to determine the mothers' previous knowledge and without any information about their prior history of breastfeeding, it would be almost impossible to determine what effect the intervention had on the breastfeeding outcome. One group posttest only designs provide a low level of evidence, and no change in nursing practice should be made based on this type of design.

Adding a comparison group slightly increases the quality of evidence found in posttest only designs. A nonequivalent groups posttest only design involves manipulation of the IV and two or more groups of subjects who are compared on the DV. For example, a researcher works in an agency where the policy is

FYI

Quasi-experimental designs lack an essential component of experimental designs. There are several types including nonequivalent control group pretest-posttest, time series designs, and preexperimental designs.

that all new mothers will receive the breastfeeding educational intervention. Because randomization of mothers is not possible, the researcher decides to compare breastfeeding knowledge of mothers from a hospital requiring the educational intervention to mothers from a hospital that does not offer that intervention. Because this is a nonequivalent groups posttest only design, it is impossible for the researcher to have any information about breastfeeding knowledge of the mothers in either group prior to the intervention. It is impossible to determine the equivalence of the two groups because the researcher does not have any pretest information. If the results of the study indicated that the mothers in the intervention group knew more about breastfeeding than the mothers in the comparison group, can the researcher conclude that the intervention was the cause of the increased knowledge? It is possible there were other factors, such as previous positive experiences with breastfeeding, increased family support, and encouragement to breastfeed by nursing staff, that were more influential in determining the results. Given that there could

TEST YOUR KNOWLEDGE 7-2

1. Quasi experimental designs include which of the following essential components.
   a. randomization, control group, and manipulation of the IV
   b. randomization and control group
   c. comparison group and manipulation of the IV
   d. randomization and manipulation of the IV

2. Experimental designs have control groups. Quasiexperimental designs have which of the following:
   a. control groups
   b. comparison groups
   c. extraneous groups
   d. peer groups

3. Rank the evidence generated from the following designs from lowest to highest:
   a. experimental designs
   b. nonequivalent control group pretest posttest
   c. one group posttest only
   d. nonequivalent groups posttest only

How did you do? 1. c, d; 2. b; 3. c, d, b, a

be many threats to internal validity, nurses should be cautious about changing practice based on data from preexperimental designs.

7.3   Nonexperimental Designs

At the end of this section, you will be able to:

< Describe the purpose of nonexperimental designs
< Identify major nonexperimental designs
< Discuss the advantages and disadvantages of various nonexperimental designs

Although experimental designs are considered to provide the strongest quantitative evidence, that is not the only type of evidence needed for nursing practice. Nurses are concerned with the whole person in interaction with the environment, and as such, they need information that is not always available from experimental studies. Information about personal phenomena such as patients' thoughts, beliefs, and subjective experiences, especially related to health care, is often most appropriately obtained using *nonexperimental designs*, which are descriptive in nature (Campbell & Stanley, 1966; Cook & Campbell, 1979). Nonexperimental designs also are important when there is little information known about a particular phenomenon, when it would be unethical to manipulate the independent variable, or when it is not practical to conduct an experiment (e.g., lack of resources or excessive burden to the subjects). The primary difference between nonexperimental and other quantitative designs is that researchers do not actively manipulate the IV. Even though the IV is not being manipulated, it is important for researchers to exert as much control as possible to avoid threats to internal and external validity. Researchers still need to protect against bias when conducting these quantitative studies. Bias can be controlled with carefully selecting the sample, having an adequate sample size to ensure sufficient statistical power, clearly defining conceptual and operational variables, using reliable and valid instruments to measure the variables of interest, and exerting control over the conditions under which the data will be collected.

Nonexperimental designs can be used for the purpose of: 1) describing a phenomenon in detail, 2) explaining relationships and differences among variables, and 3) predicting relationships and differences among variables. Because the IV is not manipulated, researchers using nonexperimental designs cannot make claims about cause and effect. Although nonexperimental designs can be categorized in many ways, they fall into two general categories: descriptive and correlational.

KEY TERM

Nonexperimental design: A research design that lacks manipulation of the independent variable and random assignment

   FYI

Nonexperimental designs are descriptive in nature and can be used to describe phenomena in detail, explain differences among variables in detail, and predict relationships and differences among variables.

Descriptive design:
Descriptive designs
provide a picture of
a situation as it is
naturally happening
without manipulation
of any of the variables

Exploratory design:
Nonexperimental
design used when
little is known about a
phenomenon

Comparative design:
Descriptive design
that compares two
or more groups or
variables

Survey design: A
descriptive design
involving data
obtained through
subjects' self report

Correlational design:
Nonexperimental
designs used to study
relationships between
two or more variables

Descriptive Designs

The purpose of *descriptive designs* is to describe in detail a phenomenon of interest. Descriptive designs provide a picture of a situation as it is naturally happening without manipulation of any of the variables. This type of design allows researchers to identify and document the different characteristics of phenomena and describe the frequency with which they occur. Because there is no manipulation of variables and no attempt to establish causality, the terms *IV* and *DV* should not be used with descriptive designs. Instead, the term *research variable* is more appropriate. Researchers use descriptive designs for a variety of purposes. These designs are often used to assess current practice. They can also be used in the early stages of theory development. Conceptual and operational definitions of the variables and possible theoretical relationships among the variables can emerge from descriptive studies. Although most descriptive designs tend to be cross-sectional, they can be conducted in any of the time dimensions as discussed previously. Descriptive designs are often called by a variety of names, such as *exploratory*, *comparative*, and *survey designs*. The term *exploratory* is used because descriptive designs are used when little is known about a phenomenon, so exploration is required. For example, an exploratory design could be used to determine factors associated with nurses' willingness to discuss sexual concerns with their patients. The term *comparative* is used if the purpose of the study is to describe phenomena by comparing two or more groups or two or more variables. For example, a researcher could use this type of design to describe nurses' willingness to discuss sexual concerns with patients and compare oncology nurses to cardiology nurses. Another approach a researcher might take could be to study oncology nurses and compare their willingness to discuss sexual concerns with patients to variables such as the nurses' age, level of education, and years of experience. The term *survey* is used to indicate that data are obtained through subjects' self-report about variables such as their attitudes, perceptions, and behaviors. Surveys can be conducted by having subjects respond to face-to-face or telephone interviews. Questionnaires are a popular method used to collect descriptive data. They can be completed face to face, through the mail, or online.

A well-controlled descriptive study offers a number of advantages over other types of quantitative designs. Descriptive designs have flexibility in the methods that can be used to collect data, often leading to more rapid collection of data and cost savings. The major disadvantage of this type of design is the inability to establish causality.

Correlational Designs

Correlational designs are used when researchers are interested in establishing relationships between two or more variables. When reviewing the evidence from correlational studies, it is important for nurses to remember that correlation does not prove causality. Because correlational designs do not involve manipulation of the IV, no causal statements can be made. For example, for some individuals there is a correlation between their symptoms of arthritis and changes in the weather. Before a change in weather, individuals may experience joint pain. However, one cannot conclude that joint pain causes the weather to change even though there is a strong correlation between the two phenomena. The best way to interpret a correlation is to understand that correlations simply mean that the variables *covary*—that is, when there is a change in one variable, there will be an associated change in the other. Evaluating statistical data will provide information about the strength of the relationship, the direction of the relationship (positive or negative), and whether the relationship is statistically significant. There are three types of correlational designs that are commonly reported in the literature: 1) descriptive-correlational, 2) predictive correlational, and 3) model-testing.

Descriptive Correlational Designs

Descriptive correlational designs build on comparative descriptive designs. Comparative descriptive designs simply describe the phenomena as they occur in two or more groups or among two or more variables associated with the phenomena. Descriptive correlational designs are used when researchers are interested in explaining the degree and characteristics of relationships that exist among the variables or groups. For example, in the case of nurses' willingness to discuss sexual concerns with their patients, the researcher can use a descriptive correlational design to determine the extent to which level of education or years of experience is related to the nurses' comfort with discussing sexual issues.

Predictive Correlational Designs

Sometimes there is insufficient empirical or theoretical literature for researchers to be able to assume the degree or direction of the relationships among the variables. Researchers use descriptive correlational designs to test nondirectional hypotheses. Like descriptive studies, there is no IV or DV, and the variables are simply referred to as "research" variables. In other situations, researchers have sufficient evidence to be able to predict the expected direction of relationships that will be found among the variables. When this is the case, a *predictive correlational design* is used. Researchers hypothesize which variables are predictors and which are outcomes. Although researchers may be able to predict a statistically significant relationship, the design is still correlational and causality cannot be assumed. Therefore, even though it is common to see the terms *IV* and *DV* used with this type of design, this is not techni-

KEY TERMS

Covary: When change in one variable is associated with change in another variable

Descriptive correlational design: Correlational design used to explain the relationship among the variables or groups using a nondirectional hypothesis

Predictive correlational design: Correlational design when researchers hypothesize which variables are predictors or outcomes cally correct. The variables should be referred to as predictor and outcome. There are two major aims of predictive designs. First, and most commonly seen in nursing, researchers attempt to determine the amount of variance in an outcome variable that can be explained by multiple predictor variables. For example, a researcher is interested in determining what factors are most likely to predict the quality of life (QOL) in patients receiving dialysis treatments. The researcher could conduct a study to determine the relationship between the hypothesized predictor variables of emotional distress, functional status, marital status, employment status, age, and length of time on dialysis. The researcher could then use statistical tests to determine the amount of variance in QOL scores that could be predicted by this group of predictor variables. Suppose the researcher finds that emotional distress accounts for a large portion of QOL scores, and employment status accounts for only a small portion of QOL scores. Using this evidence to determine best practice, nurses should recognize that interventions directed toward alleviating emotional distress would have a greater influence on dialysis patients' perceptions of QOL than interventions directed toward altering employment status. Sometimes researchers want to know how accurately a group of predictor variables can determine group membership. Determining group membership is the second aim of predictive correlational designs. For example, this type of design could be used if a researcher wanted to determine to what degree the predictor variables of age, self-efficacy, level of education, and level of general stress predict whether or not a woman will smoke during pregnancy. Data will allow the researcher to calculate the odds that a woman will be a smoker versus the odds that she will be a non-smoker. The outcome variable is the group membership because women are either predicted to be in the group of smokers or in the group of nonsmokers. While correlational studies are considered to produce a lower level of evidence, odds ratios are growing in popularity as a way to inform practice.

Model-Testing Correlational Designs

A third type of correlational design is *model-testing*. Researchers use this type of design to test a hypothesized theoretical model. All related variables are identified, and specific hypothesized relationships are stated. Researchers create graphic representations or paths to show the relationships among the variables (see **Figure 7-1**). Then statistical analysis is done to test all of the relationships at one time. The analysis will determine how well the data collected actually "fit" the hypothesized model. The better the fit of the model to the analysis, the more likely it is that the predicted theoretical relationships are true in reality. Often the term *causal modeling* is used for model-testing designs, but this is misleading. Although model-testing designs provide a rigorous test of predicted relationships among multiple variables based on theory, they can only provide a suggestion of causality, not true evidence of

FIGURE 7-1 **Diagram of a Path of Analysis**

RaLES: Racism and Life Experience Scale: β = standardized coefficient of path relationship between variables; † squared multiple correlation (variance explained); ***p<.001
Source: Benkert, Peters, Clark, & Keves-Foster (2006).

causality. Model-testing and predictive designs, while establishing predictive links between variables, is not the same as being able to say that variable X causes variable Y. True causality can be only established with an experimental design. However, because in nursing it is often unethical to manipulate IVs, model-testing designs provide the strongest nonexperimental evidence regarding the relationships among variables.

TEST YOUR KNOWLEDGE 7-3

True/False

1. In nonexperimental designs, researchers manipulate the IV to determine cause and effect relationships.

2. Nonexperimental designs can be used to develop and test theories.

3. The purposes of nonexperimental designs are to describe, explain, and predict relationships.

4. Descriptive data are usually cross-sectional and can be collected through surveys and questionnaires.

5. Researchers use correlations to determine if there are differences between two groups.

How did you do? 1. F; 2. T; 3. T; 4. T; 5. F

7.4   Specific Uses for Quantitative Designs

At the end of this section, you will be able to:

‹ Define translational research, community-based participatory action research, and health services research.

KEY TERM

Translational research: Research for the purpose of linking research findings to the point of care

Quantitative designs are often used to answer research questions involving translational research, community-based participatory action research, and health services research.

Sometimes research is categorized by its design and purpose. Quantitative designs are often used to answer research questions involving translational research, community-based participatory action research, and health services research. Because there are commonalities among these types of research, a study may fit in more than one of these categories.

Translational research "transforms scientific findings or discoveries from basic laboratory, clinical, or population studies into new clinical tools, processes, or applications" (Grady, 2010, p. 164). The purpose of this type of research is to link basic research to the point of care, ultimately improving patient outcomes. Like EBP, translational research is the study of how nurses and other healthcare providers can apply scientific findings to address real clinical problems (Grady; Woolf, 2008). Recall the cycle of scientific development introduced in Chapter 1 (Figure 1-3). Translational research occurs when research findings are disseminated and subsequently applied. For example, if a cure for the common cold were discovered through basic research, translational research could be used to determine the best way to distribute the treatment to individuals. Application of findings provides feedback for further development of theory and research. For example, if the cure is distributed and side effects are identified, additional research may be indicated to improve the product. Funding for translational research is increasing because of the recognition that failure to adopt new innovations thwarts the cycle of science. The Agency for Healthcare Research and Quality (AHRQ), committed to the support of trans-

---

CRITICAL THINKING EXERCISE 7-2

A researcher is interested in studying the effect of different medications on the pain of fractures in children admitted to the emergency department. The researcher wants to compare IV morphine, oral ibuprofen, and oral Tylenol with codeine. What kind of design do you think should be used? Why?

lational research, is the federal agency accountable for disseminating research findings for clinical decision making (AHRQ, 2008).

An alternative to traditional research approaches is *community-based participatory action research* (CBPAR; Schmittdiel, Grumbach, & Selby, 2010). CBPAR is based on a philosophy that when users of research are involved from the start of the research process, findings that are practical and relevant to community needs are more likely to result. Critical principles for CBPAR include engaging in collaborative, equitable partnerships, building on resources and goals present in the community, creating long-term sustainable partnerships, and using dynamic processes where ideas flow between researchers and community members (Schmittdiel et al.). For example, nurses traveled to a Central American community to offer health care. Using a CBPAR model, nurses first met with community leaders to determine the needs, priorities, strengths, and desired outcomes. The research team and community members mutually agreed upon the purpose and methods used. By working together, they created an intervention that fit with the community's culture and was sustainable when the research was completed.

The goals of *health services research* are to determine strategies to effectively organize, manage, finance, and deliver high quality care. Research topics include ways to reduce medical errors and improve patient safety (AHRQ, 2010). Studies often involve multidisciplinary teams. For example, a study might be conducted to determine how Internet communications can be used to connect healthcare providers practicing in rural areas to specialists around the world.

KEY TERMS

Community-based participatory action research: Active involvement of community members throughout the research process

Health services research: Research involving phenomena related to the delivery of health care

TEST YOUR KNOWLEDGE 7-4

1. A researcher is conducting a study to determine if a radio advertisement about the importance of early detection for colorectal cancer increases the attendance of middle-aged men at a free screening. This is an example of

    a. basic research

    b. community-based participatory action research

    c. health services research

    d. translational research

How did you do? 1. c, d

7.5 Keeping It Ethical

At the end of this section, you will be able to:

< Discuss ethical issues related to quantitative designs

When researchers plan studies using quantitative designs, they must incorporate mechanisms to safeguard the rights of subjects. In nursing and other health research, no subject can receive less than what is considered to be the standard of care. Even if subjects withdraw from studies, they must continue to receive standard of care. Providing standard of care protects subjects' rights to fair treatment. For example, in a study testing the effects of several educational programs on patient outcomes, it would be unethical for subjects in the control group to receive no education because the standard of care is to provide all patients with education about their care. When studies involve the use of placebos, decisions about their use must be scrutinized carefully because it is unethical to withhold treatment while testing a new intervention.

To protect the autonomy of individuals, they must be made aware of the benefits and risks of participating in a study so that they can make informed decisions about participating. All institutional review boards require that a description of benefits and risks be provided on consent forms. Most researchers also provide verbal explanations of the benefits and risks when recruiting subjects.

When designing quantitative studies, researchers must assess the associated benefits and risks of any intervention or test that they plan to use. To protect subjects from harm, the goal is to maximize the benefits while minimizing the risks. For example, suppose a researcher is testing radiation doses in women with breast cancer. Ideally, the researcher should select the dose of radiation that obtains the desired effect with the least amount of side effects. It would be unethical to irradiate women with unusually large doses of radiation even though it could be hypothesized that larger doses would be more effective because there are known complications associated with high doses. Consideration must be given to potential psychological harm as well. For example, suppose a researcher plans to interview women shortly after their miscarriages. Because miscarriage is an emotional incident for most women, the researcher must use sensitive language in consent forms and during interviews. Referring to the product of conception as a baby may cause undue emotional stress for some subjects.

In some studies, the risk of harm remains high regardless of strategies incorporated by researchers. For example, a researcher is testing a new medication for a serious condition. Regardless of whether subjects are assigned to the control or experimental groups, they are at risk for harm. When it is identified that one treatment is better than another, all subjects should be offered the best intervention. At times, unanticipated adverse reactions to interventions occur. When researchers discover that subjects are having adverse reactions, they should be reported immediately. Careful consideration should be given to discontinuing a study if this occurs.

Researchers have an obligation to minimize subject burden—that is, to place as few demands as possible on subjects. For example, a researcher is studying the effects of diet on cholesterol. Careful consideration should be given to the length of the study and the number of times subjects need to have blood samples drawn. If subjects perceive their participation in a study to be too burdensome, there is greater likelihood that they will not complete the study.

Although it is important to exert control to reduce threats to validity, researchers must ensure that strategies used are sensitive to the rights of subjects. When recruiting subjects, care must be taken to follow selection criteria to reduce selection bias. Sometimes subjects express a desire to be placed in a particular treatment group. Researchers cannot be swayed by these requests, and they must adhere to protocols about assigning subjects to groups. When subjects are enrolled in studies, it can be tempting to coerce subjects to remain in a study to limit threats related to mortality, but this is unethical. Subjects must feel free to withdraw at any time without consequences.

FYI

When designing quantitative studies, researchers must assess the associated benefits and risks of any intervention or test that they plan to use. To protect subjects from harm, the goal is to maximize the benefits while minimizing the risks.

TEST YOUR KNOWLEDGE 7-5

Which of the following situations is unethical?

1. A researcher tells a subject that he will not receive as high quality care if he withdraws from the study.

2. A research assistant carefully explains in English, without using an interpreter, the benefits and risks of being in a study to a woman who speaks only Spanish.

3. After discovering that subjects are experiencing adverse reactions to an intervention, researchers agree to discontinue the study.

How did you do? 1. Unethical; 2. Unethical; 3. Ethical

APPLY WHAT YOU HAVE LEARNED

[www]

You've come a long way in your understanding of how evidence is applied to practice. You are now ready to enter information about the designs used in Fowler, Sohler, and Zarillo (2009), Kliger, Blegen, Gootee, and O'Neil (2009), and Mark, Salyer, and Wan (2003) into the design column of your grid available on the companion website. Look at the examples and note how the types of designs are listed. Indicate the IVs and DVs if applicable.

RAPID REVIEW

- Experimental designs provide the best evidence of cause and effect relationships. These types of designs must include three features: randomization, control, and manipulation. There are six types of experimental designs: two group pretest-posttest, two group posttest only, Solomon four group, multiple experimental groups, factorial, and crossover.

- Quasi-experimental designs involve manipulation of the IV but do not meet one of the other criteria for experimental designs. Three common quasi-experimental designs are nonequivalent control group pretest-posttest, time series designs, and preexperimental designs.

- In nonexperimental designs, the IV is not manipulated; therefore cause and effect cannot be established. These types of designs are used to explore phenomena when the information is scant. Descriptive designs and correlational designs are two major types of nonexperimental designs.

- Researchers must consider maintaining standards of care and the benefits and risks of study participation when designing quantitative studies.

- Quantitative designs can be used in translational research, community-based participatory action research, and health services research.

REFERENCES

Agency for Healthcare Research and Quality. (2008). *AHRQ profile. Advancing excellence in healthcare.* Retrieved August 15, 2010, from http://www.ahrq.gov/about/profile.htm

Agency for Healthcare Research and Quality. (2010). *Quality and patient safety.* Retrieved December 16, 2010, from http://www.ahrq.gov/qual/

Benkert, R., Peters, R. M., Clark, R., & Keves-Foster, K. (2006). Effects of perceived racism, cultural mistrust and trust in providers on satisfaction with care. *Journal of the National Medical Association, 98*, 1532–1540.

Campbell, D. T., & Stanley, J. C. (1966). *Experimental and quasi-experimental designs for research*. Chicago: Rand McNally.

Cook, T. D., & Campbell, D. T. (1979). *Quasi-experimentation: Design and analysis issues for field settings*. Boston: Houghton Mifflin.

Fowler, S. B., Sohler, P., & Zarillo, D. F. (2009). Bar-code technology for medication administration: Medication errors and nurse satisfaction. *MEDSURG Nursing, 18*, 103–109.

Grady, P. A. (2010). Translational research and nursing science. *Nursing Outlook, 58*, 164–166.

Kliger, J., Blegen, M. A., Gootee, D., & O'Neil, E. (2009). Empowering frontline nurses: A structured intervention enables nurses to improve medication administration accuracy. *The Joint Commission Journal on Quality and Patient Safety, 35*, 604–612.

Mark, B. A., Salyer, J., & Wan, T. T. H. (2003). Professional nursing practice: Impact on organizational and patient outcomes. *JONA, 33*, 224–234.

Schmittdiel, J. A., Grumbach, K., & Selby, J. V. (2010). System-based participatory research in health care: An approach for sustainable translational research and quality improvement. *Annals of Family Medicine, 8*, 256–259.

Woolf, S. H. (2008). The meaning of translational research and why it matters. *JAMA, 299*(2), 211–213.

At the end of this chapter, you will be able to:

< Define qualitative research
< Describe sampling techniques in qualitative research
< Discuss the three major sources of qualitative data
< Explain analysis and interpretation methods with qualitative data
< Describe techniques used to meet the four elements of evaluation
< Distinguish among the four major types of qualitative research
< Explain the focus of phenomenological inquiry

< Give an example of grounded theory used in nursing
< Name a major nurse contributor to the advancement of ethnographic research
< List two hypothetical examples of historical research in nursing
< Discuss how qualitative studies can be used to create evidence-based practice (EBP)
< Discuss ethical considerations that are unique to qualitative methods

audit trail	etic	participant observation
bracketing	fieldwork	participants
confirmability	focus groups	peer debriefing
credibility	gatekeeper	persistent observation
data reduction	grounded theory	phenomenology
data saturation	historical	purposive
dependability	informants	referential adequacy
emic	key informants	snowball sampling
ethnography	lived experience	strategic sampling
ethnonursing	member checks	transferability
ethnoscience	memoing	

CHAPTER 8

Qualitative Designs: Using Words to Provide Evidence

Kristen L. Mauk

8.1   What Is Qualitative Research?

At the end of this section, you will be able to:

< Define qualitative research
< Describe sampling techniques in qualitative research
< Discuss the three major sources of qualitative data
< Explain analysis and interpretation methods with qualitative data
< Describe techniques used to meet the four elements of evaluation

Qualitative research was first used by disciplines such as the social and psychological sciences. It is used to answer questions related to the hows and whys of behavior that are not easily explained through quantitative methods, to investigate topics about which little is known, or to generate theory. Nursing, although using qualitative research since the 1970s, has only recently begun to embrace qualitative methods as an equally valuable means to explore certain topics while advancing the science and providing foundational evidence for best practice. Unfortunately, in the EBP process, qualitative research is still considered to be far less compelling than quantitative research because of the subjective nature of data analysis and interpretation.

In contrast to quantitative research, qualitative research focuses on words instead of numbers, on understanding and giving meaning to a phenomenon or an event. Data often stem from telling stories, describing events, and examining context, all of which emphasize words versus numbers and statistics. Qualitative research is more exploratory and inductive, while quantitative research aims to reach conclusions by deduction and hypothesis testing. Table 1-5 in Chapter 1 summarizes some important differences between quantitative and qualitative methods. You may wish to review this table to review these differences. In deciding whether or not qualitative methods would be appropriate to the topic being studied, Patton (2003) suggests a checklist such as the one found in **Table 8-1**.

Qualitative researchers often discover those important aspects of inquiry that would be easily missed if relying completely on quantitative data. Qualitative research is often the most appropriate method of inquiry for subjects that have been scarcely studied or those topics about which the researcher wishes to obtain a different viewpoint. For example, if a nurse was interested in ex-

TABLE 8-1 Example of a Qualitative Evaluation Checklist

1. Determine the extent to which qualitative methods are appropriate given the evaluation's purposes and intended uses.

2. Determine which general strategic themes of qualitative inquiry will guide the evaluation. Determine qualitative design strategies, data collection options, and analysis approaches based on the evaluation's purpose.

3. Determine which qualitative evaluation applications are especially appropriate given the evaluation's purpose and priorities.

4. Make major design decisions so that the design answers important evaluation questions for intended users. Consider design options and choose those most appropriate for the evaluation's purposes.

5. Where fieldwork is part of the evaluation, determine how to approach fieldwork.

6. Where open-ended interviewing is part of the evaluation, determine how to approach the interviews.

7. Design the evaluation with careful attention to ethical issues.

8. Anticipate analysis—design the evaluation data collection to facilitate analysis.

9. Analyze the data so that the qualitative findings are clear, credible, and address the relevant and priority evaluation questions and issues.

10. Focus the qualitative evaluation report.

Source: Patton, 2003.

ploring the healthcare practices of a culture different from his or her own, and one that had not been referenced in the research literature, a type of qualitative research method would be the logical place to begin. One would not expect to be able to develop an appropriate questionnaire or instrument to measure healthcare practices in a culture about which nothing had been previously written or studied. So qualitative methods are useful to answer descriptive and exploratory questions.

The Basics of Qualitative Research

Before nurses can apply findings from qualitative studies to nursing practice, they must have the ability to critically appraise and evaluate qualitative studies. Understanding the basics of sampling, collecting data, analyzing and interpreting data, and evaluation is necessary so that nurses can ensure that qualitative evidence is trustworthy.

Sampling

In qualitative research, the volunteers who participate in a study are called *participants* rather than subjects. Participants are also known as *informants*. The sampling method used is *purposive* rather than random, which is preferred in quantitative methods. That is because in qualitative methods, the researchers wish to obtain information from specific persons who could provide inside information about the subject being studied. Such people are sometimes referred to as *key informants* because they have intimate knowledge of the subject being investigated and are willing and able to share this with the researcher. A purposive sample is one selected intentionally, yet is comprised of volunteers who are willing to tell their stories.

Another type of sampling often used alone or in combination with purposive is called *snowball sampling*. This refers to the accumulation of participants based on word-of-mouth or referrals from other participants. For example, if a researcher interviewed a participant in his home and he mentioned that he attended a support group with others who might wish to talk with the researcher, this could be an additional source of participants for the study. If those from the support group knew others who might be included in the study, the number of participants has snowballed by referrals from the existing sample itself. Qualitative researchers often find this to be an effective way to identify key informants.

The number of participants in a qualitative research study is also different from quantitative methods. A smaller number is generally involved (often 6 to 10 in many studies). Instead of being determined by the number of variables one might have in a quantitative study, sample size in qualitative designs is

KEY TERMS

Participants: Individuals in a qualitative study; informants

Informants: Individuals in a qualitative study; participants

Purposive: Sampling method to recruit specific persons who could provide inside information

Key informants: Individuals who have intimate knowledge of a subject

Snowball sampling: Recruitment of participants based on word of mouth or referrals from other participants

FYI

Qualitative research in nursing has only recently begun to embrace qualitative methods as equal in value to quantitative research to advance the science and provide foundational evidence for best practice. However, qualitative research is still gaining acceptance in the EBP process because of the subjective nature of data analysis and interpretation.

KEY TERMS

Data saturation: No new information is being obtained and there is a repetition of information

Fieldwork: Time researchers spend interacting with participants

determined by the information being provided by the participants. Data collection stops when no new information is being obtained and repetition of information is consistently heard. This is called *data saturation.*

Collecting Data

There are three main sources of data in qualitative research. They are: 1) in-depth interviews, 2) direct observation, and 3) artifacts such as written documents, photographs, and physical objects. Each of these sources of data provides rich information for researchers. The data come from *fieldwork,* which is a term used to describe the time researchers spend interacting with participants through interviews, observations, and detailed records. These records include field notes, methodological logs, and reflective journals. Field notes include notations made before, during, and after contacts with participants to record observations about such things as the participant's mood, environment, and others in the setting. Methodological logs are used to document decisions made by the researcher about the study, such as changing an interview question or coding data. Researchers also use a reflective journal to record personal feelings and insights as studies progress. These records provide important mechanisms for keeping the researcher true to the data. The researcher must continually refer back to the data in these records as analysis and interpretation progress.

The interview is often the key source of data in qualitative research. Interview questions are generally open ended, allowing the participant to respond freely and provide the most information possible. The researcher may use an unstructured interview, following up with questions as the informant leads. However, most researchers have a set of questions that have arisen from reviewing the literature or from previous interviews that will guide the discussion with interview participants. The skill of the researcher as an interviewer is quite important in qualitative research. A common quote used is "in qualitative inquiry the researcher is the instrument" (Patton, 1990, p. 14). This means that the qualitative researcher should be skilled in the art of communication and be able to pick up on key words, phrases, thoughts, or ideas mentioned during the interview. Researchers use themselves as tools to solicit information from key informants to obtain the most accurate and useful data for the study.

Researchers must avoid common pitfalls of qualitative research (Easton, McComish, & Greenberg, 2000). This means that attention should be given to seemingly simple details such as bringing backup batteries for the tape recorder, having plenty of space on the video recorder to complete an interview that runs longer than expected, being sure there is a power source available if using electricity, and the like. A quiet place where the interview can be conducted without interruption is essential. One must anticipate every problem that could occur and have a plan in place. The normal interruptions of daily life make it difficult enough to conduct an interview, even without common problems interfering.

Recruiting volunteers who are willing to be interviewed can present a challenge. Nurse scientists may find participants from advertising in newspapers or newsletters, visiting support groups, using the media such as television or radio, putting up fliers in places where potential participants might be found, or partnering with a healthcare facility that services patients who may volunteer. For example, a nurse who wishes to recruit older people for a study about their attitudes toward living arrangements might find participants in independent living homes, church groups, senior centers, long-term care facilities, intergenerational care centers, or even the grocery store. In addition, snowball sampling may work well with this population. Whichever method of recruiting participants is used, it is essential that the researcher maintain integrity, obtain informed consent, and have institutional review board (IRB) approval to protect the rights of participants and maintain scientific rigor.

Interviews are generally audio- or videotaped as unobtrusively as possible. The interview must be sufficiently long to allow participants to share all essential information. A typical interview may last between 30 and 90 minutes. Open-ended responses and direct quotations are basic sources of data. The researcher also keeps notes during or immediately after the interview to record thoughts, ideas, and reflection on the interview itself. This provides additional contextual data from which to view the results.

The researcher continuously compares information obtained from various interviews, documents, or other sources. Unlike in quantitative research, the interview questions may even change over time as the researcher collects additional data that prompt exploration in other directions. The researcher must keep in mind that the purpose of the interview is to obtain as much pertinent information as possible about the phenomenon being studied and that the person with this information is the participant.

After an interview is complete, it is transcribed verbatim and printed for review. Another pitfall should be avoided here (Easton et al., 2000). Simple mistakes during transcription can change the meaning of a phrase, even making it read the opposite of what the participant actually said. Although most researchers have support personnel who may assist with transcribing, if the transcriber is unfamiliar with the jargon or slang used by the participant, common errors can occur. The researcher is ultimately responsible to be certain that the tapes are correctly transcribed. Researchers typically read over the line-by-line transcriptions many times prior to analysis and interpretation.

FYI

The interview is frequently used as the key source of data in qualitative research. Interview questions are generally open ended, allowing the participant to respond freely and provide the most information possible so that there is an abundance of data from which to draw interpretations.

Participant observation is the term most often used to describe the role of the researcher in qualitative data collection (Spradley, 1979). Entire books have been written on this subject because of its importance to the data collection process. The researcher is not merely an observer but also a participant during data collection. Because researchers are considered to be tools for obtaining information, they cannot be merely a detached observer in most cases. For example, a nurse scientist studying how prostate cancer survivors cope with urinary incontinence after surgery might choose to sit in on a support group for these patients. As a participant observer, the nurse might ask questions of the group while keeping notes on their interactions and the main topics of concern. The nurse would be a part of the support group for that day rather than a nonparticipating attendee. The members of that support group may even later become key informants to the nurse's study of this subject. The role of participant observer takes on an even greater meaning if the researcher has personally experienced the phenomenon being studied. In the case above, if the researcher had experienced surgery for prostate cancer and suffered the complication of urinary incontinence, he might participate within such a group at a deeper level. In such a case, however, the researcher must be careful not to allow the bias of personal experience to cloud the results that arise from the data being collected from others.

Artifacts provide an additional source of data in qualitative research. This is particularly true in historical research when the main source of data is governmental reports, journals, books, memos, photographs, letters, or diaries. When using these sources, it is important for researchers to remember that they can provide only a snapshot in time. Furthermore, the researcher must determine the authenticity of these sources of evidence. There is always room for discussion about the interpretation of findings (Kirby, 2004).

Analyzing and Interpreting Data

Although data analysis techniques may vary somewhat depending upon the type of qualitative method used, some general comments can be made. Data analysis in qualitative research involves description, data reduction, analysis, and interpretation. Unlike quantitative methods where analysis occurs only after data collection is completed, qualitative data analysis occurs as data are collected. Immersion refers to the data collection process in which the researcher "lives" with the data over time. The researcher should constantly reflect on the data and make comparisons with existing data as new information is obtained. Reading and rereading the text that has been transcribed verbatim are essential. The researcher should live with the data for a significant time, comparing every piece of data with the other. Researchers use a technique called *memoing* to record ideas that come to them as they live with data. Researchers must keep paper and pencil or their tape recorder handy because ideas may occur at any moment. It is important to memo ideas as they occur because it is difficult to recreate them after a period of time. Researchers use self-reflection to explore personal feelings and experiences to minimize their biases. This is important because analysis and interpretation are inherently subjective in qualitative research. *Bracketing* is a strategy used by researchers to set aside their personal interpretations to avoid bias. *Data reduction* occurs when the researcher begins to simplify the large amounts of data obtained from interviews and/or other sources. Terms, ideas, or quotations from transcribed interviews are identified to help the researcher focus on the common themes and patterns that will emerge. The researcher attaches meanings to certain portions of the data that seem to best represent what the majority of participants have reported. Data segments may be coded and indexed by identifying categories in the data. Repeated words or common ideas are noted. Computer software may be of great assistance in managing these data and helping to assign codes, numbers, colors, or other distinguishing marks to sets of data as the researcher attempts to group the data into meaningful segments.

After the data have been reduced in some fashion, the researcher identifies themes, patterns, and relationships. Essential to analysis and interpretation is that the themes, categories, or patterns that are ultimately chosen to represent the data do just that—represent what most of the participants in the study said. In qualitative research, one must be "true to the data" and build in continuous checks and rechecks to be certain that the labels assigned to various themes or patterns reflect what participants have told the researcher. Oftentimes, words used by the study participants form the basis for categories assigned.

The final phase of managing the data is interpretation. Interpretation is critical because it brings the message of the participants to the public for reading and application. The researcher uses interpretation to provide meanings that can be used in EBP. Interpretation is open to subjectivity because it is likely that no two researchers would interpret the meaning of the data in exactly the same way. However, to establish scientific rigor, other nurse scientists should be able to follow the paper trail and analysis of the researcher and agree that the interpretation and results reported are true to the data obtained from the participants.

In some types of qualitative research, theory development is an expected outcome. In this case, the researcher must identify concepts and find links or relationships among them to form a theory. The theory is then shared with participants to ensure that it reflects or captures what they experienced or felt.

KEY TERMS

Bracketing: Setting aside personal interpretations to avoid bias

Data reduction: Simplification of large amounts of data

KEY TERMS

Credibility:
Believability of
findings

Transferability:
Application of
findings to a different
situation

Dependability:
Findings are reflective
of data

Confirmability:
Findings can be
substantiated by
participants

**Persistent
observation:**
Spending quality
time with participants
attempting to
thoroughly describe
the phenomenon

Peer debriefing:
Researcher enlists
the help of a peer to
discuss the data and
findings

**Referential
adequacy:** When
multiple sources of
data are compared
and the findings hold
true

Member checks:
Researcher shares
the results with
participants to ensure
the findings reflect
what participants said

Remember that theories just provide a blueprint or framework from which to view a phenomenon and that they need to be tested and refined.

Evaluation

Guidelines have been established for evaluating qualitative research. Because qualitative methods are so different from quantitative methods, terms such as "validity" and "reliability" are not useful. Lincoln and Guba (1985) provided what remains the standard for evaluation of qualitative research. There are four essential elements of evaluation: *credibility, transferability, dependability*, and *confirmability*. Credibility is the qualitative equivalent of validity in quantitative research. It refers to the truth or believability of the findings (Leininger, 1985). Credibility is established through many strategies that are built into qualitative research. Strategies include *persistent observation, peer debriefing, referential adequacy*, and *member checks*.

Persistent observation means that the researcher has spent a good deal of quality time with the participants attempting to describe and capture the essence of the phenomenon being studied. The nature of qualitative research requires prolonged engagement. Thus, it is not considered to be a quick form of research.

Peer debriefing is when the researcher enlists the help of another person who is educationally prepared at a similar level to the researcher and would be considered a peer. The researcher meets on at least several occasions with the peer debriefer, who has consented to assume this role, throughout the study. The researcher and peer debriefer discuss the data and findings, as well as the researcher's reflections, feelings, and struggles. The peer debriefer provides another pair of eyes to examine the consistency of the researcher's interpretation of the data, thus holding the researcher accountable during this process. This is an excellent strategy for new researchers, particularly doctoral students, in that it provides support as well as validation for the student.

Referential adequacy and member checks are additional ways to establish credibility of qualitative research (Lincoln & Guba, 1985). Referential adequacy is satisfied when a researcher can refer to other sources of data, such as photos or journals, for comparison and have the results hold true when referencing these other data. Member checks involve the researcher going back to study participants either during or after the study, or both, and sharing the results with them to be sure that the end product reflects what the participants said.

Transferability relates to whether the findings from one study can be transferred to a similar context. The goal of qualitative research is understanding a particular phenomenon (Leininger, 1985) rather than generalizing to a population as in quantitative methods. Transferability is accomplished through techniques such as eliciting thick descriptions, adequate sampling, and achieving data saturation. Thick descriptions involve rich, written comments and narrative related to the situation being studied. Journals and mementos that help to enlighten the process can be kept. Deep and detailed description is needed to establish the scientific rigor of the study. Therefore, researchers must maintain an *audit trail* that can demonstrate the researcher's decision making throughout the study. Adequate sampling means that the researcher took enough time to be sure that data saturation was reached. That is, enough subjects were interviewed so that consistent patterns and themes emerged prior to stopping data collection. When no new information is being obtained, data saturation is said to have been achieved.

The criterion of dependability is satisfied when the researcher has established sufficient audit and paper trails through accurate and detailed journaling and logs. Record keeping and reflective writing are essential in this type of research. Other people, such as peer debriefers, should be able to look at the researcher's writings and see that the theory or results accurately reflect the data.

Confirmability means that the researcher made rigorous attempts to be objective and that audit trails were kept to document the research process. Evaluating interview questions to ensure that they are open ended and not leading is important for ensuring confirmability. The reader must be satisfied that the researcher has revealed that data were confirmed with the participants through member checks. The researcher's written records should reveal a detailed review of the data, careful analysis and coding, and detailed logs and field notes.

KEY TERM

Audit trail:
Documentation of the research process and researcher's decision making

CRITICAL THINKING EXERCISE 8-1

Which of the three types of data collection would you use to answer each of the following questions? How would you defend your choice of data collection method for each of these items? Would a combination of methods be appropriate for any of the questions below? If so, why?

1. What factors influence a student nurse's decision in choosing his/her first job after graduation?

2. How did Florence Nightingale choose which elements to focus on when she began to formalize nursing as a profession?

3. What influences whether or not a nurse reports a medication error to his/her supervisor?

TEST YOUR KNOWLEDGE 8-1

1. Which of the following terms are associated with qualitative sampling?

   a. snowball

   b. random

   c. purposive

   d. subjects

2. Which of the following are techniques for maintaining scientific rigor in qualitative studies?

   a. achieving saturation

   b. thick descriptions

   c. peer debriefing

   d. generalizing to populations

How did you do? 1. a, c; 2. a, b, c

8.2   The Four Major Types of Qualitative Research

At the end of this section, you will be able to:

< Distinguish among the four major types of qualitative research

< Explain the focus of phenomenological inquiry

< Give an example of grounded theory used in nursing

< Name a major nurse contributor to the advancement of ethnographic research

< List two hypothetical examples of historical research in nursing

< Discuss how qualitative studies can be used to create EBP

There are four major types of qualitative research: *phenomenology, grounded theory, ethnography,* and *historical.* Each of these types of research has distinguishing characteristics, so it is important for a researcher to select a method appropriate to the question. **Table 8-2** provides a comparison of these four major types.

TABLE 8-2 Comparisons of Qualitative Methods		
Type of Qualitative Research	**Focus**	**Example Question**
Phenomenology	Lived experience	What is the lived experience of a woman dying from breast cancer?
Grounded theory	Process	What is the process of recovery following breast cancer?
Ethnography	Culture	What are the self-care practices of the Athabascan Indians in Glenallen, Alaska?
Historical	The past	What were the ancient Romans' basic beliefs regarding hygiene and hand washing?

Phenomenological Research: Studying the Lived Experience

Phenomenology is the method used when one wishes to study *lived experience*. The general question being asked is: What is the meaning of . . . ? The goal is to achieve understanding of an experience from the perspective of the participants.

Method

Using purposive sampling, phenomenological studies more than likely will have small sample sizes, depending upon the phenomenon being studied. For example, in Su and Chen's (2006) study of women terminating treatment after in vitro failure, the sample size was 24. Women were selected from a common area and clinics because they were likely to have shared similar experiences. Case studies can also provide a description of the lived experience. For example, Galvin, Todres, and Richardson (2005) described one individual's experience caring for a spouse with Alzheimer's disease. However, it is important to keep in mind that one person's experience may be unique and not totally reflective of the experiences of others.

Data Collection and Management

Most of the data for phenomenological research are obtained from fieldwork, particularly interviews with people who have experienced the phenomenon being examined. Marshall and Rossman (1995) stated that "phenomenological interviewing is a specific type of in-depth interviewing grounded in the theoretical tradition of phenomenology. Phenomenology is the study of experiences and the ways in which we put them together to develop a worldview" (p. 82). Interviews are transcribed verbatim and read multiple times by the researchers. Significant statements are identified; items are coded and analyzed for themes and patterns. Statements may link together to form common themes. The researcher identifies broad themes with categories and subcategories that are consistent among participants. There may be several core themes or one broad theme with associated categories. Benner (1984) described three interpretive research steps of phenomenology: thematic analysis, analyzing exemplars, and identifying paradigms. During thematic analysis, the reasons, feelings, and thoughts of participants are explored. Meanings of the categories are analyzed and integrated into a theme or themes. Step two involves analyzing exemplars. This is when researchers repeatedly read data for possible new categories, corrections of thematic or categoric assignments, and analysis of differences among the data. Lastly, according to Benner, the researcher identifies paradigms, checking the themes and categories to be sure that they are representative of the responses from all participants.

Examples of Nursing Research Using This Method

There are many examples of nursing research using phenomenology. Some of the better known nursing theories coming from this type of research are Parse's (1991) theory of human becoming and Watson's (1989) theory of caring. Probably the best known research of this type is Benner's work *From Novice to Expert* (1984) in which she identified five stages of nursing competence that are still used to guide practice. Dr. Benner based her work on dialogue with nurses who were interviewed individually or in small groups. Her research offers examples of excellence in nursing practice and a framework demonstrating the development of nurses as they move through five stages: novice, advanced beginner, competent, proficient, and expert. This is indeed an example of how qualitative research translates into EBP as nurses all over the world study ways in which nurses develop into expert clinicians. In many healthcare facilities, professional promotion and clinical ladders are based on this model.

Grounded Theory Research: Creating Theory Through Induction

Grounded theory is the method of choice when the researcher wants to discover the process of something. The general question being asked is: What is the process of . . . ? This method is most commonly used in areas where there is little or no previous research. The grounded theory method was originated by Glaser and Strauss in 1967 when they looked at the way people approach the process of dying. They specified a systematic set of procedures that are used to inductively create a theory that is grounded in the data about a phenomenon (Strauss & Corbin, 1990). These theories can be useful in explaining and predicting phenomena (Glaser & Strauss, 1967).

Method

There are a few characteristics that make grounded theory different from other qualitative methods. The most important difference concerns the review of literature. In most research methods, an extensive review of literature is done prior to beginning the study to shed light on the phenomenon in question and identify gaps in the literature. In grounded theory, just enough literature is examined to identify the gaps in the literature, but a more extensive review of literature is done only after the research is completed (Glaser, 1978). The purpose of this approach is to avoid bias because a grounded theory must emerge from the data and never be forced by preconceived notions. Writing in a reflective journal is an effective strategy for raising self-awareness, thus reducing bias. After the theory has been generated, a thorough review of the literature is done, and the researcher compares the theory with other research. Known as comparative analysis, Glaser and Strauss (1967) listed the following steps: 1) obtaining accurate evidence, 2) making empirical generalizations, 3) specifying a concept, 4) verifying theory, and 5) generating theory. Grounded theory is dynamic and subject to change as new data become available. One could almost say that a grounded theory is never really finished but that it can be constantly validated and refined.

Data Collection and Management

Data are gathered mainly through interviews. As with other qualitative methods, the face-to-face interviews are video- or audiotaped and conducted using open-ended questions. The researcher keeps detailed field notes and methodological logs to record observations and reflections. The interview questions may become more focused as the study progresses so the researcher can discover the major processes taking place. Another unique aspect of grounded

KEY TERM

Focus groups: A strategy to obtain data from a small group of people using interview questions

theory is that researchers may use the literature as data. Both the technical and nontechnical literature can be used for this purpose (Glaser, 1992; Strauss & Corbin, 1990). Technical literature includes research reports or theoretical/philosophical papers of a scholarly nature. Nontechnical literature may include biographies, diaries, reports, newsletters, and records. Literature could be used as primary data or to supplement data gathered from interviews. There is no set sample size for grounded theory. The researcher obtains data until data saturation is reached. This may be as few as 10 interviews or more than double that depending on the data obtained. The use of *focus groups*, a strategy often used in qualitative research, lends itself well to grounded theory. Focus groups are useful to generate ideas and help formulate interview questions to be used later with key informants. Generally, a focus group consists of six to eight people with a common interest but who do not know each other well. The researcher may act as a facilitator by using open-ended questions to begin the discussion and guide the group to provide sought-after information. Or the researcher may be a participant–observer in a focus group, such as attending a breast cancer support group to gain insight. Focus groups have the added benefit of being an excellent way to identify key informants for one-on-one interviews later (Easton, 1999a). Another difference between grounded theory and other qualitative methods is the use of constant comparison. Comparisons are continuously made among the data. In this way, both data gathering and analysis occur somewhat simultaneously. The researcher records ideas, thoughts, possible emerging themes and patterns, questions for follow-up, and potential categories for data coding. As data are coded and clustered, the researcher continues to explore commonalities as interviewing and data collection continues. Negative case examples and conflicting information are also noted. All of these data form the basis for the final categories that are generated to reflect the process described by participants. As more interviews are conducted, the emerging theory is confirmed and refined as the researcher asks more focused questions. In addition, new subconcepts may be added or deleted to further refine the categories identified.

Examples of Nursing Research Using This Method

Folden (1994) used a grounded theory approach to describe how stroke survivors managed multiple functional deficits produced by stroke. The process was labeled "ensuring forward progress" (p. 81). Folden indicated that each person defined recovery "as the accomplishment of personal goals" (p. 81). Her findings were consistent with other findings in the stroke literature at the time, adding credibility to her work. Although Folden's work added much to nursing knowledge about stroke, the published articles stopped short of proposing a complete theory with assumptions and relational statements. Using the same population, stroke survivors, Mauk, who published earlier as Easton, sought to answer the question: What is the process of stroke recovery? (Easton, 1999b). From her research, a grounded theory emerged for post-stroke recovery that was labeled the post-stroke journey: from agonizing to owning. Mauk used writings and videotapes from stroke survivors to identify concepts and generate a theory. She then conducted face-to-face interviews with 18 stroke survivors to refine the theory. The end result of this grounded theory research showed that stroke survivors reported six major phases in the process of recovery: agonizing, fantasizing, realizing, blending, framing, and owning (Mauk, 2001; 2006). Nursing interventions targeted to each phase of recovery are being developed and explored but have yet to be tested. These two studies illustrate that grounded theory can be used by nurses to explore a phenomenon about which little is known. In the examples above, the process of stroke recovery was one that had to be discovered from survivors themselves. Theories can be used to develop practice guidelines. By listening to, documenting, and explaining the process that patients go through, nurses will provide better care because they are sensitized to patients' situations.

Ethnographic Research: Understanding Culture

Spradley (1979), considered to be a leading expert in ethnography, defined the method as "the work of describing a culture" (p. 3). He further stated that instead of just studying people, ethnography involves learning from people. Spradley (1980) suggested three basic aspects of human experience that researchers needed to discover: cultural behavior (what people do), cultural knowledge (what people know), and cultural artifacts (what people make and use). "The goal of inquiry is rounded, not segmented understanding. It is comprehensive in intent" (Hughes, 1992, p. 443). Ethnographic research involves studying groups and making collective observations. It is the method of choice for studying cultures.

Additional related methods that grew out of ethnography, *ethnoscience* and *ethnonursing*, warrant mention here. Ethnoscience is a method used in anthropology to discover nursing knowledge. Ethnonursing is the systematic study and classification of nursing care beliefs, values, and practices in a particular culture (Leininger, 1985; Welch, 2002). Cultural representatives share knowledge acquired through their language, experiences, beliefs, and value systems regarding nursing phenomena such as care, health, and environment. Because the focus is on nursing, studies using these methods are usually not as broad in scope and depth as studies conducted to explain an entire culture. Therefore, obtaining information may not require one to live in the culture

KEY TERMS

Ethnoscience: A method used in anthropology to discover nursing knowledge

Ethnonursing: Systematic study and classification of nursing care beliefs, values, and practices in a particular culture

KEY TERMS

Gatekeeper: Person who facilitates or hinders entry of the researcher into a particular group or setting

Emic: The insider's or participant's perspective

Etic: The outsider perspective of the researcher

for an extended period of time. These methods were used by Madeleine Leininger (1985), founder of transcultural nursing. Leininger, a noted professor and prolific author and theorist, earned a doctorate in cultural and social anthropology, which influenced her research related to nursing. She derived her theory of culture care diversity and universality from work in anthropology and nursing. Leininger firmly believed that quantitative methods had limited use in studying cultures and health and that ethnographic methods provided the clearest information when researching other cultures.

Method

A few techniques distinguish ethnographic research from the other methods previously discussed in this chapter. Because participant observation is a key strategy in this type of research, gaining access to a group, particularly if it is one to which the researcher is not attached, has unique challenges. Gaining access to a particular group often requires that the researcher go through a *gatekeeper*. This is a person who facilitates the entry of the researcher into the particular group being studied. For example, if a Caucasian researcher wished to study the culture of a particular tribe of Native Americans, the researcher might first need to identify a person from that tribe who would invite him to be a participant observer because it is highly unlikely that the researcher would gain access without assistance. The gatekeeper is generally a person with some authority in the group.

When obtaining information from key informants, the researcher is striving to discover the *emic* perspective, or the informant's perspective (i.e., the "inside" scoop; Boyle, 1994). Conversely, the researcher has an *etic*, or outside, perspective. In ethnography, discovering the emic perspective is essential. The researcher needs to record and observe both what key informants say and what they do, looking for consistencies or inconsistencies between these perspectives.

Data Collection and Management

Researchers using ethnographic methods study people in their natural environments over long periods of time to gain a comprehensive view of their culture (Leininger, 1995). There is direct personal involvement with the study of participants over time, usually several months to years (Boyle, 1994). This method takes prolonged engagement and patience. Along with participant observation, the researcher will conduct in-depth interviews with key informants. As with any method using interviews, the skill of the researcher will largely influence the quality and credibility of the results. Interviews should begin with open-ended questions to allow the informant to provide as much information as possible, keeping in mind the grand tour question, or the major question that the researcher is trying to answer. Spradley (1979) believed that the ethnographic interview should be like sharing a friendly conversation. He identified three important elements to the interview: 1) explicit purpose, 2) ethnographic explanations, and 3) ethnographic questions. First, the researcher must make the purpose of the interview perfectly clear and gradually take the lead in directing the questions and conversations to discover the knowledge of the informant. The researcher must also give repeated explanations to the informant throughout interviews about information that needs to be obtained. The informant may need to be reminded to speak from his own perspective and not "translate" for the researcher. Interviews are usually conducted over weeks during numerous encounters so that the researcher can gradually guide the informant toward providing relevant information. Spradley listed more than 30 kinds of ethnographic questions that could be used during an interview (see **Table 8-3**). Easygoing conversation should be interspersed with questions that the researcher wishes to have answered. One can see from this style of interviewing that the researcher needs to gain skill through practice and experience to be able to conduct such interviews effectively. **Table 8-4** summarizes some key points for ethnographic interviewing. In this method, as with many others, keeping detailed field notes is essential along with in-depth ethnographic interviews. The researcher should also collect artifacts or symbols of the culture, employ maps and diagrams, and obtain family trees and the like to help understand the culture. The importance of language cannot be overemphasized. Words convey various meanings in context, so the meanings of words and the situations in which they are used is essential to record and understand. Body language, vocal inflection, and tone in the context of the

TABLE 8-3 Examples of Ethnographic Questions

Type of Questions	Focus	Example
Descriptive	Sample of language	Could you describe a typical day at the mill?
Structural	How participants organize	What are all the activities you do at the mill?
Contrast	For a participant to	You mentioned earlier that ____ is a habit that only a "millrat" does. Would a ____ do that? Would ____ do that? Who wouldn't do that?

Source: Adapted from Spradley, 1979.

TABLE 8-4 Suggestions for Ethnographic Interviewing

- Explain the purpose of the interview clearly.
- Obtain informed consent and assure confidentiality and anonymity.
- Gain entry into the culture through a gatekeeper.
- Identify key informants.
- Develop a rapport with the participants.
- Practice and study techniques related to ethnographic interviewing.
- Allow sufficient time for prolonged engagement to observe and participate in the culture.
- Keep detailed field notes, records, and reflective journals.
- Collect significant artifacts.
- Keep in mind the "grand tour question."
- When interviewing, begin with open-ended questions and progress to more focused questions over time and in repeated interviews.
- Be sure all equipment is working and that you have a plan for malfunctions of tape recorders, etc.
- Keep interviews conversive and friendly even when trying to elicit specific information.
- Pay special attention to the language of the participants and the use of key words.
- Clarify the meanings of terms using contrast questions.
- Constantly compare and contrast data with each other during the collection process.
- Record all interviews and transcribe them verbatim.
- Be true to the data.

Source: Adapted from Spradley, 1979.

situation should be recorded and analyzed. Slang or jargon should be noted and explored.

As with grounded theory, the constant comparison method is often used so that data collection and data analysis may occur somewhat simultaneously. Thick descriptions are used in each area of data collection. The researcher may log an example of a typical day within the group, focus on specific unique events, or develop a story with a plot and characters (Leedy & Ormrod, 2001). Several logs or journals may be kept to organize data and observations.

The data are coded and grouped according to their meanings. Patterns and categories are identified. When presenting the findings, the researcher often uses a more personal reporting style. Researchers must strive to have objectivity when analyzing and interpreting the data. Bias can occur as a result of the closeness that the researcher typically gains with the culture when living among the people. The ultimate goal is to present a detailed picture of a culture that an outsider could read to obtain a better understanding and gain empathy for a specific group. Ethnographic research is an excellent way to increase sensitivity to those whose culture is different from our own.

Examples of Nursing Research Using This Method

Nurses have used ethnography in many unique ways to understand cultures related to health or the health practices of other cultures (Roper & Shapira, 2000). For example, Rosenbaum (1990) used Leininger's theory of culture care as a framework to uncover the cultural care needed for older Greek Canadian widows. The sample contained 12 key informants and 30 general informants, and the researcher collected data using participant observation and interviews. Rosenbaum found that for these widows, health meant a state of well-being, ability to perform activities in their role, and avoidance of pain and illness. These findings could stimulate future nursing interventions for EBP related to caring for widows in this culture and perhaps others. Pasco, Morse, and Olson (2004) used a focused ethnography to study the relationships among nurses and Filipino Canadian patients. Their sample consisted of 23 Filipino Canadian patients, and they obtained data from interviews, field notes, and diaries. The researchers discovered that for nurses to communicate with and care effectively for patients of this cultural background, they needed to understand the languages of "words, gaze, touch, and food and their levels of interaction" (p. 239). This study is a good example of how research is required to gain the knowledge and insight necessary to provide culturally competent care to a unique group of patients. It demonstrates how ethnography is a useful and preferable method of discovering the emic perspective to enhance care provided.

Kayser-Jones (2002) used ethnography to investigate the end-of-life care that was provided to people who were dying in nursing homes. The researchers found that "lack of attention to cultural needs, cognitive status, inadequate staffing, and inappropriate and inadequate communication between health care providers and nursing home residents and their families were the predominant factors that influenced the experience of dying" (p. 11). Findings show that an increased focus needs to be given to people in long-term care facilities who cannot speak for themselves regarding their end-of-life care decisions.

Another example of nurses using ethnography is a study by Shambley-Ebron and Boyle (2006) that explored self-care and mothering in African American women with HIV/AIDS. The researchers studied 10 African American mothers and found themes related to disabling relationships, strong mothering, and redefining self-care, with a cultural theme of creating a life of meaning. The researchers concluded that their study pointed out the strengths of African American women and helped to generate theory that will promote better care for this population.

Street (1992) conducted a study that became a book entitled *Inside Nursing: A Critical Ethnography of Clinical Nursing Practice*. She studied nurses and the culture of nursing at a large hospital in Australia. Street's background was social theory and feminism rather than nursing. Nonetheless, her work provided great insight into the politics, power struggles, and frustrations reported by nurses that challenged the traditional view of nursing at the time.

These studies demonstrate that culture does not have to be merely defined in terms of one's ethnic group, but that culture embodies the feelings, beliefs, attitudes, values, and behaviors of a group of people and can be conducted on a variety of topics in different settings. Today's nurse researchers "would be well-served by describing specific cultural patterns in order to develop targeted interventions to best meet increasingly diverse patient needs" (Oliffe, 2005, p. 397).

Historical Research: Learning from the Past

Historical research is based on documentation of sources that are used to retrospectively examine events or people. The questions being asked are: Who are we? Where did we come from? Why did we do this? How did we get to this point? The goal of this type of research is to explain and understand the past with the hope of guiding the present and future.

Method

KEY TERM

Strategic sampling: Sampling in historical research to locate a small group of either witnesses or participants to the phenomenon

One unique type of sampling used in this method is called *strategic sampling*. This is when the researcher locates a small group of people who were either witnesses or participants to the phenomenon being studied. In such a sample, there are often no restrictions as to age or gender except as delineated by the phenomenon being studied. There is no set sample size, but an accumulation of facts continues until no new data are obtainable. For example, Harmon (2005) studied nursing in a state hospital between 1950 and 1965. This researcher used oral history methods to describe the experiences of eight American nurses who worked in psychiatric hospitals before and during the introduction of antipsychotic medications.

Data Collection and Management

The major sources of data in historical research are eyewitness accounts and documentation. Although interviews with participants are possible, they would be reflecting on past events, and data are based on their recollections. A common criticism of the method is that data may not always be reliable because data are based on the memories of the participants. Accurate and detailed documentation on the part of the researcher is needed to maximize credibility. Some of the documentation sources that nurses might use in historical research include government reports, professional journals, oral evidence, books, memos, photographs, letters, newsletters, newspapers, diaries, journals, videos, films, official publications, written responses to surveys, and memorabilia. After the researcher has obtained all sources of data, including the verbatim transcription of personal accounts or oral histories, central themes are identified from "disciplined reflection" (Galvin et al., 2005, p. 3). The analysis and interpretation should be logical and easy to follow, flowing smoothly from the data. Most historical research tells a story of events over time. The usefulness to nursing lies in allowing the past to illuminate and positively influence the future. The following examples of historical research in nursing provide thought-provoking ways for nursing to examine the evidence on which we base our practice.

Examples of Nursing Research Using This Method

Lusk (2005), one of the proponents of nurses using historical research, used this method to study nurses who cared for patients with cancer between 1920 and 1950. She used primary sources from U.S. archives, nursing procedure books, annual reports, and even minutes from meetings. Her secondary sources included textbooks and journal articles. Lusk chronicled the development of cancer as a specialty in nursing and revealed the discomfort nurses experienced when hiding a cancer diagnosis from patients. Kirby (2004) used oral evidence and documents to provide a historical perspective of nurse researchers. By exploring the difficulties of pioneer nurse researchers, she showed that they developed formal and informal support networks. Kirby suggests that nurse researchers of today could learn from these early scientists.

Hunter (2005) examined nursing and care for the elderly in Victoria, Australia, during the 1950s to 1970s. Her research pointed out the possibilities that

CRITICAL THINKING EXERCISE 8-2

Consider a time when you may have been exposed to a new culture. What were the emic perspectives? How did these compare to your etic perspectives?

existed to improve care for the elderly but that were never realized by nursing. Changes in the law were made that allowed the care of sick elderly individuals to come under the auspices of nursing practice rather than medicine. However, nursing leadership did not take advantage of these legal changes. Nurses missed the opportunity to become leaders in geriatrics because they failed to adopt new behaviors made possible by the change in the law. Hunter's aim was to raise questions for further research rather than to explain why nurses failed to act. This research shows how identifying past behavior can be used as a basis to inform decisions about nursing practice in the present and future.

TEST YOUR KNOWLEDGE 8-2

1. Which method would you choose to answer the question, what process do older adults use when they quit smoking?

    a. ethnography

    b. historical

    c. phenomenology

    d. grounded theory

2. Match the following terms with one of the four types of qualitative methods

    a. constant comparison

    b. strategic sampling

    c. lived experience

    d. emic

How did you do? 1. d; 2. a. grounded theory, b. historical, c. phenomenology, d. ethnography

8.3   Keeping It Ethical

At the end of this section, you will be able to:

‹ Discuss ethical considerations that are unique to qualitative methods

Qualitative researchers are held to the same ethical standards as researchers using other methods. Participants have the same rights as individuals who volunteer for research involving quantitative measures. Researchers must provide informed consent, protect confidentiality, allow volunteers to withdraw from the study at any time, and avoid harm to individuals who participate. Because of their noninvasive nature, most qualitative studies qualify for exempt status from the IRB.

There are, however, some ethical considerations that are unique to qualitative research. These considerations fall into two major categories: those that have to do with the relationship between the researcher and participant and those that involve procedures to handle the data.

When conducting qualitative research, the researcher spends a prolonged time in contact with participants, and relationships are formed. It is not uncommon for researchers and participants to move from a formal (stranger) relationship to one that is more personal (friend) (Leininger, 1985; 1995). For example, a participant may share information in the context of a friendship, never expecting it to be study data. Other consequences of prolonged engagement may include the difficulty of assuring ongoing informed consent or allowing a participant to withdraw from the study if indicated. Another dilemma can occur when the subject matter is emotional for participants. They may become upset and begin to cry during an interview while sharing their experiences. When this occurs, the appropriate response for the researcher is to ask if the tape recorder should be turned off until the participant regains composure. Researchers must examine the appropriateness of responding with

 FYI

Some ethical considerations are unique to qualitative research. These fall into two major categories: the relationship between the researcher and participant and the procedures to handle the data.

CRITICAL THINKING EXERCISE 8-3

Review Table 8–2. Devise one research question for each of the four methods that could be answered by appropriately applying phenomenological, grounded theory, ethnographic, or historical research.

TABLE 8-5 Ethical Principles for Consideration With Participants

Protect the participants' rights and interests.
Put participants' interests first.
Clearly communicate the goals of the research.
Obtain informed consent.
Ensure privacy.
Avoid exploitation.
Share results and reports.
Source: Adapted from Spradley, 1980.

therapeutic use of self versus maintaining the role of researcher. In addition, researchers must avoid taking advantage of a friendship. For example, the researcher may be tempted to prolong the length of an interview past the agreed-upon time or to ask for a second interview when this was not included in the original plan. Researchers are obligated to report suspicions of abuse, neglect, or criminal activity if this is revealed. Therefore, it is essential that the consent form indicates to participants that this is the case. Spradley (1979) lists ethical principles that must be considered when working with participants. These are summarized in **Table 8-5**. There are some important strategies that must be

TEST YOUR KNOWLEDGE 8-3

Indicate if the following statements are true or false:

1. Qualitative researchers do not have to adhere to the usual protection of human subjects because most studies are noninvasive.

2. Qualitative findings must be shared with participants.

3. When a nurse researcher suspects abuse, it is unethical to report it because this information was obtained during a research interview.

4. Fictitious names should be used when transcribing data so that actual participants remain unknown to others.

How did you do? 1. F; 2. T; 3. F; 4. T

implemented when handling qualitative data to safeguard participants' rights. When audiotapes are transcribed, all identifying information such as name, address, place of employment, and phone numbers must be replaced with fictitious information. Participants are often assigned gender-appropriate code names that progress alphabetically. Audio- and videotapes must be treated as confidential and kept secured until the conclusion of the study when they are destroyed. If a participant withdraws from the study, the researcher may still use the data, provided that the participant agrees to this. A unique feature of qualitative research is that sharing findings with participants is expected as part of the research process. It is appropriate to share categories, themes, and theories with participants; however, transcripts, audio- and videotapes, and participant names must never be shared.

RAPID REVIEW

Qualitative research focuses on words instead of numbers to give meaning to a phenomenon or events.

Qualitative research uses induction to inquire about topics with little evidence and/or to develop a theory.

Individuals who volunteer for qualitative studies are known as participants. Purposive sampling is used to obtain a sample.

Sampling continues until data saturation is achieved. Typically, sample sizes are small in qualitative studies.

The three main sources of data in qualitative research are in-depth interviews, direct observation, and artifacts.

Data come from fieldwork and can involve participant observation.

Analysis and interpretation are conducted simultaneously with data collection.

The four essential elements of evaluation are credibility, transferability, dependability, and confirmability.

Strategies to maintain scientific rigor include bracketing, persistent observation, peer debriefing, referential adequacy, member checks, and audit trails.

The four major types of qualitative research are phenomenology, grounded theory, ethnography, and historical.

APPLY WHAT YOU HAVE LEARNED

The committee has found one qualitative study about medication errors. Read Schwappach, Hochreutener, and Wernli (2010) and enter information into the first two columns and complete the design column of the grid on the companion website as you have done previously for other articles. As you complete this exercise, consider if the following were consistent with what you learned in the chapter:

< Sampling method and size
< Data collection methods
< Analysis and interpretation
< Strategies used to maintain scientific rigor
< Ethical considerations

⚡ Phenomenology describes the lived experience and has provided the foundation for some nursing theories.

⚡ Grounded theory uses constant comparison to create theories about processes.

⚡ Ethnography is the method of choice when studying a culture. Ethnoscience and ethnonursing are methods used to study cultural interpretations of nursing phenomena such as care, health, and environment.

⚡ The emic perspective provides the "inside" scoop while the etic perspective is the outsider's viewpoint.

⚡ Historical research examines past events or people with the purpose of guiding the present and future. Strategic sampling can be used to obtain participants.

⚡ Findings from qualitative studies contribute to EBP by sensitizing nurses to patient experiences and providing theories to explain various processes.

⚡ Qualitative researchers are held to the same ethical standards as researchers using other methods; however, there are some unique ethical considerations associated with qualitative methods.

REFERENCES

Benner, P. (1984). *From novice to expert: Excellence and power in clinical nursing practice.* Menlo Park, CA: Addison-Wesley.

Boyle, J. S. (1994). Styles of ethnography. In J. M. Morse (Ed.), *Critical issues in qualitative research methods*. Thousand Oaks, CA: Sage.

Easton, K. L. (1999a). Using focus groups in rehabilitation nursing. *Rehabilitation Nursing, 24*, 212–215.

Easton, K. L. (1999b). The post-stroke journey: From agonizing to owning. *Geriatric Nursing, 20*(2), 70–75.

Easton, K. L., McComish, J., & Greenberg, R. (2000). The pitfalls of qualitative data collection and transcription. *Qualitative Health Research, 10*(5), 703–707.

Folden, S. L. (1994). Managing the effects of a stroke. *Rehabilitation Nursing Research, 3*(3), 79–85.

Galvin, K., Todres, L., & Richardson, M. (2005). The intimate mediator: A carer's experience of Alzheimer's. *Scandinavian Journal of Caring Science, 19*, 2–11.

Glaser, B. G. (1978). *Theoretical sensitivity: Advances in the methodology of grounded theory*. Mill Valley, CA: Sociology Press.

Glaser, B. G. (1992). *Emergence vs. forcing: Basics of grounded theory analysis*. Mill Valley, CA: Sociology Press.

Glaser, B. G., & Strauss, A. L. (1967). *The discovery of grounded theory*. Chicago: Aldine.

Harmon, R. B. (2005). Nursing care in a state hospital before and during the introduction of antipsychotics, 1950–1965. *Issues in Mental Health Nursing, 26*, 257–279.

Hughes, C. C. (1992). Ethnography: What's in a word—Process? Product? Promise? *Qualitative Health Research, 4*, 439–450.

Hunter, C. (2005). Nursing and care for the aged in Victoria: 1950s to 1970s. *Nursing Inquiry, 12*, 278–286.

Kayser-Jones, J. (2002). The experience of dying: An ethnographic nursing home study. *The Gerontologist, 42* (Special Issue III), 11–19.

Kirby, S. (2004). A historical perspective on the contrasting experiences of nurses as research subjects and research activists. *International Journal of Nursing Practice, 10*, 272–279.

Leedy, P. D., & Ormrod, J. E. (2001). *Practical research: Planning and design*. Upper Saddle River, NJ: Merrill Prentice Hall.

Leininger, M. M. (1985). Ethnography and ethnonursing: Models and modes of qualitative data analysis. In M. M. Leininger (Ed.), *Qualitative methods in nursing* (pp. 33–71). New York: Grune & Stratton.

Leininger, M. M. (1995). *Transcultural nursing: Concepts, theories, and practice*. Columbus, OH: McGraw-Hill College Custom Series.

Lincoln, Y. S., & Guba, E. G. (1985). *Naturalistic inquiry*. Newbury Park, CA: Sage.

Lusk, B. (2005). Prelude to specialization: U.S. cancer nursing, 1920–1950. *Nursing Inquiry, 12*(40), 269–277.

Marshall, C., & Rossman, G. B. (1995). *Designing qualitative research.* Thousand Oaks, CA: Sage.

Mauk, K. L. (2001). *The post-stroke journey: From agonizing to owning.* Unpublished doctoral dissertation, Wayne State University, Detroit, MI.

Mauk, K. L. (2006). Nursing interventions within the Mauk model for post-stroke recovery. *Rehabilitation Nursing, 31*, 259–267.

Oliffe, J. (2005). Why not ethnography? *Urologic Nursing, 25*, 395–399.

Parse, R. R. (1991). Parse's theory of human becoming. In I. E. Goertzen (Ed.), *Differentiating nursing practice: Into the twenty-first century* (pp. 51–53). Kansas City, MO: American Academy of Nursing.

Pasco, A. C. Y., Morse, J. M., & Olson, J. K. (2004). Cross-cultural relationships between nurses and Filipino Canadian patients. *Journal of Nursing Scholarship, 36*, 239–246.

Patton, M. Q. (1990). *Qualitative evaluations and research methods.* Newbury Park, CA: Sage.

Patton, M. Q. (2003). *Qualitative evaluation checklist.* Retrieved October 25, 2010, from http://citeseerx.ist.psu.edu/viewdoc/summary?doi=10.1.1.135.8668

Roper, J. M., & Shapira, J. (2000). *Ethnography in nursing research.* Thousand Oaks, CA: Sage.

Rosenbaum, J. N. (1990). Cultural care of older Greek Canadian widows within Leininger's theory of culture care. *Journal of Transcultural Nursing, 2*(1), 37–47.

Schwappach, D. L. B., Hochreutener, M. A., & Wernli, M. (2010). Oncology nurses' perceptions about involving patients in the prevention of chemotherapy administration errors. *Oncology Nursing Forum, 37*, E84–E91.

Shambley-Ebron, D. Z., & Boyle, J. S. (2006). Self-care and mothering in African American women with HIV/AIDS. *Western Journal of Nursing Research, 28*(1), 42–69.

Spradley, J. P. (1979). *The ethnographic interview.* Orlando, FL: Harcourt, Brace, Jovanovich College Publishers.

Spradley, J. P. (1980). *Participant observation.* Orlando, FL: Harcourt, Brace, Jovanovich College Publishers.

Strauss, A., & Corbin, J. (1990). *Basics of qualitative research: Grounded theory procedures and techniques.* Newbury Park, CA: Sage.

Street, A. (1992). *Inside nursing: A critical ethnography of clinical nursing practice.* Albany, NY: University of New York Press.

Su, T. J., & Chen, Y. C. (2006). Transforming hope: The lived experience of infertile women who terminated treatment after in vitro fertilization failure. *Journal of Nursing Research, 14*(1), 46–54.

Watson, J. (1989). Watson's philosophy and theory of human caring in nursing. In J. Riehl-Sisca (Ed.), *Conceptual models for nursing practice* (3rd ed., pp. 219–236). Norwalk, CT: Appleton & Lange.

Welch, A. Z. (2002). Madeleine Leininger: Culture care: Diversity and universality theory. In A. M. Tomey & M. R. Alligood (Eds.), *Nursing theorists and their work* (pp. 501–526). St. Louis, MO: Mosby.

www

At the end of this chapter, you will be able to:

< Identify factors that should be considered when planning for data collection

< Discuss reasons for piloting data collection

< Describe various methods to measure and collect quantitative data

< Discuss advantages and disadvantages to data collection methods

< Identify levels of measurement

< Examine strategies used to address issues associated with quantitative data collection methods

< Identify types of random and systematic measurement errors

< Define validity and reliability

< Name strategies that researchers use to establish reliability and validity of various measures

< Recognize questions used to appraise quantitative data collection methods

< Identify the researcher as the most important data collection instrument

< Describe various methods used to collect qualitative data

< Discuss the advantages and disadvantages of qualitative data collection methods

< Recognize questions used to appraise qualitative data collection methods

< Discuss the importance of protecting human subjects during data collection

alternate form
case studies
categorical data
concurrent validity
construct validity
content validity
continuous data
convergent testing
correlation coefficient
criterion-related validity
Cronbach's alpha
dichotomous
direct observations
divergent testing
equivalence
face validity
factor analysis
focus groups

hypothesis testing
internal consistency
interrater reliability
interval
interviews
item to total correlation
known group testing
Kuder-Richardson
    coefficient
levels of measurement
Likert scales
measurement error
methodological
multitrait-multimethod
    testing
nominal
observation
ordinal

parallel form
physiological measures
predictive validity
psychometrics
questionnaires
random error
ratio
reliability
scales
split-half reliability
stability
systematic error
test-retest reliability
unstructured observations
validity
visual analog scale

CHAPTER 9

Collecting Evidence

Jan Dougherty

9.1 Data Collection: Planning and Piloting

At the end of this section, you will be able to:

< Identify factors that should be considered when planning for data collection
< Discuss reasons for piloting data collection

Data collection is a key component in all research studies. Just as it is essential to use a theoretical or conceptual model to ask the important research questions, there must be a solid plan for collecting and managing the data to study and ultimately to answer research questions. Many nurses may be intimidated as they read the methods section of a research article. Words describing study designs, such as double-blind, quasi-experimental, and ethnography can be overwhelming for those with limited research background. Additionally, terms discussing reliability, validity, and level of significance may further intimidate or overwhelm nurses (Schmelzer, 2000). Many readers may be tempted to skim this information or to bypass it completely. However, because practice decisions will be made based on the findings of the data, it is important for nurses to be able to understand and critically evaluate methods used by researchers. Accurate data collection methods are more likely to yield valid findings. These findings will provide or support the evidence that can be trusted by nurses when making evidence-based practice (EBP) decisions. In EBP, quantitative studies are considered to produce the strongest evidence. Yet, in health care, many clinical and cultural phenomena are better studied using qualitative research. Many nursing and health research studies draw upon both quantitative and qualitative measures. In both types of methods, it is imperative that the same rigor be employed when collecting data.

Planning for Data Collection

Researchers are often very excited to begin collecting data. Most often they have spent months working on their overall framework and/or research questions and have organized pertinent literature to further support the study at hand. They have also carefully selected and developed data collection methods. This requires that researchers detail the data collection plan from the time consent is obtained from subjects to the actual completion of the data collection period. A timeline should be included along with a comprehensive budget that accounts for costs such as salaries of research staff, mileage, meals, data collection materials and instrumentation, fees related to the recruitment of subjects, and data input and interpretation. A plan for how data will be managed should also be included. A haphazard approach to collecting data, planning the timeline and budget, and managing data can lead to serious problems for researchers. Therefore, when appraising research studies, it is important for nurses to carefully read and determine if the data collection methods support the framework and are appropriate for the study questions. If appropriate data collection methods are not used, the findings can easily be challenged and the evidence may not support the desired changes in practice (Havens, 2001).

Researchers begin by determining the type of data that need to be collected. This includes when and how data will be collected, who will collect the data, and what type of data collection methods or instruments will be used. There are many factors that affect data collection. Such factors may include availability and access to preexisting instruments or data collection sites, personnel needed to collect data, the amount of data to be collected, and the sample size. Budget considerations are key because researchers are accountable to stay within the planned budget. Data collection can be one of the most costly parts of conducting a research project.

Piloting Data Collection Methods

Many researchers will conduct a pilot study using a scaled-back version of the data collection method. This is very helpful to evaluate the instruments and process so that unexpected problems can be identified. Additionally, a pilot study helps confirm the study's feasibility and allows for revisions to be made. Researchers do not want to get midway into projects only to find that the instruments are flawed, the projected sample size is unachievable, there is a need for additional research assistants, or the study cannot be completed within the budget. All of these issues can cause serious problems and ultimately jeopardize the study.

TEST YOUR KNOWLEDGE 9-1

1. Factors to consider when planning data collection include which of the following?
   a. time frame
   b. budget
   c. training of personnel
   d. availability of preprinted questionnaires

2. A pilot:
   a. is a small version of the study
   b. confirms feasibility of the study
   c. critiques the conclusions from a study
   d. is the small stipend that subjects receive for participating in a study

How did you do? 1. a, b, c, d; 2. a, b

9.2   Collecting Quantitative Data

At the end of this section, you will be able to:

< Describe various methods to measure and collect quantitative data
< Discuss advantages and disadvantages to data collection methods
< Identify levels of measurement
< Examine strategies used to address issues associated with quantitative data collection methods

Collecting Numbers

Quantitative methods are used to test stated hypotheses and call for researchers to use formal, objective, and systematic procedures and instruments that produce numerical data (Havens, 2001). Data from quantitative studies are the highest level of evidence on which clinicians can base EBP decisions. For example, studies involving meta-analyses of multiple randomized controlled trials are considered to be the strongest level of evidence while those based on case reports and opinions of experts and authorities are considered to be the lowest level of evidence (Myers & Meccariello, 2006). In quantitative studies, research questions and hypotheses are derived from theories. The study design reflects the objectives of the study. Researchers must decide how each variable will be operationalized and what types of data will need to be gathered. The main methods used in quantitative research include *questionnaires*, *observation*, *scales*, and *physiological measures*. Table 9-1 provides an overview of data collection methods that are associated with various quantitative research designs.

Questionnaires

Questionnaires are commonly used in quantitative research and can provide an inexpensive way to gather numerical data from a potentially large number of respondents. Although questionnaires may be inexpensive to administer, when compared to other data collection methods, they can be expensive in terms of design time and interpretation. It is essential that each question is monitored for clarity, sensitivity to the respondent, reading level, and absence of bias (Havens, 2001).

The formatting and length of the questionnaire is an important detail. The questionnaire should include only essential questions because shorter questionnaires are more likely to be completed. Whenever possible, the questions

KEY TERMS

Questionnaires: Printed instruments used to gather numerical data

Observation: A technique to gather data

Scales: Used to assign a numeric value or score a continuum

Physiological measures: Data obtained from biological, chemical, and microbiological phenomena

TABLE 9-1 Quantitative Research Designs and Data Collection Methods

Quantitative Research Design	Data Collection Method
Exploratory/Descriptive (answers what questions; describes frequency of occurrence)	Questionnaire Scales
Correlational (examines relationships among variables)	Questionnaire Scales Biophysiological
Quasi-experimental (examines why certain effects occur)	Questionnaire Scales Biophysiological
Experimental/Clinical Trial (examines causes of certain effects)	Questionnaire Scales Biophysiological

---

FIGURE 9-1   **Example of Easy, Consistent Survey Design**

1. Nursing research is interesting to me.   Yes ____   No____

2. I have to study a lot in my nursing research course.   Yes ____   No____

3. I understand how evidence can be used to improve practice.   Yes ____   No____

---

using numbered answers should be either circled or checked and should use a consistent pattern throughout (**Figure 9-1**). There should be a balance among positive and negative questions to decrease biased responses in subjects (Merchant & Mateo, 1993). Each research subject is assigned a research identification number that should be on each page of the questionnaire in case the pages get separated.

Questionnaires can be administered in person, via mail, and increasingly via e-mail. Confidentiality is necessary to ensure that respondents not only participate in the study but also answer questions honestly and without fear of reprisal. It is desirable to have a good response rate, which is the percentage of questionnaires that are returned. Low response rates can lead to bias because samples may not be representative. A variety of factors can influence if subjects complete a questionnaire. Not all subjects are able to respond to questionnaires. For example, young children, the blind, and many frail or cognitively impaired elders may have difficulty completing questionnaires. Questionnaires that are long, hard to understand, or time consuming are not likely to be completed. Using appropriate colors, fonts, and white space can improve the likelihood that individuals will complete a questionnaire.

Observation

Structured observations provide a way to quantify an explicit feature of the phenomenon under observation. For example, a researcher could count the number of people who wash their hands after using a public restroom. Researchers serve as objective observers and follow systematic methods using specific directions during a scheduled period of time. In the hand washing example, the researcher may observe individuals during dinner time at a popular restaurant. Not only do researchers outline what observations are made, but they also note how observations are recorded and coded. The researcher in this example may record tallies under three columns: no hand washing, water only, or soap and water. Establishing a detailed protocol is extremely important if researchers use research assistants.

FIGURE 9-2   Example of Likert-type Scale

When several Likert scales are used in a questionnaire, the positive numbers or indicators should consistently be in the same position, for example 1 = strongly disagree, 2 = disagree, 3 = neutral, 4 = agree, 5 = strongly agree.

Scales

Scales are used to assign a numeric value or score along a continuum. They are frequently incorporated into a questionnaire or interview. Numerous types of scales have been developed to measure social and psychological concepts specific to nursing. Researchers choose scales based on the ability to measure identified concepts. Ideally, it is best to choose scales that have already been tested. If a scale does not exist, researchers can develop and test a new scale (Havens, 2001). Scales can be designed to measure either a single or multidimensional concept. For example, the Marwit-Meuser Caregiver Grief Inventory is a 50-item multidimensional scale that measures grief reactions by current caregivers of people with progressive dementias (Marwit & Meuser, 2002). Because there are three subscales that compose the total grief score, it is a multidimensional scale. Each subscale measures a specific part of the caregiving experience as detailed in the Caregiver Grief Model (Meuser & Marwit, 2001).

You may already be familiar with *Likert scales*, which are frequently used to collect data. The scale consists of statements on which respondents indicate whether they agree or disagree on a continuum of seven points. Seven points allows for a neutral opinion. Some researchers find a neutral response hard to interpret. Therefore, researchers may adapt the scale to eliminate the neutral point by having an even number of points. Scales containing fewer than seven points are known as Likert–type scales (see **Figure 9-2**).

Another type of scale is the *visual analog scale* (VAS) (see **Figure 9-3**). Researchers use this type of scale to measure the intensity of sensations and

FIGURE 9-3 Example of a VAS to Measure Pain

Line length = 100 mm

No Pain   Worst Pain

CRITICAL THINKING EXERCISE 9-1

A nurse researcher is interested in testing an intervention on the quality of life of individuals with lung cancer. What methods do you think the nurse researcher should use to collect data?

feelings. The VAS is a 100 mm line that is anchored on each end with words or symbols. Subjects mark a line across the VAS to indicate the intensity of their feelings or attitudes along the continuum represented. In nursing, VAS scales are frequently used to collect data about pain, fatigue, quality of life, and health status. This type of scale can be completed easily and quickly and is understood by most people. To score the VAS, researchers measure the distance of the mark from the end of the scale in millimeters. Usually the low end of the scale is used as the zero point.

Physiological

Physiological measures provide a wide range of biological, chemical, and microbiological data. Measures of blood pressure, cardiac output, and weight are examples of biological variables. Chemical measures include electrolytes, hormones, and cholesterol, while microbiological measures include the bacterial counts obtained from urine and blood cultures. There are many advantages to using these objective measures because they tend to be accurate. Some physiological data are typically accessible in most healthcare settings, allowing for ease of data collection with minimal or no cost to the researcher. Researchers must specify measurement protocols that include specific equipment used for measurement, frequency and methods for calibration of equipment, training for data collectors, specific times to obtain measurements, procedures for measuring and recording data, and any special storage or handling considerations (Merchant & Mateo, 1993).

Issues in Quantitative Data Collection

Regardless of how the data are collected, researchers must consider a variety of issues to ensure a high quality study. They must have a written plan that outlines the process for data collection, particularly when additional data collectors are employed. Research assistants must be trained to collect data in a very consistent manner (i.e., instruments should be administered in the same order for all subjects, in the same context and setting, using the same set of directions). Interrater reliability must also be established when more than one person is involved in making observations. Interrater reliability is the extent to which two or more individual raters agree. While it is necessary for multiple observers or raters to achieve interrater reliability, this may slow the process of observational methods. Interrater reliability should be monitored periodically throughout the study to increase the degree of confidence in the data (Casey, 2006). Researchers may choose to prepare a code book to organize the raw data prior to collection and to assign numerical values to data obtained during data collection. For example, researchers may assign a numerical value of one to females and two to males (Wolf, 2003).

Data collection plans should detail a time frame. It is not uncommon for researchers to encounter unplanned obstacles when gathering data. Frequently data collection requires at least twice as long as the researcher anticipates. Issues such as slow enrollment of consented subjects, heavy workloads, or staff turnover are common causes of delay. Plans should include strategies to manage attrition of subjects as a result of death, dropout, or relocation. Plans also must address decisions about missing data. For example, subjects may fail or refuse to respond to particular questions.

Many studies are funded by federal grants, state grants, or private foundation monies. A budget is necessary to consider all of the factors involved in data collection, including any delays that may be anticipated. Time extensions may be requested by researchers because of delay, and this subsequently requires researchers to account for any changes in budgeting. If the project is cut back as a result of delays or exceeding the budget, the research can be seriously compromised (Anastasi, Capili, Kim, & Chung, 2005).

Levels of Measurement

Measurement is the process of assigning numbers using a set of rules. There are four categories that are used to describe measurements: *nominal*, *ordinal*, *interval*, and *ratio*. These categories are more commonly known as *levels of measurement*. When researchers collect data, they must know which level of measurement is used to select appropriate statistical tests for analyzing data. Nurses must be able to identify levels of measurement correctly to appraise evidence. Nominal measurement is the weakest level of measurement. The word "nominal" is derived from the word "name." Researchers use nominal measurement to classify or categorize variables, also referred to as *categorical data*. The numbers assigned to each category are just labels and do not indicate any value. For example, responses of "yes" and "no" on a survey are often assigned numbers one and two. The value of these numbers has no meaning because one cannot claim that a "no" response is higher than a "yes" response. The arbitrary numbers are assigned for the purpose of coding, recording, and entering data for collection and analysis. Questionnaires will often utilize nominal measures

KEY TERMS

Nominal: The lowest level of measurement whereby data are categorized simply into groups

Ordinal: A continuum of numeric values where the intervals are not meant to be equal

Interval: A continuum of numeric values with equal intervals but lacks an absolute zero

Ratio: Highest level of measurement that involves numeric values that begin with an absolute zero and have equal intervals

Levels of measurement: Classifying measurements according to a hierarchy of measurement and the type of statistical tests that are appropriate

Categorical data: Lowest level of measurement whereby data are categorized simply into groups

FIGURE 9-4   **Examples of Nominal Level Measurement**

Gender: Male = 1;	Female = 2
Race:	African American = 1
	Asian = 2
	Caucasian = 3
	Hispanic = 4
	Native American = 5
	Other = 6
Type of Dementia:	Alzheimer's disease = 1
	Lewy body dementia = 2
	Vascular dementia = 3
	Frontotemporal
	dementia = 4
	Unknown = 5

to record a variety of categorical data and/or closed-ended questions with fixed responses such as gender, race, and diagnosis (see **Figure 9-4**). *Dichotomous* is the term used when there are only two possible fixed responses, such as true or false, yes or no, and male or female. Ordinal measurement represents the second lowest level of measurement. A continuum of numeric values is used with small numbers representing lower levels on the continuum, while larger numbers represent higher values. However, while the values are ordered or ranked, the intervals are not meant to be equal. For example, in a marathon the distance and time among those who finish in first, second, and third is not equal; however, there is value to the number assigned. Many questionnaires and scales use ordinal measurements. **Figure 9-5** provides examples of ordinal measures. Interval measurement is a third level of measurement and uses a continuum of numeric values, also known as *continuous data*. In this level, the values have meaning and the intervals are equal. In interval scales, the zero point is arbitrary and not absolute. The zero is not an indication of the true absence of something. The best example of this is the Celsius scale. When measuring temperature in Celsius, 0 does not mean the absence of temperature. In fact, it is quite cold. Other examples of interval scores include intelligence measures, personality measures, and manual muscle testing.

Continuous data are also collected using ratio measurement, which is the highest level of measurement and uses a continuum of numeric values with

KEY TERMS

Dichotomous: Nominal measurement when only two possible fixed responses exist

Continuous data: Interval or ratio-level data that use a continuum of numeric values with equal intervals

---

FIGURE 9-5 **Examples of Ordinal Level Measurement**

To what extent are you satisfied with the quality of care you received?

Extremely Dissatisfied	Very Dissatisfied	Somewhat Satisfied	Very Satisfied	Extremely Satisfied
1	2	3	4	5

Put the following in order of importance to you. Assign 1 to the most important and 5 to the least important.

_____ Time with family
_____ Satisfaction with work
_____ Income
_____ Health
_____ Personal appearance

---

equal intervals and a zero point that is absolute. Age, weight, height, and income are good examples of this type of measurement. VAS also provide ratio measurement along with many other biochemical and physiological measures.

TEST YOUR KNOWLEDGE 9-2

1. Which of the following are advantages that questionnaires have over interviews?
   a. Take less time to administer
   b. Provide for anonymity
   c. Allow for more in-depth responses
   d. Minimize socially desirable responses

2. Which of the following are physiological measures?
   a. blood pressure
   b. grades on an exam
   c. digoxin levels
   d. mini mental status exam

3. Match the terms
   a. Nominal   1. intake and output measurement
   b. Ordinal   2. pH of urine
   c. Interval   3. type of cancer
   d. Ratio   4. strength of contractions (mild, moderate, strong)

How did you do? 1. a, b, d; 2. a, c; 3. 1, c 2. d 3. b 4. a

9.3   Validity and Reliability

At the end of this section, you will be able to:

< Identify types of random and systematic measurement errors
< Define validity and reliability
< Name strategies that researchers use to establish reliability and validity of various measures
< Recognize questions used to appraise quantitative data collection methods

Measurement Error

While it may seem that creating surveys and instruments is easy, researchers actually spend a significant amount of time designing them. They do this to reduce *measurement error* so that they know the measurements provide a true reflection of the sample characteristics. In any measurement, the goal is for the observed measurement to be as close to the true measurement as possible. The equation $O = T + E$ will help you to understand this concept. O stands for the observed score. This is the actual number or value that is obtained from the instrument regarding the characteristic. T stands for the true score, the actual amount of the characteristic. If $O = T$, there would be a perfect instrument, but this is never the case because error (E) is always present during measurements. Error can be either *random error* or *systematic error*. Random error is error that occurs by chance. It is difficult for researchers to control for random error because it results from transient factors. Random error can be attributed to subject factors, instrumentation variations, or environmental factors. For example, have you ever made the mistake of answering a test question by filling in the wrong bubble? While you knew the correct answer, something occurred that caused a mistake. In this example, the observed score (your test score) indicates that you did not know the content, while your true score would indicate otherwise.

KEY TERMS

Measurement error: The difference between the true score and the observed score

Random error: Error that occurs by chance during measurement

Systematic error: Error that occurs in the same way with each measurement

CRITICAL THINKING EXERCISE 9-2

What if you were to take an exam two times? The first time would be in a comfortable room sitting at a desk in a nice chair. The second time you are expected to stand with a clipboard in a hot, stuffy room. Which observed score is likely to be closer to your true score? Why?

Systematic error occurs when the same kind of error occurs repeatedly. Also known as consistent error, it can result from subject, instrumentation, and environmental factors. For example, a researcher is measuring body temperatures after an intervention. The researcher assumes that the electronic thermometer is measuring accurately; however, the device has not recently been calibrated. Body temperatures are being reported a half degree lower than the actual temperatures. Because every temperature measured is affected, this is systematic error.

If there is error in all measurement, how do researchers know when instruments are useful? Instruments can be tested using a variety of strategies to identify error. Researchers conduct *methodological* studies to test instruments. The nursing literature, as well as literature from other disciplines, contains such reports. Another term, *psychometrics*, is also associated with instrument testing. Psychometrics refers to the development of measures for psychological attributes.

Validity

When selecting an instrument, researchers must first ask themselves if it is valid. *Validity* refers to the degree an instrument measures what it is supposed to measure. A valid instrument reflects the characteristics or concept that is being measured. For example, a researcher might want to measure the amount of fear patients have prior to surgery. The researcher would need to carefully select an instrument that measures fear, and not anxiety, which is a similar but different concept. There are three kinds of validity: *content validity*, *criterion-related validity*, and *construct validity* (**Table 9-2**).

Content validity is established when researchers know that the instrument measures the concept intended to be measured. This requires that researchers clearly define the concept being studied to ensure that the selected instrument fits.

There are two ways researchers test for content validity: *face validity* and content validity. Both methods involve letting others examine the instruments. When researchers try to obtain face validity, they ask colleagues or subjects to examine an instrument and indicate whether the instrument appears to measure the concept. Face validity is less desirable than content validity because face validity uses an intuitive approach. To establish content validity, researchers give an instrument to a panel consisting of experts on the concept. The experts judge the instrument by rating each item for the degree to which it reflects the concept being measured. After researchers receive feedback from the panel, they make adjustments to the instrument. Items that receive high ratings are kept, and items with low ratings are altered or eliminated. For

TABLE 9-2 Validity: Does the Instrument Accurately Measure What It Is Supposed to Measure?

Type	Test	Description
Content Validity: Is the content representative of the content domain under study?	Content Validity	Experts on the topic are asked to judge each item on an instrument by assigning a rating to determine its fit with the concept being measured.
	Face Validity	Colleagues or subjects examine an instrument and are asked whether it appears to measure the concept.
Criterion-Related Validity: To what degree are the "observed score" and the "true score" related?	Concurrent Validity	New instrument is administered at the same time as an instrument known to be valid. Scores of the two instruments are compared. Strong positive correlations indicate good validity.
	Predictive	New instrument is given at two different times and scores are correlated. Strong positive correlations indicate good validity.
Construct Validity: To what extent does it measure the theoretical construct or trait?	Hypothesis Testing	Hypotheses derived from theories are tested with the new instrument.
	Convergent	New instrument is administered at the same time as an instrument known to be valid. Scores of the two instruments are compared. Strong, positive correlations indicate good validity.
	Divergent	New instrument is administered at the same time as an instrument measuring the opposite of the concept. Scores of the two instruments are compared. Strong negative correlations indicate good validity.
	Multitrait-multimethod	New instrument, established instrument of same concept, and established instrument of opposite concept are given at the same time. Strong positive and negative correlations indicate good validity.
	Known Groups	New instrument is administered to individuals known to be high or low on the characteristic being measured.
	Factor Analysis	Statistical approach to identify items that group together.

KEY TERMS

Concurrent validity:
Test for criterion-related validity where a new instrument is administered at the same time as an instrument known to be valid

Predictive validity:
Test for criterion-related validity where a new instrument is given at two different times and scores are correlated

Hypothesis testing: Collection of objectively measurable data that are gathered through the five senses to confirm or refute a hypothesis

Convergent testing:
Test for construct validity in which new instruments are administered at the same time as an instrument known to be valid

Divergent testing:
Test for construct validity in which new instruments are administered at the same time as an instrument measuring the opposite of the concept

example, when Beyer, Denyes, and Villarruel (1992) developed a pediatric photographic pain scale, they asked children, rather than adults, to rank pictures of a child experiencing pain. Children placed the pictures in order from no pain to most pain. Researchers found consensus among children regarding some photographs and eliminated others when children disagreed about the amount of pain being expressed.

Criterion-related validity is concerned with the degree to which the observed score and the true score are related. There are two ways researchers test for criterion-related validity: *concurrent validity* and *predictive validity*. Concurrent validity is tested when researchers simultaneously administer two different instruments measuring the same concept. Usually, the new instrument being developed is compared to an instrument already shown to be valid. Researchers use correlations to compare scores from the two instruments. High correlations indicate agreement between the instruments, while low correlations indicate that the instruments are measuring different concepts. Predictive validity refers to whether a current score is correlated with a score obtained in the future. For example, suppose that a class of sophomore nursing students completed an instrument measuring critical thinking today, and they will complete the instrument again one month from now. If the instrument has good criterion-related validity, their scores will be correlated.

Construct validity focuses on theory. Constructs are theoretical concepts that are tested empirically. When researchers test for construct validity, they are asking how well the instrument measures a theoretical concept. Because establishing construct validity requires empirical testing, more sophisticated strategies implemented over a longer period of time are needed. There are a number of ways to determine construct validity: *hypothesis testing*, *convergent testing*, *divergent testing*, *multitrait-multimethod testing*, *known group testing*, and *factor analysis*.

For hypothesis testing, researchers use theories to make predictions about the concept being measured. Data are gathered, and a determination is made as to whether the findings support the hypothesis. In the study by Beyer et al. (1992), they hypothesized that pain scores would be highest on the day of the surgical procedure and then gradually decrease. They found that scores were highest on the operative day and gradually decreased over the course of the hospital stay. The construct validity of the Oucher, a children's pain scale, was supported because data were consistent with predicted pain patterns.

When researchers use two or more instruments to measure the same theoretical component, they are testing for convergent validity. Convergent validity focuses on how the observed scores compare to one another. For example, Beyer et al. (1992) compared the Oucher to a VAS pain scale. Pain ratings were highly correlated, thus establishing convergent validity. Divergent validity testing involves comparing scores from two or more instruments that measure different theoretical constructs. In this strategy, it is not unusual for researchers to compare opposites, for example, depression and happiness. In this situation, negative correlations support construct validity. When convergent testing and divergent testing are combined, researchers are using a strategy known as multitrait-multimethod. This approach is especially helpful to reduce systematic error.

Another way to test for construct validity is to use the known group approach. Instruments are administered to individuals known to be high or low on the characteristic being measured. Researchers expect that there will be significantly different scores between the high group and the low group. Beyer et al. (1992) tested known groups by comparing pain scores for children who had experienced extensive surgical procedures with pain scores for children who had minor surgical procedures. Children who had spinal fusions reported significantly higher pain scores using the Oucher than children who had a cardiac catheterization.

Most concepts have more than one dimension. These dimensions are known as factors. Researchers use factor analysis, a statistical approach, to identify questions that group around different factors. Thus, items that group together as one factor will have high correlations. These items may or may not highly correlate with items around a different factor. Questions that do not fit are altered or eliminated. Because factor analyses require complex, simultaneous computations of correlations, computers are needed.

Reliability

Instruments are considered to be reliable when researchers obtain consistent measurements over time. *Reliability* must be considered in relation to validity. An instrument can be reliable but not valid. If you weighed yourself 10 times in a row on your bathroom scale this morning, you would expect the scale to show the same weight each time. You would conclude that the scale is reliable. If you are anxious about your weight, you cannot conclude that the scale measured your level of anxiety. While the scale is a valid instrument to measure your weight, it is not a valid instrument to measure your anxiety even though the scale was shown to be reliable. Estimates of reliability are usually presented in the form of a *correlation coefficient*, with +1.00 indicating a perfect reliability and 0.00 reflecting the absence of reliability. Typically, reliability coefficients of 0.80 and above are acceptable for well established instruments, while reliability coefficients of 0.70 and above are acceptable for newly developed instruments (Griffin-Sobel, 2003).

KEY TERMS

Multitrait-multimethod testing: Test for construct validity in which a new instrument, established instrument of same concept, and established instrument of opposite concept are given at the same time

Known group testing: Test for construct validity in which new instruments are administered to individuals known to be high or low on the characteristic being measured

Factor analysis: Test for construct validity that is a statistical approach to identify items that group together

Reliability: Obtainment of consistent measurements over time

Correlation coefficient: An estimate that indicates the reliability of an instrument

KEY TERMS

Stability: When instruments render the same scores with repeated measures under the same circumstances

Equivalence: Attribute of reliability where alternate forms of an instrument or alternate raters are in agreement

Internal consistency: Attribute of reliability when all items on an instrument measure the same concept

Test-retest reliability: Test for instrument reliability when new instruments are given at two different times under the same conditions

Parallel form: Test for instrument reliability where new instruments are given in two versions

Alternate form: Test for instrument reliability where new instruments are given in two versions

Interrater reliability: Test for instrument reliability when two observers measure the same event

Split-half reliability: Test for instrument reliability when the items are divided to form two instruments

When testing instruments for reliability, researchers are interested in three attributes: *stability*, *equivalence*, and *internal consistency*. Instruments are stable when the same scores are obtained with repeated measures under the same circumstances (as in the bathroom scale example). An instrument is said to be equivalent when there is agreement between alternate forms or alternate raters. Internal consistency, also known as homogeneity, exists when all items on a questionnaire measure the same concept. There are seven ways commonly used to test instruments for reliability. They are *test-retest reliability*, *parallel* or *alternate form*, *interrater reliability*, *split-half reliability*, *item to total correlation*, *Kuder-Richardson coefficient*, and *Cronbach's alpha* (**Table 9-3**).

Test-retest reliability determines stability by administering the instrument to the same subjects under the same conditions at two different times. Scores are used to calculate a Pearson *r*, a type of correlation coefficient. Parallel or alternate form testing is used to test for both stability and equivalence. Researchers create parallel forms by altering the wording or layout of items. Because the forms are similar, researchers expect high positive correlations. For example, Beyer et al. (1992) compared a pocket-sized Oucher with a poster-sized Oucher and obtained similar pain ratings.

Interrater reliability also tests for equivalence. This method is used when instruments record observations. A common way to determine interrater reliability is to have two observers score the same event. Ratings are compared, and if the ratings are similar, the instrument is considered to have strong reliability. Another way to establish interrater reliability is to have one individual make multiple observations over time.

Sometimes, researchers divide the items on a questionnaire in half to make two versions, a technique known as split-half reliability. Researchers use the Spearman-Brown formula to compare the two halves. Split-half testing is used to establish internal consistency. Item to total calculations are also used to test for internal consistency. Each item on the instrument is compared to the total score obtained. Strong items have high correlations with the total score. Items with low correlations to the total score are examined, and decisions are made to change or eliminate them. When the level of measurement is dichotomous, researchers determine internal consistency using the Kuder-Richardson (K–2R) coefficient. This correlation compares all items at the same time. Cronbach's alpha is the most common method used by nursing researchers to assess internal consistency. This method can be used when data are interval level or higher. Like the Kuder-Richardson, all items are compared simultaneously to obtain a single correlation. Computer software is required to perform these sophisticated tests.

As nurses appraise the methods section of any research article, it is important to consider the issues of validity and reliability (Roberts & Priest, 2006)

TABLE 9-3 **Reliability: Does the Instrument Yield the Same Results on Repeated Measurements?**

Type	What Is Determined?	Description
Test-Retest	Stability	New instrument is given at two different times under the same conditions. Scores are correlated. Strong positive correlations indicate good reliability.
Parallel or Alternate	Stability Equivalence	New instrument is given in two different versions. Scores are correlated. Strong positive correlations indicate good reliability.
Interrater reliability	Equivalence	Two observers measure the same event. Scores are correlated. Strong positive correlations indicate good reliability.
Split-half	Internal consistency	Divide the items to form two instruments. Give both instruments and compare the halves using the Spearman-Brown formula.
Item to total	Internal consistency	Each item is correlated to the total score. Reliable items have strong correlations with the total score.
Kuder-Richardson Coefficient	Internal consistency	Used with dichotomous items. Using a computer, all items are simultaneously compared.
Cronbach's alpha	Internal consistency	Used with interval or ratio items. Using a computer, all items are simultaneously compared.

before making practice decisions. The report should contain information about the validity and reliability of each instrument used. References for the original development of the instruments should be provided. Occasionally researchers include instruments in articles that allow readers to observe how the questions align with the concepts that were being measured.

Appraising Data Collection in Quantitative Studies

When reading the methods section of any research article, nurses should determine that each instrument is described and the reliability and validity are reported. The level of measurement should be noted for each variable measured. Nurses should also appraise if instruments represent the concepts and variables being operationalized. Interventions should be detailed so that nurses

KEY TERMS

Item to total correlation: Test for instrument reliability when each item is correlated to the total score

Kuder-Richardson coefficient: Test for instrument reliability for use with dichotomous items

Cronbach's alpha: A test for instrument reliability used with interval or ratio items

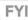 **FYI**

When selecting an instrument, researchers must first ask themselves if it is valid—whether it reflects the characteristics or concept that is being measured. There are three kinds of validity: content validity, criterion-related validity, and construct validity.

TABLE 9-4 **Assessing the Quality of Quantitative Data Collection Methods**

What are the variables being measured?
Does the data collection method fit with the study variables?
What is the intervention?
Is there sufficient detail given about the intervention and the control group?
Was the setting described?
What steps were taken to minimize measurement error?
What instruments are used? Were validity and reliability discussed for each instrument?
Was the level of measurement considered?
Were there any difficulties with enrollment, attrition, or missing data?

know what was done in the research. If a pilot was done prior to the study, its instruments, interventions, and findings should be presented. If subjects are grouped, the author should describe how grouping was accomplished.

Many quantitative studies fall short of significant findings if there are holes in the methods section. If the instruments do not adequately measure the concepts or variables or if they lack validity and reliability, the study may be flawed. **Table 9-4** lists questions that nurses should consider when appraising the methods section.

 TEST YOUR KNOWLEDGE 9-3

True/False

1. Validity is concerned with obtaining accurate and repeatable measures.

2. Content validity is established by having a panel of experts review the instruments.

3. Face validity is the strongest method to establish validity.

4. Equivalence, internal consistency, and stability are tested to ensure instrument reliability.

5. An instrument with a reported Cronbach alpha of .65 has good reliability.

How did you do? 1. F; 2. T; 3. F; 4. T; 5. F

9.4   Collecting Qualitative Data

At the end of this section, you will be able to:

< Identify the researcher as the most important data collection instrument
< Describe various methods used to collect qualitative data
< Discuss the advantages and disadvantages of qualitative data collection methods
< Recognize questions used to appraise qualitative data collection methods

Collecting Words

In recent years, the use of qualitative methods has become more common in health services research, resulting in an increase in publication of these studies in healthcare journals (Devers, Sofaer, & Rundall, 1999). Qualitative researchers collect data that are in-depth and descriptive in order to understand the phenomena being studied. The methods allow participants to express their thoughts and describe their actions and intentions in their own words (Ellett & Beausang, 2001). The researcher is the most important data collection instrument (Masters, Carlson, & Pfadt, 2006). Researchers gather qualitative data through questionnaires, *interviews*, *focus groups*, *case studies*, and *direct observations*. **Table 9-5** lists data collection strategies associated with the four major qualitative methods.

Questionnaires

Questionnaires are frequently used to collect qualitative data from individuals or groups of participants. The questionnaire is typically a list of written questions that can be self-administered. It can also be administered using the Internet or can be read to the participant by the data collector. Questionnaires can use open-ended questions, closed-ended questions, or both. Open-ended questions are used to elicit statements without providing a fixed answer. An example of an open-ended question is, "Tell about your experience as a caregiver for a person with Parkinson's disease." Closed-ended questions offer fixed choices that must be selected. For example, a closed-ended question may ask participants to respond "yes" or "no" to a list of questions. Thoughtful consideration should be given to wording questions in a clear and concise manner. A sufficient number of questions must be included so that accurate descriptions can be obtained. The font size should be large enough for easy reading.

The advantages of questionnaires are that they are usually easy to administer, can provide a wealth of data, and are relatively inexpensive. They can provide anonymity when desired; however, researchers cannot ensure that

TABLE 9-5 **Qualitative Research Methods and Instruments**

Method	Instrument/Tool
Phenomenology	In-depth interviews Diaries Artwork
Grounded Theory	Observations Open-ended question interviews with individuals or small groups
Ethnography	Participant and direct observations Open-ended question interviews Diagrams Documents Photographs
Historical	Open-ended questions Interviews Documents Photographs Artifacts

intended participants actually answered the questions. The sample may be limited to literate participants when individuals are expected to self-administer the questionnaire.

Interviews

The one-on-one nature of interviews makes them more personal than self-administered questionnaires, and researchers are able to probe more deeply with follow-up questions. Interviews can be conducted in person or over the telephone. Structured interviews emphasize obtaining answers based on carefully predetermined questions. For some qualitative methods, an in-depth interview guide is used that does not follow this structured form. Rather, a general or "grand tour" question is asked, and a dialogue between the researcher and the participant unfolds leading to more detailed information. Interviews are frequently tape recorded so they can be transcribed word for word at a later date. Researchers must take care to minimize distractions and interruptions to allow participants to focus on the topic. While interviews provide the opportunity to clarify questions and answers, they are more expensive and take more time to conduct than questionnaires. Because anonymity is impossible to achieve, participants may be inclined to answer in socially desirable ways. Face-to-face interviews provide an opportunity for researchers to assess nonverbal communication and the context in which the interview occurs. Self-reported data, whether obtained from questionnaires or interviews, provide a rich source of information. Additionally, response rates are generally high for participants who are willing to express their opinions.

Focus Groups

Focus groups are small groups comprised of usually less than 12 participants (Beyea & Nicoll, 2000). Participants are brought together to explore attitudes and thoughts about a particular subject. Through group interaction, insights are often gained that may not have emerged through individual interviews. When focus groups are used, researchers must identify and define the objectives of the focus group. A facilitator guides the group process by stating ground rules, objectives, and questions. This role is essential to keep participants comfortable and the group process flowing and on track. Facilitators must be skilled at involving all participants and ensuring that the conversation is not monopolized by one or two individuals. It is recommended that the researcher not be the facilitator of the group but rather an observer who can listen, take notes, and ask specific follow-up questions.

Focus group participants must represent the intended population identified by the researcher. There should be an adequate number of participants represented because they are not randomly selected. They should be notified in advance regarding the date, time, and location of the focus group. Focus group sessions are usually audiotaped and involve a note taker. Approximately 60 to 90 minutes are given to ask no more than 10 structured questions. Following the session, the data are transcribed and analyzed to look for trends and patterns.

There are both advantages and disadvantages to using focus groups. This data collection method is an economical way to bring participants together to gather information. Often participants selected for focus groups are pleased to offer their answers, opinions, and insights about the objectives identified for the group. However, participants must feel secure about the topic. For example, a researcher investigating the attitudes of nurses about employment practices may be wise to put nursing managers in separate focus groups from staff nurses. Like other qualitative methods, the transcription and analysis may be costly and time consuming (Beyea & Nicoll, 2000).

Case Studies

Case studies are often used to gain an understanding of the circumstances around a rare or sentinel health event. A group of individuals involved in the

KEY TERM

**Unstructured
observations:**
Phenomena of
interest are allowed
to emerge over time
as observations are
made

situation is brought together to analyze and draw conclusions about the event. Researchers use this method to examine participants' behaviors and decision making. While this method may be used less in research, it is an important method in quality improvement programs in almost every healthcare setting. For example, healthcare providers may convene when a major error is made such as amputating the wrong limb. Circumstances of the situation are examined and strategies to ensure that this type of error is avoided are identified.

Observation

Observations are another type of qualitative data collection method and must be consistent with the aims of the study (Casey, 2006). Researchers capture information in the natural and often unstructured setting either by being present or by recording on videotape to view at a later time. *Unstructured observations* use an inductive approach. Phenomena of interest are allowed to emerge over time as observations are being made. Researchers may be both observers and participants. Participants are aware of the researchers' roles and the research taking place, but researchers are also participants to gain insiders' perspectives about the phenomena (Casey).

Researchers usually make observations in settings where research projects take place. Observations can be expensive and time consuming. When more than one individual is involved in making observations, they should confer occasionally to make sure that data are being collected in the same manner. The presence of researchers may alter behaviors that are observed. Therefore, researchers may need to spend additional time in the setting so that participants feel more comfortable and the behaviors that are observed are more likely to by typical (Casey, 2006).

Preparing to Go Into the Field

After consent has been obtained from participants and researchers go into the field to collect data, they should be prepared with additional materials and anticipate needs that may arise. Researchers should come prepared with

CRITICAL THINKING EXERCISE 9-3

Recall the last time you performed a physical assessment on a client.
What type of data were you able to gather through interview? Through observation? What open-ended questions did you use? What closed-ended questions did you use?

additional consent forms should additional participants be identified, participant information sheets that explain the study, stamped self-addressed return envelopes, and additional interview guides. Because field notes are essential in qualitative research methods, it is helpful to have notebooks with extra pens and pencils available. If interviews are being conducted, extra tape recorders, additional batteries, and audiotapes need to be available as backups. Likewise, if video is being used for observations, extra video cameras, additional batteries, and extra videotapes should be available. When compensation is given to participants, researchers should also be prepared with monetary and nonmonetary rewards (Anastasi et al., 2005).

Appraising Data Collection in Qualitative Studies

As nurses read and interpret evidence from qualitative studies, it is essential that they determine if data collection methods are appropriate. **Table 9-6** outlines critical questions that can be used when appraising data collection methods of qualitative research. Data collection methods should be congruent with the research question. For example, when appraising an ethnographic study, the reader must ask if there is a broad question that is clearly stated. This question may become more focused as time is spent in the field and the

TABLE 9-6 Appraising Data Collection Methods in Qualitative Studies

Where was the setting of the study?
What was the rationale for choosing the setting?
Who were the participants and what were their roles and characteristics?
Why were they chosen?
What data collection methods were used?
What role did the researcher adopt within the setting?
Who collected the data and were they qualified for their roles?
How were data collectors trained? Was the training adequate?
Was the process of the fieldwork adequately reported?
How did the event unfold?
Was data collection continued until saturation was achieved?
Were the researchers' assumptions or biases acknowledged?

TEST YOUR KNOWLEDGE 9-4

1. Which of the following statements is true regarding the collection of qualitative data?
    a. Questionnaires are an economical way to collect anonymous data.
    b. Researchers can probe for more data when using questionnaires than when using interviews.
    c. Focus groups can be led by anyone interested in the subject.
    d. Researchers should never interact with individuals they are observing.

2. Which of the following should nurses consider when appraising qualitative data collection methods?
    a. The cost of the study
    b. The setting of the study
    c. The ages of the data collectors
    d. The role of the researcher

How did you do? 1. a; 2. b, d

researcher identifies emerging themes. Do emerging questions make sense to participants and therefore accurately reflect what they are saying? When looking at the study sample, does the particular group or individuals selected represent the experiences into which the researcher hopes to gain insight? The sample of the study should also be assessed. The setting should be adequately described so that readers may determine if the findings relate to other settings. Readers need to ask if a systematic method or procedure for data collection was described so that others could replicate the study and if enough data were collected to reach saturation. Greenhalgh and Taylor (1997) recommend that readers ask, "Have I been given enough information about the methods used?" and "Are these methods a sensible and adequate way of addressing the research question?" (p. 742).

9.5   Keeping It Ethical

At the end of this section, you will be able to:

‹ Discuss the importance of protecting human subjects during data collection

Protecting human subjects is essential throughout the data collection process. In healthcare research, subjects or participants are considered to be more vulnerable because of alterations in health status. Dilemmas can arise when advocating for the rights of individuals conflicts with the need to promote nursing science. It is not uncommon for nurses to find themselves caring for individuals involved in research studies; therefore, it is helpful for nurses to understand some basic safeguards.

Prior to data collection, informed consent must be obtained. One of the fundamental responsibilities of researchers is to make sure each person understands the nature of the research project and the implications of participating. Potential research participants should not be given too much hope that the intervention will benefit them because this could influence their decisions to participate. Individuals, or the proxy decision makers, must be able to freely decide whether or not to participate. They must be assured that they can withdraw from the study at any time without fear of reprisal. If nurses determine that potential subjects are not fully informed or lack understanding, they have an obligation to notify primary investigators. If proxy decision makers are involved in informed consent, nurses should determine that decisions are in the best interest of participants (Bross, 2003).

Sometimes research studies raise sensitive issues among nurses who feel protective of their patients. Nurses may be reluctant to identify and recruit subjects or collect only partial data. For example, Moody and McMillan (2002) reported that hospice nurses shielded their patients from a study even though the study was supported by the hospice administrative staff. Only 60 patient–caregiver dyads were enrolled despite there being 475 eligible patients. It was noted that many nurses believed that patients who were in the final stage of life should not be disturbed.

Randomized controlled trials (RCTs) also create dilemmas for nurses because subjects are randomized into treatment or control groups. Nurses must accept that randomization occurs to better understand the differences between groups, particularly when it is not known if treatments are beneficial. In blinded studies, nurses should not speculate with subjects or their families about the intervention. When nurses are informed of RCTs, they are more likely to assist researchers in recruiting, enrolling, and retaining participants (Anastasi et al., 2005; Moody & McMillan, 2002).

As the Internet becomes an accepted source of data or method to collect data, it is important for nurses to be aware of some ethical considerations, namely privacy and confidentiality. Because Internet communications leave a trail of archived records, privacy and confidentiality might be threatened. There is growing debate about whether information on the Internet is private

FYI

One of the fundamental responsibilities of researchers is to make sure each person understands the nature of the research project and the implications of participating. Potential research participants should not be given too much hope that the intervention will benefit them because this could influence their decisions to participate.

TEST YOUR KNOWLEDGE 9-5

True/False

1. When collecting data via the Internet, the rights of human subjects can be ignored since the Web is public domain.

2. Nurses should not speculate about the treatments subjects receive in a blinded RCT.

3. Data collection instruments should have codes rather than subject names to ensure anonymity.

How did you do? 1. F; 2. T; 3. T

or public. If the site is considered to be public, researchers may use information without obtaining informed consent (Ahern, 2005). There is mounting concern that data collected via the Internet could be sold to others, posing threats to individuals who are willing to meet via the Internet and share health-related experiences. When online methods are used, individuals should access the Internet via a secure site and use user names and passwords. Security issues must be monitored continuously throughout the data collection process, and researchers also need to update and upgrade security measures frequently (Im & Chee, 2006). Ahern notes that ethical guidelines for using the Internet need to be developed by professional organizations, and methods of obtaining informed consent need to be determined.

Regardless of how data are collected, researchers must implement strategies to keep data secure. Attention to data collection methods is imperative to prevent error. Researchers should not feel pressured to falsify or fabricate data because there are statistical methods to address missing data. Security measures must be in place to ensure that only authorized individuals have access to data. For example, data should be kept in secured computer files that require passwords to access. Codes, rather than names of subjects, must be used on data collection instruments such as questionnaires and laboratory reports to ensure anonymity. Raw data should be stored in locked cabinets and audiotapes should be destroyed after they are transcribed.

RAPID **REVIEW**

  Data collection takes a significant amount of time and resources when conducting research. Pilot studies can help identify unexpected problems.

Quantitative data collection methods involve measurements that gather numbers.

Questionnaires, observation, scales, and physiological measures are data collection methods used in quantitative studies.

There are four levels of measurement: nominal, ordinal, interval, and ratio. Statistical tests used in data analysis are selected based on the level of measurement.

All measurement contains error. There are two types of error: random and systematic.

Validity refers to whether an instrument measures what it should be measuring. There are three kinds of validity: content validity, criterion-related validity, and construct validity.

Reliability refers to the accuracy and consistency of an instrument. Reliable instruments have stability, equivalence, and internal consistency.

A correlation coefficient of 0.70 or greater indicates that an instrument has good reliability. Cronbach's alpha is one correlation coefficient that is commonly reported for interval and ratio data.

The purpose of qualitative data collection is to collect words.

The researcher is the most important data collection instrument in qualitative data collection. Researchers use questionnaires, interviews, focus groups, case studies, and observation to collect qualitative data.

Protecting human subjects is an important aspect of all research studies and one in which nurses play a key role.

APPLY WHAT YOU HAVE LEARNED

Read the article by Crimlisk, Johnstone, and Sanchez (2009) and note the methods used for data collection. Also consider the other articles that you have read. Fill in the measurement column on your grid found on the companion website by indicating the instruments that were used to collect quantitative data. For the qualitative study, indicate the method used to obtain data. For the articles that are not data based, indicate "not applicable" in the column. Examples are provided.

REFERENCES

Ahern, N. (2005). Using the Internet to conduct research. *Nurse Researcher, 13*, 55–70.

Anastasi, J., Capili, B., Kim, G., & Chung, A. (2005). Clinical trial recruitment and retention of a vulnerable population: HIV patients with chronic diarrhea. *Gastroenterology Nursing, 28*, 463–468.

Beyea, S., & Nicoll, L. (2000). Collecting, analyzing, and interpreting focus group data. *AORN, 71*, 22–30.

Beyer, J. E., Denyes, M. J., & Villarruel, A. M. (1992). The creation, validation, and continuing development of the Oucher: A measure of pain intensity in children. *Journal of Pediatric Nursing, 7*, 335–346.

Bross, W. (2003). Nursing and ethics: Biomedical research. *Alabama State Nurses' Association, 31*, 21.

Casey, D. (2006). Choosing an appropriate method of data collection. *Nurse Researcher, 13*, 75–92.

Crimlisk, J. T., Johnstone, D. J., & Sanchez, G. M. (2009). Evidence-based practice, clinical simulations workshop, and intravenous medications: Moving toward safer practice. *MEDSURG Nursing, 18*, 153–160.

Devers, K., Sofaer, S., & Rundall, T. (1999). Qualitative methods in health services research. *Health Services Research, 24*, 1153–1188.

Ellett, M., & Beausang, C. (2001). Introduction to qualitative research. *Gastroenterology Nursing, 24*, 10–14.

Greenhalgh, T., & Taylor, R. (1997). How to read a paper: Papers that go beyond numbers (qualitative research). *British Medical Journal, 315*, 740–743.

Griffin-Sobel, J. (2003). Evaluating an instrument for research. *Gastroenterology Nursing, 26*, 135–136.

Havens, G. A. (2001). A practical approach to the process of measurement in nursing. *Clinical Nurse Specialist, 15*, 146–152.

Im, E., & Chee, W. (2006). An online forum as a qualitative research method. *Nursing Research, 55*, 267–273.

Marwit, S., & Meuser, T. (2002). Development and initial validation of an inventory to assess grief in caregivers of persons with Alzheimer's disease. *The Gerontologist, 42*, 751–765.

Masters, C., Carlson, D., & Pfadt, E. (2006). Winging it through research: An innovative approach to a basic understanding of research methodology. *Journal of Emergency Nursing, 32*, 382–384.

Merchant, J., & Mateo, M. (1993). Accurate data: The basis of decision. *Gastroenterology Nursing, 16*, 163–169.

Meuser, T., & Marwit, S. (2001). A comprehensive, stage-sensitive model of grief in dementia caregiving. *The Gerontologist, 41*, 658–700.

Moody, L., & McMillan, S. (2002). Maintaining data integrity in randomized clinical trials. *Nursing Research, 51*, 129–133.

Myers, G., & Meccariello, M. (2006). From pet rock to rock-solid: Implementing unit based research. *Nursing Management, 37*, 24–29.

Roberts, P., & Priest, H. (2006). Reliability and validity in research. *Nursing Standard, 20*, 41–45.

Schmelzer, M. (2000). Understanding the research methodology: Should we trust the researchers' conclusions? *Gastroenterology Nursing, 23*, 269–274.

Wolf, Z. R. (2003). Teaching the code book. *Nurse Educator, 38*, 132–135.

CHAPTER OBJECTIVES

At the end of this chapter, you will be able to:

< Identify the basic concepts associated with sampling

< Differentiate between probability and nonprobability samples

< Describe various sampling methods

< Identify quantitative and qualitative research sampling strategies

< Discuss factors that should be considered when determining sample size

< Describe strategies that enhance the recruitment and retention of subjects

< Identify factors related to sampling that must be considered when appraising studies for evidence-based practice (EBP)

< Describe ethical considerations related to sampling

KEY TERMS

accessible population
anonymity
assent
attrition rate
cluster sampling
coercion
confidentiality
convenience sampling
data saturation
effect size
elements
exclusion criteria
heterogeneous
homogeneity

inclusion criteria
informed consent
nonprobability sampling
population
power analysis
probability sampling
purposive sampling
quota sampling
randomization
representativeness
sample
sampling bias
sampling error
sampling frame

sampling interval
sampling plan
significance level
simple random sampling
snowball sampling
stratified random
   sampling
subjects
systematic random
   sampling
target population
theoretical sampling
vulnerable population

CHAPTER 10

Using Samples to Provide Evidence

Ann H. White

10.1 Fundamentals of Sampling

At the end of this chapter, you will be able to:

< Identify the basic concepts associated with sampling

The ultimate goal of EBP is high quality health care with beneficial outcomes (Tolentino-DelosReyes, Ruppert, & Shioa, 2007). Nurses must believe that EBP will improve patient outcomes. Only then will there be a change in practice and an understanding of the benefits for the nurses in implementing evidence-based care (Porter-O'Grady, 2006).

A major component of collecting evidence to change clinical practice is to identify relevant nursing research on clinical topics. After research studies are identified, nurses must appraise if the research is valid and relevant to clinical practice. One consideration when appraising evidence is to determine if the sample and the sampling method were appropriately selected for the study.

Learning the Terms

When designing a research study, researchers must define the population as specified in the research question. A *population* is the entire group of elements that meet study criteria (Bloom & Trice, 2007). *Elements* are the basic unit of the population and may be people, events, experiences, or behaviors (Bloom & Trice). When elements are people, they are referred to as *subjects*. After determining the population of interest, researchers must create a *sampling plan*. They must consider the size of the sample, who will be eligible to be in the study, how individuals will be selected, and how they will be recruited. It is not economical, feasible, and time efficient to include all possible subjects in a study. An alternative is to identify a select group of subjects that is representative of all eligible subjects. These individuals constitute the *sample*.

To obtain the sample needed for the study, researchers must identify the *target population*, which is defined as all elements that meet the study criteria. For example, if a researcher is conducting a study on individuals ages 13–17 who have Type I diabetes, then every single adolescent who has Type I diabetes and is 13–17 years of age would be included in the target population. The researcher may choose to narrow the scope of the study by defining the target population as a more specific group of subjects. For example, the target population could be defined as adolescents 13–17 years of age with Type I diabetes whose care is managed by a local diabetic clinic. The researcher determines the target population based upon the purpose of the study, the design, and the type of data collection being planned.

After the target population is defined, researchers identify the *accessible population*, which is the group of elements to which the researcher has reasonable access. Typically, the accessible population is a smaller group than the target population; however, in some cases it may be the same group. In the previous example of adolescent diabetics that received care in one local clinic, the sample target population and accessible population may be the same. Regardless, researchers select subjects from the accessible population (see **Figure 10-1**). Learning these terms means using them correctly when appraising research studies. Frequently, individuals use the words "population" and "sample" interchangeably. This is not correct. The term "sample" is used appropriately when one discusses the elements of a study. The term "population" is used appropriately when one is generalizing findings to all possible elements.

CRITICAL THINKING EXERCISE 10-1 www

The next time you use the term *sample* or *population*, pause and consider whether you have used the terms correctly. Were you referring to the individuals who participated in a study or were you referring to the group of individuals to whom the findings would be generalized? Listen to how others use these terms. Are they using them correctly?

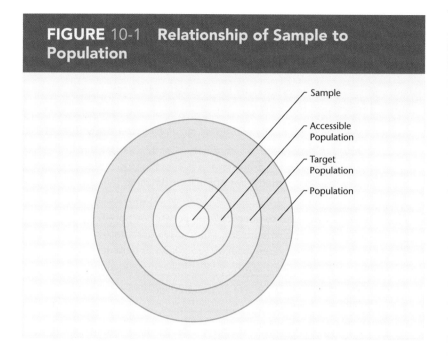

FIGURE 10-1   **Relationship of Sample to Population**

Sample

Accessible Population

Target Population

Population

FYI

In order to collect evidence that changes clinical practice, nurses must identify and appraise research that is relevant to clinical practice—key to this appraisal is determining that the sample and the sampling method are appropriate for the study and generalizable. Confidence in generalizability can be increased if samples accurately represent the target population.

The Hallmark of a Sample: Representativeness

Researchers place much importance on *representativeness*. This means obtaining representative samples so that results of studies can be generalized to target populations. Generalizability, also referred to as external validity, is the applicability of study findings to target populations. There is greater concern for generalizability in quantitative research studies than qualitative studies. Generalizabilty of study findings is a critical factor in EBP. As nurses identify and read research studies to determine best practice, they must determine if results of the studies are applicable to patients in their organizations. Confidence in generalizability can be increased if samples accurately represent the target population. This means that the elements of a sample must possess similar characteristics to the elements composing the target population. Melnyk and Cole (2005) identified a four-step method to ensure that samples are representative of target populations (see **Table 10-1**). By following this process, the potential for obtaining a representative sample is high. When the population, target population, accessible population, and sample are similar, the sample can be said to be representative. Specifying elements that can and cannot be included in a study is one way to increase representativeness.

KEY TERM

Representativeness: Degree to which elements of the sample are like elements in the population

> ## TABLE 10-1 Four Steps to Ensure Representative Samples
>
> 1. Define and clearly articulate the target population for the study by listing all of the essential characteristics of the target population or eligibility criteria for inclusion in the study.
>
> 2. Identify the population the researcher has access to for the study, taking care to verify that the accessible population closely resembles the target population by using the same eligibility criteria.
>
> 3. Develop a method to approach the accessible population. Some researchers refer to this as a sampling frame. The sampling frame is a practical method used to gain access to the population that is readily available to the researcher.
>
> 4. Select subjects from the accessible population to include in the sample.
>
> *Source:* Adapted from Melnyk & Cole (2005).

Inclusion criteria are used to determine subjects to be included in the sample. Researchers identify characteristics that each element must possess to be included in the sample. Inclusion criteria are guided by the research question and careful identification of the target and accessible populations. For example, in the study of adolescent diabetics, the researcher would first identify the essential characteristics or inclusion criteria for the target population. These characteristics could include age, a diagnosis of Type I diabetes, receiving care at a local diabetic clinic, and ability to speak English. Researchers often report inclusion criteria to clearly identify the subjects of the study.

Researchers may also designate *exclusion criteria*, which are characteristics of elements that will not be included in a sample. The use of exclusion criteria may decrease the risks of certain characteristics impacting the results of a study (Jerum & Melnyk, 2001). For example, suppose the researcher wants to study coping in adolescents with Type I diabetes. Individuals having another chronic disease such as asthma may be excluded from the study. The researcher may believe that having another chronic disease is an extraneous variable that could affect coping. If researchers choose to set exclusion criteria, the criteria must be clearly delineated, and researchers must have valid explanations to support the reasons for the exclusions.

KEY TERMS

Inclusion criteria: Characteristics that each element must possess to be included in the sample

Exclusion criteria: Characteristics of elements that will not be included in the sample

Inclusion and exclusion criteria are also important to appraise when considering evidence. When criteria are explicit, nurses can determine if results are applicable to the clinical practice topic being considered. Clearly defined inclusion and exclusion criteria tend to improve studies because the precision of sample selection is enhanced. This precision leads to stronger evidence when looking at research relevant to clinical practice (Haber, 2006).

When samples are not representative of target populations, the potential for sampling errors and bias is increased. *Sampling error* occurs when subjects in a study do not adequately represent the population. In most instances, sampling error is a result of small sample size that could not adequately represent all of the elements of the target population. *Sampling bias* occurs when the sample includes elements that over- or underrepresent characteristics when compared to elements in the target population. This is a threat to the external validity of the study.

KEY TERMS

Sampling error: Error resulting when elements in the sample do not adequately represent the population

Sampling bias: Elements of a sample over- or underrepresent characteristics of the target population

TEST YOUR KNOWLEDGE 10-1

Match the following:

1. Population

2. Target Population

3. Accessible Population

4. Sample

5. Inclusion criteria

6. Exclusion criteria

7. Representativeness

8. Element

a. The elements included in a study

b. All elements that meet a well defined set of criteria

c. Degree to which the sample reflects the population

d. Characteristics that eliminate elements from a study

e. A population that meets sampling criteria

f. Basic unit of the population

g. Population from which a researcher can sample

h. Characteristics of elements in a study

How did you do? 1. b; 2. e; 3. g; 4. a; 5. h; 6. d; 7. c; 8. f

10.2   Sampling Methods

At the end of this section, you will be able to:

‹ Differentiate between probability and nonprobability samples
‹ Describe various sampling methods
‹ Identify quantitative and qualitative research sampling strategies

Once inclusion criteria have been determined, researchers identify a method to select subjects for the sample. There are several sampling methods that researchers can use to select subjects. These methods are divided into two categories: probability and nonprobability sampling.

Probability Sampling Methods

When researchers use *probability sampling*, every element in the accessible population has an equal chance of being selected for inclusion in the study. There are three conditions that must be met in probability sampling. First, an accessible population must be identifiable. Next, the researcher must create a *sampling frame*, that is, a list of all possible elements in the accessible population. Finally, random selection must be used to choose elements from the sampling frame. The use of *randomization* is important because it reduces the threat of selection bias, which should result in a more representative sample. The probability that the characteristics of elements in the sample will be similar to elements of the population is increased (Melnyk & Fineout-Overholt, 2005). This type of sampling method is typically used with quantitative designs. There are four probability sampling methods: simple random sampling, stratified random sampling, cluster sampling, and systematic random sampling.

Each of the four probability sampling methods has advantages and disadvantages. Researchers should select a method based on the purpose of the research, the research question, and the research design. **Table 10-2** provides an overview of the assumptions, potential bias, and representativeness of probability sampling methods.

Simple Random Sampling

Simple random sampling involves randomly selecting elements from the accessible population and is considered by some authorities to be the most effective method to obtain a representative sample. If the accessible population is small, simple random sampling may be as easy as drawing names. For example, if the accessible population is 25 nursing students and the researcher needs 10

TABLE 10-2 **Overview of Probability Sampling Methods**

Type of Sampling	Assumptions	Possibility of Bias	Representativeness	Other Comments
Simple Random Sampling	1. Each subject has the same chance to be selected 2. Strategy used to select subjects upholds randomization	Low risk of bias if randomization of subjects upheld	With each subject having the same chance for selection, high probability the sample will represent the population as long as sample size is sufficient	Time consuming for researcher if the study has a large sample size
Stratified Random Sampling	1. Strata must be mutually exclusive so a subject can be assigned to only one stratum 2. Random sampling used to select subject from each stratum	Low risk of bias if randomization of subjects upheld	If assumptions upheld, high probability the sample will represent the population if the number of subjects in each stratum is sufficient	Time consuming for researcher if the study has a large sample size
Cluster Sampling	1. Simple random sampling used to first select groups or clusters and then select subjects within each cluster	Potential for bias greater if the initial clusters selected under- or overrepresent groups within the population	Greater potential for the sample to not represent the population depending upon how the initial clusters are selected	Less time consuming than the first two because the initial clusters focus the sites for subject selection
Systematic Random Sampling	1. Begin sampling with a random start. Start counting each kth subject on the list by first identifying the start location. Close eyes and point to a number on the list to start the counting	Some bias may be introduced if randomization of start location is not maintained	If bias occurs, not as representative of population as other three sampling methods	Simpler to complete than the other three forms of probability sampling

Source: Adapted from Wood and Ross-Kerr (2006) and Haber (2006).

FYI

There are several sampling methods that researchers can use to select subjects, which can be divided into two categories: probability and nonprobability sampling. Researchers should select a method based on the purpose of the research, the research question, and the research design.

students for the study, the name of each student could be placed in a container. The first name is drawn and recorded as a potential participant. This process continues until 10 student names have been selected. Should one of the selected students decline to participate in the study, another name would be selected in the same manner. When the accessible population is large, it may be easier for researchers to use a random numbers table. Such a table contains columns of digits (see **Table 10-3**). Each element in the sampling frame is assigned a number. The researcher, with eyes closed, points to a number on the random numbers table to begin the selection process. The researcher then proceeds through the table either horizontally, vertically, or diagonally. Numbers are selected until the desired sample size is achieved. Elements corresponding to the numbers selected form the sample. For example, in a study to determine student interest in creating a smoke-free campus, the accessible population is 5,500 undergraduate and graduate students. The researcher secures a list of all students enrolled in the university and assigns each name on the list a number. It has been determined that a sample of 200 students is necessary to achieve representativeness. After selecting the start point, the researcher selects additional elements by proceeding vertically through the columns until 200 subjects are selected.

TABLE 10-3 Table of Random Numbers

5	2	25	52
57	63	12	72
29	31	84	20
27	80	48	11
59	1	26	6
8	19	28	86
83	53	64	22
14	45	35	37
7	23	21	46
22	4	15	57
17	61	82	85
44	34	31	10
60	24	58	55
16	54	13	71
56	62	65	33
81	9	87	47

Stratified Random Sampling

Stratified random sampling involves selecting elements from a population that has been divided into groups or strata. Researchers identify characteristics that they want to stratify. These determinations are frequently based on what is already known about the phenomenon being studied. For example, findings show that boys and girls respond differently to pain. Therefore, a researcher may want to stratify subjects on the variable of gender to ensure that they have enough boys and girls to make comparisons.

Strata must be mutually exclusive. This means that each element can be fit into one and only one stratum (Haber, 2006). For example, if the sample is stratified according to gender, subjects can only be categorized as a boy or a girl. These strata are mutually exclusive because subjects cannot fit into both categories. After strata are established, researchers assign each element from the accessible population to a stratum. Participants are then randomly selected from each stratum. For example, the researcher may want to study nursing student attitudes toward treatment of pain. Because there are significantly fewer male than female nursing students, the researcher needs to account for gender disparity in the study. If less than 10% of the accessible population is male, the researcher uses stratified random sampling so that 10% of the sample is male. After strata are determined, subjects are randomly selected from each stratum.

One advantage to stratified random sampling is that sampling error can be reduced because elements are selected by strata that are known to represent the population. Representative samples increase the likelihood that findings can be generalized to the population. Stratifying can also decrease data collection time and costs of collecting data (Burns & Grove, 2005). However, care must be taken when using this method. Each stratum must have a sufficient number of elements. In the example above, if 50 males are needed to constitute 10% of the sample, there must be at least 50 males in the accessible population.

Cluster Sampling

Cluster sampling is also known as multistaging sampling. Cluster sampling is an effective and efficient method to collect data from large populations. A manageable sample is obtained by randomly selecting elements from larger to smaller clusters or subsets of a population. First, researchers identify all elements that could be included in a study. Then they determine logical subsets of the populations using random selection techniques. The participants are then randomly selected within those groups. For example, a researcher wants to study baccalaureate nursing education in the United States. Using cluster sampling, the researcher first randomly selects 10 states that will be included

KEY TERMS

Stratified random sampling: Selecting elements from an accessible population that has been divided into strata

Cluster sampling: Selecting elements from larger to smaller subsets of an accessible population in the study. Then all baccalaureate nursing programs in each of the 10 states are identified. The researcher then randomly selects three schools from each state and obtains the names of baccalaureate students enrolled in each of the programs selected. Sampling is concluded by randomly selecting 30% of the names on each list. While cluster sampling is an effective method to sample large populations, there are limitations. In the example above, suppose the researcher decided to select 50 students from each program rather than selecting 30%. This could result in oversampling of students from small programs and undersampling of students from large programs. Selecting a percentage of students provides a more representative sample. Sampling bias also occurs if a school is not selected because students in that program have no opportunity to participate. In addition, students from one program may have similar characteristics because they attend the same school.

Systematic Random Sampling

A fourth type of probability sampling is *systematic random sampling*. In this method, subjects are selected by creating a numbered list of elements and then selecting every *k*th element. Sometimes every odd or even numbered element may be chosen. To determine the *sampling interval*, researchers must know two things: the desired size of the sample and the size of the sampling frame. The formula for determining sample interval is:

$$k = \frac{\text{size of sampling frame}}{\text{size of sample}}$$

For example, a researcher desires to study infant feeding patterns and has access to a well baby clinic. At this clinic, 300 infants are registered as patients. The researcher needs 20 subjects for the study. Using systematic random sampling, the researcher would obtain a list of names of all infants seen in the clinic and assign each name a number. The sampling interval would be calculated by dividing 300 by 20, which equals 15. After randomly selecting a starting point on the list, every 15th (*k*th) name would be invited to participate in the study. Sampling bias may be introduced with this method. This method should not be

CRITICAL THINKING EXERCISE 10-2

Suppose you are on a task force at your university. The task force needs to survey students about attitudes toward adopting a smoke free campus. What are the advantages and disadvantages to using each of the probability sampling methods?

used if there is a pattern inherent in the list of elements. For example, if every 10th name on the list is a baby with formula intolerance, these infants would either be over- or undersampled, resulting in a biased sample.

Nonprobability Sampling Methods

A second category of sampling methods is *nonprobability sampling*. These methods do not require random selection of elements and therefore are less likely to be representative of the target population. Researchers use nonprobability sampling methods when a sampling frame cannot be determined. Because randomization is not used, the threat of selection bias is increased; therefore, samples selected using nonprobability are likely to be less representative than samples selected using probability methods (Melnyk & Fineout-Overholt, 2005). There are three nonprobability sampling methods: convenience, quota, and purposive. Table 10-4 provides an overview of nonprobability sampling methods.

KEY TERM

Nonprobability sampling: Method that does not require random selection of elements

TABLE 10-4 Overview of Nonprobability Sampling

Type of Sampling	Assumptions	Possibility of Bias	Representativeness	Other Comments
Convenience Sampling	1. Inclusion criteria identified prior to selection of subjects 2. All subjects are invited to participate	Highest probability of bias	Because sample is selected for ease of data collection, may not be representative of the target population	Seen in many nursing studies because of ease of data collection
Quota Sampling	1. Strata must be mutually exclusive so a subject can be assigned to only one stratum 2. Convenience sampling used to select subject from each stratum	May have some bias due to convenience sampling after strata identified	Because sample within each stratum is selected using convenience sampling method, may not represent the population	Similar to stratified random sampling except convenience sampling used to obtain the sample in each stratum

Type of Sampling	Assumptions	Possibility of Bias	Representativeness	Other Comments
Purposive Sampling	1. Researcher has sufficient knowledge of topic to select sample of experts 2. Researcher should identify criteria to include in selection of subjects	May have minimal bias if identification of subjects adheres to selection criteria and sample in study is homogenous	Because sample is selected by research, cannot generalize to population; generalizing the results is not an expected outcome of this type of research	Focus of this research is to learn more about and understand the phenomenon being studied
Snowball Sampling	1. Researcher selects initial subjects for study 2. Data saturation is researched	Not applicable with this type of sampling	Cannot generalize to population; generalizing the results is not an expected outcome of this type of research	Focus of this research is to learn more about and understand the phenomenon being studied
Theoretical Sampling	1. Data collection and data analysis occur simultaneously	Not applicable with this type of sampling	Cannot generalize to population; generalizing the results is not an expected outcome of this type of research	Used in grounded theory

Source: Adapted from Wood and Ross-Kerr (2006) and Haber (2006).

Convenience Sampling

In *convenience sampling*, also known as accidental sampling, researchers select elements for inclusion in the sample because they are easy to access. For example, a researcher desires to conduct a study of patients with Type II diabetes presenting for treatment at an emergency department. Because the researcher cannot predict which diabetic patients will use the emergency department over the course of the study, it is impossible for the researcher to create a sampling frame and randomly select subjects. Therefore, the researcher elects to use a convenience sample that includes all Type II diabetic patients who seek care at the emergency department. While sampling bias is a concern with this method, there are strategies that can be used to control for bias. Comparing demographic data from individuals in the sample to population demographics can help researchers determine if the sample is representative. Researchers should present a thorough description of the convenience sample in the study results and compare it to the target population. A careful explanation of why and how the sample was selected allows nurses to determine the potential for sampling bias and whether study findings should be used as evidence for clinical practice.

Quota Sampling

When researchers sample from strata without randomly selecting elements, they are using quota sampling. Like stratified random sampling, researchers select strata based on what is already known about the phenomenon being studied. The desired number, or quota, needed to fill each stratum should be proportionate to the population to obtain a representative sample. The difference between *quota sampling* and stratified random sampling is the use of random selection. In quota sampling, elements are conveniently selected from each strata rather than being randomly selected. For example, in a study about how age is related to success in nursing programs, a researcher could stratify according to age by creating three age groups: 18–22, 23–30, and over 30. Suppose 80% of nursing students are ages 18–22, 15% are ages 23–30, and 5% are over the age of 30. If the researcher needs a sample size of 100, the sampling would continue until 80 students between the ages of 18–22, 15 students between the ages of 23–30, and 5 students over the age of 30 had been recruited. By establishing proportional quotas that mirror the nursing student population, the researcher is more likely to obtain a representative sample. Convenience and quota sampling are predominantly used in quantitative research studies. They are frequently used because it is often difficult in nursing research to determine a sampling frame in advance of a study. They also are less time consuming and less costly than probability sampling methods. The ability to generalize results to the target population depends heavily on the appropriateness of the sampling method used.

Purposive Sampling

Purposive sampling, which is a nonprobability sampling method, is used in qualitative studies. Sampling methods used in qualitative research must be appropriate to allow researchers to gain insight into the experience or event being studied. There is less focus on the results of the study being generalized to the target population, and more emphasis is placed on the interpretation and understanding of the event or experience being studied (Haber, 2006). Researchers use purposive sampling in qualitative research to select a distinct

KEY TERM

Snowball sampling:
Recruitment of
participants based on
referrals from other
participants

group of individuals that either have lived the experience or have expertise in the event or experience being studied. In qualitative studies, individuals in the sample are referred to as participants. For example, researchers investigating the lived experience of women under the age of 25 who have survived a liver transplant would use purposive sampling. Because the focus of the study is so specific, the researcher can hand select women who meet the inclusion criteria. Researchers must carefully document the process used to select subjects. A strategy researchers use in purposive sampling is known as *snowball sampling*, or network sampling. When using this approach, an initial participant who meets the study criteria is identified. This participant then identifies other individuals who meet the criteria for inclusion in the study. To protect confidentiality, researchers must ascertain from the referring participant that it is permissible to contact suggested potential participants. When using snowball sampling, researchers assume that individuals will identify others who are

TEST YOUR KNOWLEDGE 10-2

1. A researcher desires to study the effect of a memory game on older adults' abilities to recall a short term task list. The researcher randomly selects 20 elders from a list of residents at a local nursing home. The sampling method used is

   a. convenience sampling

   b. quota sampling

   c. simple random sampling

   d. purposive sampling

2. Which of the following sampling methods involves randomization?

   a. systematic sampling

   b. snowball sampling

   c. stratified random sampling

   d. cluster sampling

3. In order to use random sampling, a researcher must know the

   a. sampling frame

   b. characteristics of the population

   c. exclusion criteria

   d. sampling interval

How did you do? 1. c; 2. a, c, d; 3. a

similar to themselves. Snowball sampling is a useful method to identify participants that would otherwise be difficult for the researchers to find. Suppose a researcher is investigating the lived experience of young women with eating disorders. By first identifying a small group of women who meet the criteria and then asking them to identify other young women that they know, the number of potential participants is increased.

Another sampling method used specifically in grounded theory is *theoretical sampling*. When using this sampling method, researchers collect data from an initial group of participants. After conducting some preliminary analyses of data, researchers identify additional participants for inclusion in the sample.

10.3   Sample Size: Does It Matter?

At the end of this section, you will be able to:

‹ Discuss factors that should be considered when determining sample size

‹ Describe strategies that enhance the recruitment and retention of subjects

‹ Identify factors related to sampling that must be considered when appraising studies for EBP

Determining Sample Size

After the sampling method is identified, researchers must decide how large a sample is needed. Various factors determine sample sizes for quantitative and qualitative studies. In either type of design, the sample size must be sufficient to adequately support the research purpose and design of the study. *Homogeneity* of the population is one factor that needs to be considered when determining sample size in quantitative studies. Homogeneity refers to the degree to which elements are homogenous or similar. If a population has a number of common characteristics, the sample size does not need to be as large as a more *heterogeneous*, or diverse, population. Another factor to consider when determining sample size is the purpose of the study and what is being studied. If the focus of the study is narrow, the sample may not need to be as large as a sample for a very broadly focused study. A study investigating eating habits of fifth graders is very broad and would require a large sample. A study on eating habits of fifth graders who have diabetes is narrower in focus; thus, the number of subjects needed for the study may be smaller.

KEY TERMS

Attrition rate: Loss of subjects before a study is completed

Power analysis: Statistical method to determine the sample size that will best detect the effect of the independent variable

Significance level: The alpha level established before the beginning of a study

Effect size: Estimate of how large a difference will be observed between groups

Another factor that researchers need to consider when conducting quantitative studies is *attrition rate*, also known as dropout rate. Typically, there will be subjects who agree to participate in a study and, for whatever reason, do not complete the study. Some researchers suggest that the anticipated attrition rate be added to the sample size. Melnyk and Fineout-Overholt (2005) indicated that research studies may have up to a 20% attrition rate. If that is the case and the researcher has established the need for 200 subjects, 240 subjects would need to be recruited to account for the anticipated attrition.

The design of the study also influences decisions about sample size. The number of variables being investigated is an important factor. Typically, the greater the number of variables being tested in a study, the larger the sample size needed to be able to detect changes in the variables. The sensitivity of instruments used to collect data will also affect the sample size. A very precise instrument typically requires fewer subjects than a less precise instrument (Bloom & Trice, 2007). In addition, decisions about sample size are influenced by practical matters such as cost, convenience, and feasibility.

There are two accepted rules for determining sample size when using quantitative research designs (Bloom & Trice, 2007). The rule of 30 is one rule that is used by many quantitative researchers (Burns & Grove, 2005). This rule states that in order to have a sufficient sample size to adequately represent the target population, there needs to be a minimum of 30 subjects in each group being studied. For example, in an experiment using a control group and an intervention group, a sample size of 60 would be indicated. Another well accepted rule is the rule of 10. This rule states that 10 subjects are required for each variable under study. For example, in a correlational study examining the relationships among number of symptoms, coping, self-care abilities, and quality of life in patients with multiple sclerosis, a minimum of 40 subjects would be needed.

A more powerful and accurate method to determine sample size for quantitative studies is to conduct a *power analysis*. This is fast becoming the gold standard for determining sample size, because sophisticated computer software is readily available to make these calculations. A power analysis is a statistical method used to determine the acceptable sample size to detect the true effect (Li, Melnyk, & McCann, 2004). When nurses read that a power analysis was conducted, they can have greater confidence that the sample size was appropriate for the study and be confident applying the findings to the target population (Burns & Grove, 2005).

There are two factors that must be established to conduct a power analysis: significance level and effect size. The *significance level* is the alpha level established prior to the beginning of the investigation. A vast majority of nursing researchers use $p = 0.05$ as the significance level. The *effect size* is an estimate of how large a difference will be observed between the groups (Bloom & Trice, 2007). When researchers expect that the effect size is large, fewer subjects will be needed to detect differences between the groups. If the effect of an intervention is small, a larger sample is needed to be able to statistically demonstrate that the intervention was effective (Burns & Grove, 2005). After the sample size is determined through power analysis, researchers must still account for other factors, such as attrition and instrumentation.

There are also factors that determine sample sizes in qualitative studies. These factors include the scope of the study, the phenomenon being investigated, the quality of data collected, and the study design. The size of the sample is sufficient when qualitative researchers achieve *data saturation*. Saturation means that collecting data from additional participants adds no new information to what has already been collected (Munhall, 2007). Researchers should provide information about sample selection so that nurses can make determinations about the adequacy of the sample. Because the focus is on the data collected, the richness of data, and the researchers' conclusions, qualitative studies tend to have smaller samples than quantitative studies.

Recruitment and Retention of Subjects

Effective recruitment and retention of subjects is imperative to the credibility of research studies. Failure to attend to recruitment and retention details can critically impact the size of samples. Initial contacts made by researchers may determine whether subjects will participate and remain in the study. Because researchers may have only one opportunity to encourage participation, information should be professional, informative, and culturally sensitive for the accessible population. Flyers, letters, and advertisements are all methods used to recruit subjects. Decisions about recruitment strategies are based on cost, predicted success, and appropriateness for the accessible population. Recruitment materials should include a brief description of the study purpose, inclusion criteria, and information explaining how to enroll in the study. It is helpful to indicate in recruitment materials if incentives are being offered for participation. Researchers should determine reasons that subjects elect not to

KEY TERM

Data saturation:
When no new information is being obtained and information is repetitive

 FYI

Various factors determine sample sizes for quantitative and qualitative studies, including homogeneity or diversity of the population, purpose of the study, focus of the study; design of the study, and number of variables being investigated. Sample size must be sufficient to adequately support each of these factors.

CRITICAL THINKING EXERCISE 10-3

Suppose you are in charge of designing recruitment materials for a study examining Hispanic mothers' attitudes towards breast feeding. What factors would need to be considered when designing these materials?

participate in studies. Being cognizant of who is not participating in a study should be included in the discussion of the results because selection bias affects generalizability of the results. Even with mailed, anonymous questionnaires, researchers may discover, by trending demographic data, similarities among subjects who did not respond. Researchers should be aware that certain age groups, socioeconomic groups, or ethnic groups may be underrepresented.

It is important to retain subjects after they have been recruited to participate in a study. Strategies to reduce threats of mortality can be effective in reducing subject attrition. Reasons why subjects withdraw from studies should be monitored, and conditions causing subjects to withdraw should be modified if possible.

Considerations for EBP

It is imperative that nurses use the best possible evidence to make decisions about clinical practice. When considering research studies for EBP, nurses must critically appraise if samples represent target populations. Nurses should expect detailed accounts of sampling methods, sample sizes, and recruitment and retention strategies. When critically appraising studies, nurses should look for discussion about power analyses in quantitative studies and data saturation in qualitative studies. By carefully examining attributes of samples and sampling methods, nurses can make decisions about the applicability of findings to clinical practice (Newman & Roberts, 2002; Welk, 2007).

10.4 Keeping It Ethical

At the end of this section, you will be able to:

< Describe ethical considerations related to sampling

Individuals who participate in research have fundamental rights that must be protected. The American Nurses Association (ANA) code of ethics and human rights guidelines direct researchers to protect the rights of each and every subject (ANA, 2001). The ANA (2001) code addresses five human rights that mandate protection when conducting research. These rights include the right to anonymity and/or confidentiality, the right to self-determination, the right to privacy, the right to fair treatment, and the right to protection from discomfort and harm.

Researchers have a responsibility to protect all subjects, especially those who are considered to be in a *vulnerable population*. Children, pregnant women, the unborn, frail elderly, prisoners, and individuals with some level of mental incapacity are considered to be members of vulnerable populations. In some situations, factors such as ethnicity, gender, socioeconomic status, education, and language may create potential vulnerability for certain subjects (Anderson & Hatton, 2000). To ensure subject protection, researchers maintain *anonymity* and *confidentiality*. Anonymity means keeping the names of the subjects separated from the data so that no one, not even the researcher, knows their identities. In some studies, it is not possible for subjects to remain anonymous. In these situations, confidentiality must be protected. Confidentiality refers to protecting subjects' identities. One way identities are protected is to keep a master list with the names of subjects and the codes assigned to the data collected. The list is locked away from other data and destroyed after all data are collected. Another way to ensure confidentiality is by reporting results as group data, not as individual data. Actions such as these are in accordance

KEY TERMS

Vulnerable population: Special groups needing protection because of their limited ability to provide informed consent or risk for coercion

Anonymity: Concealing the identity of subjects, even from the researcher

Confidentiality: Protection of subjects' identities from everyone except the researcher

CRITICAL THINKING EXERCISE 10-4 [www]

Check out the Health Insurance Portability and Accountability Act (HIPAA) regulations at http://www.hhs.gov/ocr/privacy/hipaa/understanding/index.html How do these guidelines provide direction to researchers about protecting confidentiality of subjects?

Informed consent:
Obtaining voluntary
participation by
subjects after they
have been informed
of possible risks and
benefits

with the ANA code of ethics and human rights guidelines (2001), as well as the HIPAA guidelines.

Another major responsibility of researchers is maintaining subjects' rights to self-determination by obtaining *informed consent*. Prior to beginning a research study, institutional review board (IRB) approval must be obtained. This board consists of individuals who review research proposals to ensure that research is conducted in an ethical manner and that the rights of subjects are not violated. The IRB pays particular attention to the process of informed consent and ensures that mandatory content is included in consent forms. See **Table 10-5** for a list of essential components of consent forms. Subjects must be informed that they may choose to participate or not participate in the study and that they may withdraw at any time without harm or consequences. There must be a clear and concise explanation of the study and what subjects will be asked to do in the study. There should also be a discussion of the potential benefits and risks of participation in the study. If there are monetary benefits, there must be a description of the amount of money participants will receive and what is required to receive that monetary amount. If there are risks to subjects, those risks must be clearly detailed and include any physical, emotional,

 FYI

When inviting
subjects to
participate
in studies,
researchers must
obtain informed
consent, with
particular regard
for vulnerable
populations.
With children,
nurses should
obtain assent.
Nurses should
also maintain
anonymity and
confidentiality
as well as avoid
coercion when
sampling.

TABLE 10-5 Mandatory Components of Consent Forms

Title of study
Invitation to participate
Basis for subject selection
Purpose of study
Explanation of procedures
Benefits and risks
Alternatives to participation
Financial obligations
Confidentiality assurance
HIPAA disclosure
Subject withdrawal
Offer to answer questions
Consent statement
Identification of researchers

Source: Adapted from Code of Federal Regulations: Protection of Human Subjects (1983).

spiritual, economic, social, or legal risks. There are other factors to consider when obtaining informed consent. Informed consents should be written in simple language. If subjects cannot read, forms should be read to potential subjects. For subjects who speak English as a second language, consent forms should be read by an interpreter or written in their native language. Subjects should have sufficient time to carefully think about whether or not to participate. Both subjects and researchers must sign consent forms after assuring that participation is voluntary. Consent forms should not be kept with data. This protects subjects' confidentiality. A copy of the signed form should also be given to subjects.

One reason that considerable attention is given to the process of obtaining informed consent is that it is unethical for subjects to feel coerced into participating in research. *Coercion* is the threat of harm or the offer of an excessive reward with the intent to force an individual to participate in a research study. Healthcare providers must be extremely careful when conducting clinical research to ensure that patients do not feel coerced into participating in studies. Patients may feel particularly vulnerable if they decline participation because they may fear that treatment may be withheld (Wood & Ross-Kerr, 2006). Coercion can also be a factor in studies involving nursing education. Faculty who conduct research involving nursing students must be careful that students do not feel coerced into participating.

KEY TERM

Coercion: Threat of harm or offer of reward to force an individual to participate in a study

TEST YOUR KNOWLEDGE 10-4

Indicate whether the following actions are ethical or unethical?

1. Allowing a subject who does not speak English to sign a consent form without providing an interpreter.

2. Allowing a nursing administrator to see group data from surveys conducted in the organization.

3. Keeping a folder for every subject that contains a signed consent form and raw data.

4. Providing subjects with money to reimburse their travel to the data collection site.

5. Promising health care for life to individuals if they choose to participate in a study.

How did you do? 1. Unethical; 2. Ethical; 3. Unethical; 4. Ethical; 5. Unethical

Children, because they are minors, cannot give consent to participate in research; however, researchers are obligated to obtain *assent* when possible. Children may have difficulty understanding what a study involves, and they may agree to participate to please adults. Typically, children 7 years of age and older must give oral assent while children 12 years and older must sign an assent form. Regardless of the age, parents or legal guardians must sign consent forms.

Despite the importance placed on adherence to IRB guidelines and informed consent, there usually is little discussion about the process used to ensure that subjects' rights were not violated. In research articles, authors typically state that IRB approval was obtained and that the rights of subjects were protected. When such a statement is made, nurses can assume that ethical principles were upheld.

 RAPID **REVIEW**

 Sampling methods are determined by the research purpose and the research design.

 There are two major types of sampling: probability and nonprobability.

 Probability sampling and selected nonprobability sampling are used in quantitative research. Fundamental to probability sampling, but not nonprobability sampling, is random selection of subjects.

 Probability sampling methods include simple random sampling, stratified random sampling, cluster sampling, and systematic random sampling.

 Nonprobability sampling methods include convenience sampling, quota sampling, purposive sampling, snowball sampling, and theoretical sampling.

 In quantitative research, the goal of sampling is to select a representative sample by identifying subjects that reflect the same characteristics as the population.

 The more representative the sample, the more confidence there is generalizing to the population.

 Nonprobability sampling is used in qualitative research.

 Sample size is determined by homogeneity of the population, purpose of the study, attrition rate, design, number of variables being investigated, and the sensitivity of instruments used.

APPLY WHAT YOU HAVE LEARNED

As your committee has progressed in its assignment to identify strategies that reduce medication errors, you have been challenged to apply research principles for the purpose of establishing best practices. The next step is to review your articles, paying particular attention to details about the sample. Fill in the sample column on your grid found on the companion website by including details such as sample characteristics, sampling method, and size. Consult the examples already done.

 Power analysis is used to calculate the minimal number of subjects required in a quantitative study.

 Sample size for qualitative research continues until saturation is achieved.

 When making decisions about EBP, critical appraisal of the sampling method and sample size is desirable.

 Researchers must attend to many factors to ensure that the rights of subjects are protected. Researchers must ensure that informed consent is obtained and that individuals choose freely, without coercion, to participate in studies.

 Vulnerable populations must be especially protected by researchers.

REFERENCES

American Nurses Association. (2001). *Code of ethics for nurses with interpretative statements.* Washington, DC: American Nurses Association.

Anderson, D. G., & Hatton, D. C. (2000). Accessing vulnerable populations for research. *Western Journal of Nursing Research, 22,* 244–252.

Bloom, K. C., & Trice, L. B. (2007). Sampling. In C. Boswell & S. Cannon (Eds.), *Introduction to nursing research: Incorporating evidence based practice* (pp. 121–143). Sudbury, MA: Jones and Bartlett.

Burns, N., & Grove, S. (2005). *The practice of nursing research: Conduct, critique and utilization* (5th ed.). St. Louis, MO: Elsevier Saunders. Code of Federal Regulations: Protection of human subjects, 45 CFR 46, *OPRR Reports*, Revised March 8, 1983.

Haber, J. (2006). Sampling. In G. LoBiondo-Wood & J. Haber (Eds.), *Nursing research: Methods and critical appraisal of evidence-based practice.* St. Louis, MO: Mosby.

Jerum, A., & Melnyk, B. M. (2001). Evidence-based practice: Effectiveness of interventions to prevent obesity and obesity-related complications in children and adolescents. *Pediatric Nursing, 27,* 606–610.

Li, H., Melnyk, B. M., & McCann, R. (2004). Review of intervention studies for families with hospitalized elderly relative [Electronic version]. *Journal of Nursing Scholarship, 36*(1), 54–59.

Melnyk, B. M., & Cole, R. (2005). Generating evidence through quantitative research. In B. Melnyk & E. Fineout-Overholt (Eds.), *Evidence-based practice in nursing and healthcare* (pp. 239–281). Philadelphia: Lippincott Williams & Wilkins.

Melnyk, B. M., & Fineout-Overholt, E. (2005). Evidence-based practice: Rapid critical appraisal of randomized control trials (RCTs): An essential skill of evidence-based practice (EBP). *Pediatric Nursing, 31,* 50–52.

Munhall, P. (2007). *Nursing research: A qualitative perspective* (4th ed.). Sudbury, MA: Jones and Bartlett.

Newman, M., & Roberts, T. (2002). Critical appraisal 2: Can the evidence be applied in your context? In J. Craig & R. Smith (Eds.), *The evidence-based practice manual for nurses* (pp. 114–135). Edinburgh, Scotland: Churchill Livingstone.

Porter-O'Grady, T. (2006). A new age for practice: Creating the framework for evidence. In K. Malloch & T. Porter-O'Grady, *Introduction to evidence-based practice in nursing and health care* (pp. 5–27). Sudbury, MA: Jones and Bartlett.

Tolentino-DelosReyes, A. F., Ruppert, S. D., & Shioa, S. P. (2007). Evidence-based practice: Use of the ventilator bundle to prevent ventilator-associated pneumonia. *American Journal of Critical Care, 16*(1), 20–27.

Welk, D. S. (2007). How to read, interpret, and understand evidence-based literature statistics. *Nurse Educator, 32*(1), 16–20.

Wood, M., & Ross-Kerr, J. (2006). *Basic steps in planning nursing research: From question to proposal* (6th ed.). Sudbury, MA: Jones and Bartlett.

www

At the end of this chapter, you will be able to:

< List the 5Ss in the pyramid of evidence

< Discuss the types and purposes of other sources of evidence

< List interdisciplinary databases that can provide evidence for practice

< Use the 5Ss to locate evidence in a logical fashion

< Discuss one ethical dilemma when using other sources of evidence

case studies
concept analyses
integrative review
meta-analysis
meta-synthesis
nonpropositional
   knowledge

practice guidelines
propositional knowledge
studies
summaries
synopses

syntheses
systematic review
systems
traditional literature
   review

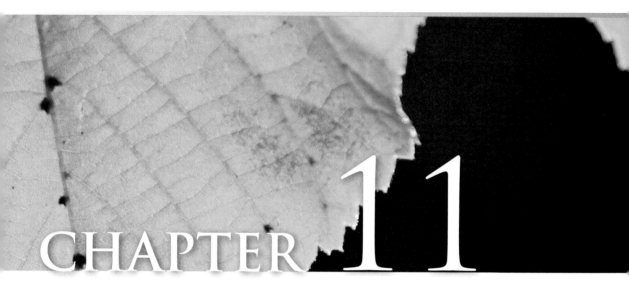

CHAPTER 11

Other Sources of Evidence
Cynthia L. Russell

11.1 The Pyramid of Evidence: The 5 Ss

At the end of this section, you will be able to:

< List the 5 Ss in the pyramid of evidence
< Discuss the types and purposes of other sources of evidence

Nursing is both an art and a science. We learn and practice nursing by using both propositional knowledge and nonpropositional knowledge. *Propositional knowledge* is the science of nursing or knowledge that is "formal, explicit, derived from research and scholarship and concerned with generalisability" (Rycroft-Malone et al., 2004, p. 83). For example, the knowledge we gain from research studies is propositional knowledge. *Nonpropositional knowledge* is the art of nursing or knowledge that is "informal, implicit and derived primarily through practice (Rycroft-Malone et al., p. 83). When we learn to prepare adhesive tape before dressing a wound, we are gaining nonpropositional knowledge. Both of these ways of knowing must come from many sources, be critically evaluated by experts, and integrated into the evidence that guides nursing practice.

An organizing framework to explain the importance and contribution of various levels of information to evidence-based healthcare delivery has been developed (Haynes, 2006). The framework is organized in a pyramid with five levels including *studies*, *syntheses*, *synopses*, *summaries*, and *systems* (see **Figure 11-1**). These levels are known as the 5Ss (Haynes). Research studies form the base of the pyramid. The use of

KEY TERMS

Propositional knowledge: Knowledge obtained from research and scholarship

Nonpropositional knowledge: The art of nursing or knowledge obtained through practice

Studies: Pyramid of evidence level containing quantitative and qualitative studies, case studies, and concept analyses

Syntheses: Level in the pyramid of evidence containing a whole depiction of a phenomenon

Synopses: Level in the pyramid of evidence containing brief descriptions of evidence

Summaries: Level in the pyramid of evidence containing detailed descriptions of evidence

Systems: Level in the pyramid of evidence involving electronic medical records integrated with practice guidelines

Case studies: A description of a single or novel event

Concept analyses: Scholarly papers exploring the attributes and characteristics of a concept

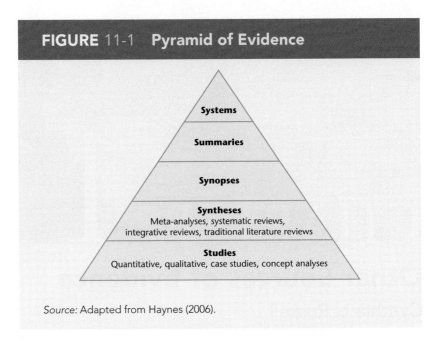

FIGURE 11-1 Pyramid of Evidence

Source: Adapted from Haynes (2006).

research studies as one source of evidence has been presented previously. Additional types of evidence that form this bottom layer of the pyramid include *case studies* and *concept analyses*. Haynes identifies subsequent layers of the information pyramid moving upward. These levels are syntheses or systematic reviews, synopses or brief evidence-based journal abstracts, summaries such as evidence-based textbooks, and finally systems such as computerized decision support systems.

The First S: Studies

The case study report can expand and generalize theory, represent a typical case, and provide great detail about a phenomenon for which little information is known (Yin, 2003). Yin notes that a case study "is an empirical inquiry that investigates a contemporary phenomenon within its real-life context, especially when the boundaries between the phenomenon and context are not clearly evident" (p. 13). What does this mean? In nursing, case studies are frequently used to report the story of one patient including details such as diagnosis, nursing care, and influential environmental factors. The case study report provides enough detail so that the reader feels informed about that particular situation. The case study approach, which originated from sociology, informs nurses about phenomena through the information that it provides. Case studies can be exploratory, but they are typically descriptive or explanatory and answer research questions that ask "how" or "why" (Yin). The case or cases that are selected for study are based upon their representativeness of a particular situation. Cases may also be selected for their potential to describe or explain a theory. Case studies involve direct observation of the situation and are best used as a research approach when studying events that are currently happening and when the researcher has little or no control over these events. Yin notes that "the case study's unique strength is its ability to deal with a full variety of evidence—documents, artifacts, interviews, and observations" (p. 8). Just like research studies, the merit of the case study must be evaluated to determine its contribution to the evidence. **Table 11-1** lists criteria for evaluat-

FYI

An organizing framework, or pyramid of evidence, explains the importance and contribution of various levels of information to evidence-based healthcare delivery. It has five levels, known as the 5Ss: studies, syntheses, synopses, summaries, and systems.

TABLE 11-1 Criteria for Evaluating a Case Study

Does the case study answer a "how" or "why" question?

Is the purpose of the case study appropriate?

Are study propositions or theories identified, if appropriate?

Is the research question adequately specific so that the unit of analysis is clear?

Is a theoretical framework presented for the case study?

Is construct validity addressed?

Are multiple sources of evidence used?

< Is a chain of evidence made explicit?

< Was a draft of the case study reviewed by the informants?

Is internal validity adequately addressed? (only appropriate for explanatory case studies)

< Does the author make plausible inferences?

< Have all other explanations been considered?

< Does all of the evidence point to the same conclusion?

Is external validity adequately addressed?

Is the case study protocol reliable?

< Was the case study described in such detail that an auditor could repeat the procedures and obtain the same results?

Is the case study investigator adequately prepared to conduct the case study?

Is the rationale for selection of the case study subject clearly described?

Is an analysis strategy clearly identified and followed?

Does the analysis strategy lead to answering the proposed research question?

Source: Adapted from Yin (2003).

ing a case study. Although the findings from case studies are not regarded as highly as findings from research studies, in some instances case study findings can provide insight and understanding when little evidence is available. For example, when a novel innovation is implemented, a case study may be the only published information about it.

Other sources of evidence in the first S of the pyramid are concept analyses. Rogers and Knafl (2000) define concepts as being "formed by the identification of characteristics common to a class of objects or phenomena and the abstraction and clustering of these characteristics, along with some means of expression (most often a word)" (p. 78). For example, pain is an important concept in patient care. One way to define pain is an uncomfortable feeling, but this definition is problematic because it is too broad and other concepts, such as itching, could be defined the same way. Therefore, concepts must be described, understood, and communicated so they can be used for building theory. Concept analyses provide for the exploration of the attributes and characteristics of a concept (Walker & Avant, 2005). Specific steps for concept analyses have been described (Walker & Avant). Understanding these steps will assist you in evaluating concept analyses for application to evidence-based practice (EBP). The author of the concept analysis should begin by clearly stating the aims of the analysis. The contribution of the concept analysis to research and practice should be clearly described. Assumptions made about the concept may also be presented and assist in understanding the perspective of the author's analysis. Possible uses of the concept should be presented, including definitions and descriptions found in all types of literature. Related and interchangeable concepts may also be described. This further assists in clarifying the concept being studied. After this, the author can state specific characteristics of the concept known as defining attributes. Antecedents, or conditions that must precede the concept, are also presented. For example, a person must have functioning neurons to feel pain. Next, the consequences, or outcomes, of the concept should be discussed.

The most interesting part of the concept analysis is the presentation of various cases. In the pain example, one case would describe pain, another may describe itching, and yet another may describe pleasure. These cases

FYI

Within the 5 Ss there are several types of evidence, including case studies, concept analyses, meta-syntheses, systematic reviews, traditional literature reviews, integrative reviews, meta-analyses, practice guidelines, and abstracts.

CRITICAL THINKING EXERCISE 11-2

Read a concept analysis article on a concept that is of interest to you.
How does the report increase your understanding of the concept?
Describe how the concept analysis report helped you clarify the "edges" of the concept.

represent, almost represent, and do not represent the concept. Critiquing the rigor with which the author has approached the concept analysis report is of utmost importance in determining the contribution of the report to evidence. When the author has carefully and thoughtfully followed the concept analysis steps, the results and implications for practice and research can contribute to the development of evidence.

Although qualitative findings are considered lower level evidence, they do provide the patient perspective for EBP. When a systematic review contains only qualitative studies, it is known as a *meta-synthesis*. Authors use a systematic approach to search for both published and unpublished qualitative studies (Beck, 2009).

The Second S: Syntheses

Syntheses integrate various pieces of evidence to present a whole depiction of a phenomenon. A *systematic review* is a common type of synthesis found in nursing. It is a rigorously conducted process of obtaining and reviewing the literature to answer preestablished theoretical or practice questions. The word "systematic" is the key to understanding the nature and intent of a systematic review. "Systematic" means "done methodically or carried out in a methodological and organized manner" (Encarta Dictionary, n.d.). A systematic review of the literature includes both a systematic approach to obtaining the literature and also a systematic approach to conducting the review of the literature after it is obtained. Understanding the critical steps to these two processes assists in evaluating the quality of a systematic review.

Before beginning the systematic review process, the author of the review clarifies the problem and the questions to be answered (Cooper, 1998). Questions that can be answered by a systematic review include, What is the state of the theoretical knowledge in this area?, What are the methodological gaps in the current studies?, What is the impact of interventions on patient outcomes from these studies?, What should be the focus of the next research study?, and How are two bodies of literature related or unrelated? Because the systematic review can assist in answering many types of questions, the author must define

KEY TERMS

Meta-synthesis:
When a systematic review contains only qualitative studies

Systematic review:
Rigorous synthesis of research findings about a clinical problem

what variables and/or concepts are important to the problem or question. Furthermore, the author may also identify the relationships between variables if these relationships are important to the problem being investigated.

The author must decide what kinds of studies to include in the systematic review. Therefore, inclusion and exclusion criteria must be established based upon the problem and question to be answered. For example, if the question relates to a particular age group, then research reports that include that particular age group would only be included in the systematic review. If studies with a particular design are the target, for example a randomized controlled trial, then only reports with this design would be included. The inclusion and exclusion criteria must logically flow from the problem and questions.

After the problem and question to be answered by the systematic review are clarified and the inclusion/exclusion criteria are identified, relevant literature is obtained by the author (Cooper, 1998). This begins the data collection phase of the systematic review. Through an exhaustive process, both published and unpublished literature is sought for the review. Because most published studies have significant findings, including unpublished literature helps to decrease bias. Computerized databases are searched, including *Cumulative Index to Nursing and Allied Health Literature* (CINAHL), MEDLINE, PsycINFO, Health-STAR, the Cochrane Library, and Dissertation Abstracts Online. Keywords are used to query the databases. Additional computerized databases may also be used, depending upon the selected topic. For example, if the author were conducting a systematic review on a topic related to geriatric nursing, the AgeLine Database would be included. The author of the review should consult with expert health science information specialists during the search. These specialists can locate more studies than less experienced researchers (Conn, Valentine, Cooper, & Rantz, 2003; Cook, Guyatt, & Ryan, 1993). The author must also search for additional published literature through the ancestry approach. This strategy is completed when the reference lists of articles are carefully reviewed for any additional articles that are pertinent to the review. Hand searches of journals in which other eligible articles have been found should also be completed. Locating all pertinent research reports is critical to enhancing external validity of the systematic review. External validity is the ability to generalize the findings from a study, in this case a systematic review, to another situation (e.g., your clinical practice).

The next phase of the systematic review involves evaluation of the literature (Cooper, 1998). Each piece of literature can be conceptualized as a subject, much like a subject in primary research. Each piece of literature is evaluated for its contribution to the problem and posed questions. A typical approach for data evaluation involves a data collection tool similar to the grid on the companion website that you are developing in the Apply What You Have Learned exercise. A table such as this is often created, where each evaluation criterion is listed and data that are extracted from each report are placed into the format. Depending upon the question to be answered by the systematic review, data evaluation may include gathering author, year, study purpose, research question/hypothesis, variables studied, sample size, sample age, setting, research design, research instruments used to measure each variable, instrument psychometrics, procedures used for data collection, and study results.

The next phase of the systematic review process is data analysis (Cooper, 1998). This stage is defined as "reducing the separate data collection points collected by the inquirer into a unified statement about the research problem" (Cooper, p. 104). The goal of the systematic review determines the data analysis approach used. On one hand, reviews of concepts, definitions, and methods are best summarized qualitatively. On the other hand, if the body of reports is still relatively small and quantitative results are reported, then descriptive statistics can be applied to the group of studies.

The final step of the systematic review is interpretation of the data and dissemination of the results (Cooper, 1998). The stated results should flow logically from the data presented in the systematic review. The problem and research questions should be answered from the data. Systematic reviews are written using a format similar to that used in primary research reports, including the introduction, methods, results, and discussion. Most often a table of the data collected from each study is included in the systematic review article.

There are two additional types of syntheses that are less rigorous than systematic reviews. These include the *traditional literature review* and the *integrative review*. A traditional literature review differs from a systematic review because when a literature review is conducted, the author typically does not go to the extreme lengths of obtaining all possible literature on a topic. When conducting a traditional literature review, the author may include only literature that supports a particular point, excluding reports that have conflicting findings. You are very familiar with the traditional literature review because this is the type of paper you write for many of your nursing courses.

CRITICAL THINKING EXERCISE 11-3

Locate a systematic review of the literature that addresses a topic pertinent to your patients. Evaluate the rigor of the study using the information presented in Table 11.1. How will you use the results of the systematic review to enhance the evidence that you use to provide the best care possible?

KEY TERMS

Meta-analyse:
Combination of
results of studies
that statistically
estimates the
effects of proposed
interventions

Practice guidelines:
Systematically
developed statements
for specific clinical
circumstances

Integrative reviews are more rigorous than traditional literature reviews but are not as rigorous as systematic reviews. Authors of integrative reviews seek only published reports, while systematic reviewers use a more rigorous method of obtaining both published and unpublished reports. Authors follow very methodical approaches for both types of reviews. Because the scope of integrative reviews is narrower, the findings are less likely to have external validity than the findings from a systematic review.

When the body of reports is large and homogeneous, a *meta-analysis* can be conducted. Meta-analysis is the most sophisticated synthesis of evidence. It is highly regarded because this method synthesizes a significant number of studies about the same phenomenon. In a meta-analysis, results of many studies are integrated through a statistical analysis process (Glass,1976). Like the systematic review, the author obtains both published and unpublished evidence. Authors may even contact researchers for their data to perform the analyis.

In nursing and other practice disciplines, an important kind of synthesis is *practice guidelines*. They are "systematically developed statements to assist practitioner and patient decisions about appropriate health care for specific clinical circumstances" (Institute of Medicine [IOM], 1990, p. 8). These guidelines are systematically created by a group of experienced experts and key affected groups who read, critique, and prioritize the pertinent evidence. Practice guidelines have been introduced into practice for several reasons. These consensus recommendations are developed for use in practice to improve patient and system outcomes. These tools seek to reduce variations in practice, resulting in more consistent care delivery by those who use the guidelines. Guidelines also enhance efficient use of resources that frequently result in reducing the cost of care delivery. Guidelines should have the following characteristics (IOM):

< Validity
< Reliability/reproducibility
< Clinical applicability
< Clinical flexibility
< Clarity

Nursing practice guidelines can be found at the Registered Nurses' Association of Ontario Nursing Best Practice Guidelines Program (www.rnao.org), the National Guideline Clearinghouse (www.guideline.gov), and the Royal College of Nursing (www.rcn.org.uk). Clinical practice guidelines may also be written and made available to educate and enhance decision making for the public. The guidelines can be very helpful to the layperson who is faced with making choices about health care.

CRITICAL THINKING EXERCISE 11-4

Locate a nursing clinical guideline and explore the process that was used to develop the guideline. How do you think the guideline changes practice patterns?

Understanding the process of clinical practice guideline development will assist in evaluating the merit of clinical practice guidelines. Depending upon the area of practice, the team of experts may be multidisciplinary in nature. Guidelines are typically focused on patient problems that involve many disciplines working toward similar patient goals. Practice guidelines may be created locally, nationally, or internationally. Often they are developed by professional organizations or federal agencies. Examples of professional organizations that have developed guidelines include the Gerontological Nursing Interventions Research Center (www.nursing.uiowa.edu/excellence/nursing_interventions), the Association of Women's Health, Obstetric and Neonatal Nurses (www.awhonn.org/awhonn/), the American Pain Society (www.ampainsoc.org), and the Oncology Nursing Society (www.ons.org). Systematic reviews of the literature are frequently used to assist a group of experts with integrating the larger body of literature pertinent to the practice guideline development. If current systematic reviews of the literature are not available, the experts must use the rigorous systematic review process for assimilating the body of literature to create practice guidelines. As new evidence is generated from primary research reports, systematic reviews of the literature and practice guidelines must be revised and updated. The Agency for Healthcare Research and Quality has developed a series of questions that can be used to guide systematic review updates (2007).

The Third S: Synopses

A synopsis is a brief description of evidence. Abstracts obtained through CINAHL and MEDLINE are essentially synopses. Within the last few years, a variety of evidence-based journals have emerged that provide synopses of valid and clinically useful studies (DiCenso et al., 2005; Melnyk & Fineout-Overholt, 2005; Straus, Richardson, Glasziou, & Haynes, 2005). While most of these require subscriptions, many websites allow guests access to some full-text articles. The medication alerts you may receive on your personal digital assistant (PDA) as updates to your drug book are another example of synopses.

The Fourth S: Summaries

Integrative summaries are addressed in the fourth level in the pyramid of evidence (Haynes, 2006). These can be found in several summary services such as BMJ Clinical Evidence (www.clinicalevidence.com/ceweb/index.jsp), the Agency for Healthcare Research and Quality's National Guideline Clearinghouse (www.guideline.gov), and Physicians' Information and Education Resource (pier.acponline.org/index.html?jhp; Haynes).

The Fifth S: Systems

If you deliver nursing care in a healthcare organization that has an integrated computerized decision support system, you have the system in place to implement evidence-based care (Haynes, 2006). This system model uses an electronic medical record that has integrated practice guidelines with patients' specific characteristics. Most healthcare providers do not practice in such an advanced healthcare system. Imagine a future when you would open the electronic medical record and you would receive pop-ups (like when surfing the Web) that you could click on to link to synopses of evidence that pertain to your patient.

TEST YOUR KNOWLEDGE 11-1

1. Which of the following are considered to be at the bottom of the pyramid of evidence?
   a. meta-analyses
   b. concept analyses
   c. synopses
   d. systems

2. The systematic review involves which of the following?
   a. methodical review of the literature
   b. obtaining published and unpublished sources
   c. creating a grid for summarizing data collection
   d. establishing inclusion criteria

How did you do? 1. b; 2. a, b, c, d

11.2 Using the Pyramid for EBP

At the end of this section, you will be able to:

< List interdisciplinary databases that can provide evidence for practice
< Use the 5Ss to locate evidence in a logical fashion

Because the purpose of EBP is to answer clinical questions, and the goal is to efficiently find information, nurses should begin the search for information at the top of the pyramid and work down the various levels. The best option is having a system already in place that brings the information to the nurse. However, because such systems are not very common, the next best source of evidence is integrative summaries. If you are unable to locate summaries of the evidence, you should attempt to locate synopses of the evidence in *Evidence-Based Nursing* (ebn.bmjjournals.com) or another selected evidence-based journal. If you are unable to find what you need there, you should look for systematic and other types of reviews of the literature. The Cochrane Library (www.cochrane.org) is a good place to begin. When none of these are available, you must rely on individual studies, case studies, and concept analyses. **Table 11-2** presents a multidisciplinary list of online resources that can assist in accessing all levels of evidence.

FYI

Because the purpose of EBP is to answer clinical questions, and the goal is to efficiently find information, nurses should begin the search for information at the top of the pyramid and work down the various levels. The best option is having a system already in place that brings the information to the medical record.

TABLE 11-2 Databases to Search for Evidence

BMJ Clinical Evidence

http://www.clinicalevidence.com/ceweb/index.jsp

BMJ Clinical Evidence presents summaries that address common or important clinical conditions seen in primary and hospital care and benefits and harms of preventive and therapeutic interventions. A rigorous process of developing the summaries is described. Drug safety alerts and links to national guidelines are included.

Physicians' Information and Education Resource (PIER)

http://pier.acponline.org/index.html?jhp

This site provides evidence-based guidance to improve clinical care. It is available to the American College of Physician members only. Topics include diseases, screening and prevention, complementary/alternative medicine, ethical/legal issues, procedures, quality measures, and drug resources.

Agency for Healthcare Research and Quality (AHRQ)

http://www.ahrq.gov

AHRQ works with 12 Evidence-Based Practice Centers that develop evidence reports and technology assessments on topics relevant to clinical, social science/behavioral, economic, and other healthcare organization and delivery topics. Professional societies, health plans, insurers, employers, and patient groups can nominate topics. AHRQ sponsors a National Guideline Clearinghouse at www.guideline.gov.

Evidence-Based Nursing

http://ebn.bmj.com/

Evidence-Based Nursing presents abstracts of selected research with an expert commentary on its clinical application.

Evidence-Based Medicine

http://ebm.bmj.com/

Evidence-Based Medicine presents abstracts of international medical journals with commentary on its clinical application to primary medicine.

The Cochrane Library

http://www.thecochranelibrary.com

The Cochrane Library provides systematic reviews related to clinical topics. The complete reviews are available by subscription, either on CD-ROM or via the Internet. Abstracts of the reviews are available on the website.

The Community Guide to Preventive Services

http://www.thecommunityguide.org

The Community Guide to Preventive Services is a multidisciplinary, independent, nonfederal group that develops evidence-based practice guidelines for community preventive services.

U.S. Preventive Services Task Force

http://www.ahrq.gov/clinic/uspstfix.htm

The U.S. Preventive Services Task Force, sponsored by AHRQ, systematically reviews the evidence of effectiveness of a wide range of clinical preventive services, including screening tests, counseling, immunizations, and chemoprophylaxis.

DynaMed

http://www.ebscohost.com/dynamed/

DynaMed provides clinically organized summaries of nearly 1,800 evidence-based topics for use at the point of care via the Internet and/or PDA.

First CONSULT

http://www.firstconsult.com/fc_home/public/

FirstCONSULT supports clinical decision making by providing concise, readable summaries of evidence that relates to patient care.

UpToDate

http://www.uptodate.com/

UpToDate provides evidence-based clinical information to a variety of clinicians on the Internet, CD-ROM, and Pocket PC.

InfoPOEMs

http://www.infopoems.com/index.cfm

InfoPOEMs (Patient-Oriented Evidence that Matters) is a searchable database from the *Journal of Family Practice*. POEMs are summaries similar to ACP Journal Club articles in methodology and format that are targeted at family practitioners.

Health Services/Technology Assessment Text

http://www.ncbi.nlm.nih.gov/books/bv.fcgi?rid=hstat

The Health Services/Technology Assessment Text is a free, Web-based resource of full-text documents including guidelines that provide health information and support healthcare decision making for healthcare providers, health service researchers, policymakers, payers, consumers, and the information professionals who serve these groups.

National Research Register

http://www.dh.gov.uk/en/Aboutus/Researchanddevelopment/AtoZ/DH_4002357

The National Research Register is a database of ongoing and recently completed research projects funded by, or of interest to, the United Kingdom's National Health Service.

Physiotherapy Evidence Database
http://www.pedro.org.au/
PEDro is the Physiotherapy Evidence Database, which was developed to provide rapid access to bibliographic details and abstracts of randomized controlled trials, systematic reviews, and evidence-based clinical practice guidelines in physiotherapy.

Primary Care Clinical Practice Guidelines
http://medicine.ucsf.edu/education/resed/ebm/practice_guidelines.html
This site, compiled by Peter Sam at the UCSF School of Medicine, includes all guidelines, evidence-based, consensus, practice parameters, protocols, and other resources such as integrative studies, meta-analyses, critically appraised topics, and review articles.

SUMSearch
http://sumsearch.org/
SUMSearch provides references to answer clinical questions about diagnosis, etiology, prognosis, and therapy (plus physical findings, adverse treatment effects, and screening/prevention) by searching sources such as Merck Manual, MEDLINE, National Guideline Clearinghouse from AHRQ, Database of Abstracts of Reviews of Effects, and PubMed.

TRIP Database
http://www.tripdatabase.com/index.html
This site supports evidence-based practice by presenting evidence summaries for healthcare providers.

Joanna Briggs Institute
http://www.joannabriggs.edu.au/about/home.php
The Joanna Briggs Institute is an International Research and Development Unit of Royal Adelaide Hospital, and an Affiliated Institute of the University of Adelaide that supports the development and dissemination of international systematic reviews and summaries of best practices to consumers, healthcare professionals, and all levels of the healthcare systems, governments, and service provider units.

CRITICAL THINKING EXERCISE 11-5

Consider each of the types of evidence and how to locate each type. How will you integrate the use of these other sources of evidence into your practice?

TEST YOUR KNOWLEDGE 11-2

1. Put the following sources of evidence in order, beginning at the top of the pyramid of evidence.

   a. synopses

   b. systems

   c. studies

   d. summaries

   e. syntheses

How did you do? 1. b, d, a, e, c

11.3   Keeping It Ethical

At the end of this section, you will be able to:

< Discuss one ethical dilemma when using other sources of evidence

Fortunately, few ethical dilemmas arise when considering use of evidence. Care must be taken to label evidence correctly and to be true to the process of review. Shortcuts should not be taken when searching for evidence, and attention to detail is critical. On occasion, an author might mislabel the type of review conducted because there are many commonalities. Authors sometimes generalize beyond the scope of the evidence or ignore limitations of studies. It is therefore important for you to critically read and be familiar with the various types of review to determine for yourself the usefulness of the findings.

FYI

Fortunately, few ethical dilemmas arise when considering use of evidence. When finding evidence that can be applied to practice, changes must be considered carefully because lives are at stake; however, it is unethical to *not* adopt practice guidelines when the evidence is clear.

TEST YOUR KNOWLEDGE 11-3

True/False

1. Nurses are ethically obligated to follow practice guidelines.

2. Authors who publish their work in professional journals never draw conclusions beyond their findings.

How did you do? 1. T; 2. F

It is normal to become excited when finding evidence that can be applied to practice. Such enthusiasm makes providing nursing care stimulating. On one hand, practice changes must be considered carefully because lives are at stake. On the other hand, it is unethical to not adopt practice guidelines when the evidence is clear. Our nursing efforts must focus on providing the best care to achieve optimum patient outcomes, with the least variation in practice, in a resource conscientious manner while integrating the evidence with patient preferences. Using other sources of evidence upon which to base your nursing practice will enhance your abilities to achieve these goals.

 RAPID **REVIEW**

- Propositional knowledge is the science of nursing, and nonpropositional knowledge is the art of nursing.

- The pyramid of evidence is an organizing framework that explains the importance of various levels of evidence. It uses the 5Ss: studies, syntheses, synopses, summaries, and systems.

- Syntheses include case studies, concept analyses, systematic reviews, traditional literature reviews, integrative reviews, and meta-analyses.

- Case studies provide great detail about phenomena for which little is known.

- Concept analyses are an example of a synthesis. Nurses use them to clarify understanding about concepts that are important in patient care.

- Meta-syntheses combine the results of multiple qualitative studies about the same topic.

- While all reviews require searching for evidence, the amount and kind of evidence included varies among the types of reviews.

APPLY WHAT YOU HAVE LEARNED

Your committee has found some additional articles. They are not reports about research studies, yet they contain some very pertinent information about medication errors. The article by Benjamin (2003) provides case studies that vividly illustrate the ramifications of making a medication error. The systematic review by Lanksbear, Sheldon, and Maynard (2005) summarizes findings from several international studies about medication errors. A very interesting strategy is presented in the Web-based article by Murphy (2006). Read these articles and complete the grid on the companion website for each of them. Look to the Rich (2005) article as an example.

Practice guidelines are developed by experts who systematically review the literature and develop recommendations about patient care.

Nurses can use synopses, summaries, and systems to efficiently obtain evidence for practice.

To avoid ethical dilemmas, nurses must critically read and be familiar with the various types of review to determine the usefulness of the findings.

REFERENCES

Agency for Healthcare Research and Quality. (2007). *Updating systematic reviews.* Retrieved September 12, 2010, from http://www.ahrq.gov/clinic/tp/sysrevtp.htm

Beck, C. T. (2009). Metasynthesis: A goldmine for evidence-based practice. *AORN, 90,* 701–702, 705–710.

Benjamin, D. M. (2003). Reducing medication errors and increasing patient safety: Case studies in clinical pharmacology. *Journal of Clinical Pharmacology, 43,* 768–783.

Conn, V. S., Valentine, J. C., Cooper, H. M., & Rantz, M. J. (2003). Grey literature in meta-analyses. *Nursing Research, 52,* 256–261.

Cook, D. J., Guyatt, G. H., & Ryan, G. (1993). Should unpublished data be included in meta-analyses? *JAMA, 269,* 749–753.

Cooper, H. M. (1998). *Synthesizing research: A guide for literature reviews* (3rd ed., Vol. 2). Thousand Oaks, CA: Sage.

DiCenso, A., Ciliska, D., Marks, S., McKibbon, A., Cullum, N., & Thompson, C. (2005). Evidence-based nursing. In S. E. Straus, W. S. Richardson, P. Glasziou, & R. B. Haynes, *Evidence-based medicine: How to practice and teach EBM* (3rd ed.; electronic media). Edinburgh, Scotland: Churchill Livingstone.

Encarta Dictionary. (n.d.). *MSN Encarta*. Retrieved November 8, 2010, from http://encarta.msn.com/encnet/features/dictionary/DictionaryResults.aspx?lextype=3&search=systematic

Glass, G. V. (1976). Primary, secondary, and meta-analysis of research. *Educational Researcher, 5*, 3–8.

Haynes, R. B. (2006). Of studies, syntheses, synopses, summaries, and systems: The "5S" evolution of information services for evidence-based health care decisions [Editorial]. *ACP Journal, 145*(3), A8.

Institute of Medicine. (1990). *Clinical practice guidelines: Directions for a new program*. Washington, DC: National Academies Press.

Lanksbear, A. J., Sheldon, T. A., & Maynard, A. (2005). Nurse staffing and healthcare outcomes: A systematic review of the international research evidence. *Advances in Nursing Science, 28*, 163–174.

Melnyk, B. M., & Fineout-Overholt, E. (2005). *Evidence-based practice in nursing and healthcare: A guide to best practice*. Philadelphia: Lippincott Williams & Wilkins.

Murphy, K. (2006, October 31). What pilots can teach hospitals about patient safety. *New York Times*. Retrieved September 12, 2010, from http://www.nytimes.com/2006/10/31/health/31safe.html?ex=1319950800&en=a64123f3e689ea9f&ei=5088&partner=rssnyt&emc=rss

Rich, V. L. (2005). How we think about medication errors: A model and a charge for nurses. *AJN, 105*(3) (Suppl.), 10–11.

Rogers, B. L., & Knafl, K. A. (2000). *Concept development in nursing: Foundations, techniques, and applications* (2nd ed.). Philadelphia: Saunders.

Rycroft-Malone, J., Seers, K., Titchen, A., Harvey, G., Kitson, A., & McCormack, B. (2004). What counts as evidence in evidence-based practice? *Journal of Advanced Nursing, 47*(1), 81–90.

Straus, S. E., Richardson, W. S., Glasziou, P., & Haynes, R. B. (2005). *Evidence-based medicine: How to practice and teach EBM* (3rd ed.). Edinburgh, Scotland: Churchill Livingstone.

Walker, L., & Avant, K. (2005). *Strategies for theory construction in nursing* (4th ed.). Upper Saddle River, NJ: Pearson Prentice Hall.

Yin, R. K. (2003). *Case study research: Design and methods* (3rd ed.). Thousand Oaks, CA: Sage.

Decision

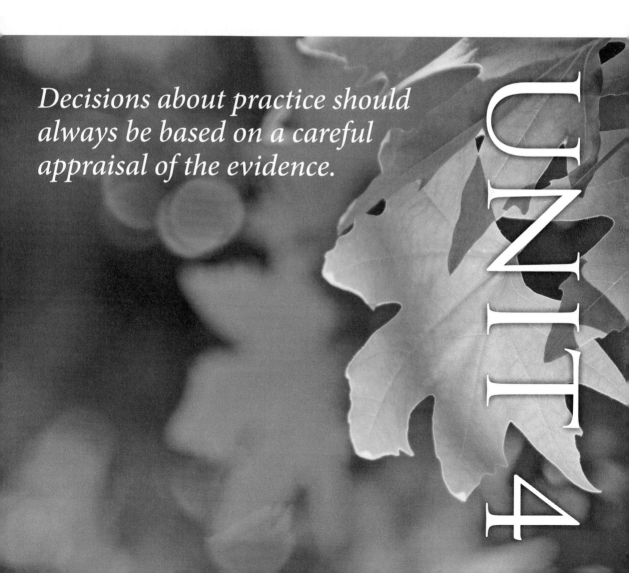

Decisions about practice should always be based on a careful appraisal of the evidence.

UNIT 4

CHAPTER OBJECTIVES

At the end of this chapter, you will be able to:

< Define statistics
< Differentiate between descriptive and inferential statistics
< Identify how frequencies can be graphically depicted
< Describe measures of central tendency and their uses
< Name patterns of data distribution correctly
< Describe measures of variability and their use
< Discuss the purpose of inferential statistical tests
< Explain how statistical testing is related to chance
< Distinguish between type I and type II errors
< Describe alpha levels commonly used in nursing research
< Match common notations with associated statistical tests

< Identify common statistical tests as parametric or nonparametric
< Describe tests used to determine statistically significant differences among groups
< Discuss tests used to determine statistically significant differences among variables
< Assign commonly used statistical tests to examples based on type of research question and level of measurement
< Interpret data reported in statistical tables
< Differentiate between statistical significance and clinical significance
< Appraise data analysis sections of an article
< Discuss ethical considerations when conducting statistical analyses

KEY TERMS

alpha level
amodal
analysis of variance
bimodal
bivariate analysis
Chi square
coefficient of variation
confidence intervals
correlated t test
correlation coefficients
degrees of freedom
descriptive statistics
direction
heterogeneous
homogeneous
independent t test
inferential statistics
kurtosis
magnitude

mean
measures of central tendency
measures of variability
median
modality
mode
multiple regression
negatively skewed
nonparametric
nonsignificant
normal distribution
parametric
Pearson's r
percentage distributions
percentile
population parameters
position of the median
positively skewed

probability.
range
Rule of 68-95-99.7
sample statistics
sampling distribution
sampling error
semiquartile range
skewed
standard deviation
statistically significant
statistics
Statistics
t statistic
tailedness
type I error
type II error
unimodal
univariate analysis
z scores

CHAPTER 12

What Do the Quantitative Data Mean?

Rosalind M. Peters, Nola A. Schmidt, and Moira Fearncombe

12.1   Using Statistics to Describe the Sample

At the end of this section, you will be able to:

< Define statistics
< Differentiate between descriptive and inferential statistics

Originally the term *statistics* referred to information about the government because the word is derived from the Latin "statisticum," meaning "of the state." It was given its numerical meaning in 1749 when Gottfried Achenwall, a German political scientist, used the term to designate the analysis of *data* about the *state* (Wikitionary, 2007). Currently there are two meanings of the term "statistics." *Statistics*, with a capital S, is used to describe the branch of mathematics that collects, analyzes, interprets, and presents numerical data in terms of samples and populations, while *statistics*, with a lowercase s, is used to describe the numerical outcomes and the probabilities derived from calculations on raw data.

There are two types of statistics: descriptive and inferential (Munro, 2004). Oftentimes both types are presented in research reports. *Descriptive statistics* deal with the collection and presentation of data used to explain characteristics of variables found in a sample. As its name implies, descriptive statistics describe, summarize, and synthesize collected data. Calculations and information presented with

Statistics: Describes the branch of mathematics that collects, analyzes, interprets, and presents numerical data in terms of samples and populations

statistics: Describes the numerical outcomes and probabilities derived from calculations on raw data

Descriptive statistics: Collection and presentation of data that explain characteristics of variables

Inferential statistics: Analysis of data as the basis for prediction related to the phenomenon of interest

Population parameters: Characteristics of a population inferred from characteristics of a sample

Sample statistics: Numerical data describing characteristics of the sample

Univariate analysis: The use of statistical tests to provide information about one variable

Bivariate analysis: The use of statistics to describe the relationship between two variables

descriptive statistics must be accurate. *Inferential statistics* involve analysis of data as the basis for predictions related to the phenomenon of interest. Inferential statistics are used to make inferences or draw conclusions about a population based on a sample. They are used to develop *population parameters* from the *sample statistics*. For example, a researcher conducted a study on the efficiency of vitamin C in preventing the common cold. Descriptive statistics would be used to report that 60% of subjects in the experimental group had fewer colds than subjects receiving the placebo. The researcher would then use inferential statistics to determine if the difference in the number of colds between the two groups was statistically significant. If it was, then it could be inferred that taking vitamin C would be advantageous. Descriptive statistics are used to provide information regarding univariate or bivariate analyses.

Univariate analysis is conducted to present organized information about only one variable at a time and includes information regarding frequency distributions, measures of central tendency, shape of the distribution, and measures of variability, sometimes known as dispersion. *Bivariate analysis* is performed to describe the relationship between two variables that can be expressed in contingency tables or with other statistical tests.

The results of descriptive analysis are frequently presented in table format, and scientific notations are often used. Therefore it may be helpful to review common notations used in tables as shown in **Table 12-1**.

TABLE 12-1 **Statistical Symbols for Descriptive Statistics**

Symbol/Abbreviation	Definition
f	Frequency
M	Mean
Mdn	Median
n	Number in subsample
N	Total number in a sample
%	Percentage
SD	Standard deviation
z	A standard score

TEST YOUR KNOWLEDGE 12-1

1. To describe the frequency of the single variable myocardial infarction in adults ages 30–49, which of the following could be used?

    a. descriptive statistics

    b. inferential statistics

    c. univariate analysis

    d. bivariate analysis

How did you do? 1. a, c

FYI

There are two types of statistics: descriptive and inferential. Descriptive statistics describe, summarize, and synthesize collected data, while inferential statistics involve analysis of data as the basis for predictions related to the phenomenon of interest.

12.2   Using Frequencies to Describe Samples

At the end of this section, you will be able to:

‹ Identify how frequencies can be graphically depicted

Information about the frequency, or how often, a variable is found to occur may be presented as either ungrouped or grouped data. Ungrouped data are primarily used to present nominal and ordinal data, while grouped data are used to present interval and ratio level data. **Table 12-2** provides an example of how categorical data about a sample may be presented in ungrouped format.

Ungrouped data are rarely presented when reporting on continuous variables such as age, scores on scales, time, or physiologic variables (e.g., temperature, blood pressure, cell counts). For example, if readers of an article were presented with a set of ages for 20 different patients, it would be difficult to make sense of this raw data (see **Table 12-3**). However, if the numbers were arranged in a frequency distribution and graphed, they would make much more sense to the readers. Before a graph can be constructed, the researcher must create a frequency distribution table. First, the raw data are sorted, usually in ascending order. Next, the number of times each value occurs is tallied, and the frequency of each event is recorded in the table. Table 12-3 shows how the raw data can be organized to more clearly present the information. The table shows how raw data are tallied and the resulting frequencies and percentages

TABLE 12-2 **Example of Categorical Data Presented in Ungrouped Format**

Variable	n(P)
Gender	
Men	14 (41)
Women	20 (59)
Annual income	
<$10,000	4 (11.7)
$10,000–24,999	7 (20.6)
$25,000–49,999	7 (20.6)
> $50,000	9 (26.5)
No answer	7 (20.6)
Self-care behaviors	
Current smoker	7 (18)
Alcohol > 1 drink/day	0 (0)
Exercise	
No regular exercise	9 (27)
1–2 days/week	10 (29)
3–4 days/week	8 (24)
≥ 5 days/week	5 (15)

are recorded. The left-hand side of the table shows the frequency with which individual age data occur. Because all possible data points are presented, it is still somewhat difficult to comprehend this presentation of the ungrouped data. The right-hand side of the table shows a grouped frequency and percentage distribution with the ages grouped in 2-year increments. It should be obvious that the grouped data are more meaningful than either the raw or ungrouped data.

While there are few fixed rules regarding how and when to group data, it is imperative that there be no overlap of categories. Each group must have a well defined lower and upper limit so that the groups are mutually exclusive, yet the groups must include all data collected. For example, if the groupings in Table 12-3 had been 18–20 and 20–22, people who are 20 years old would have been counted in both groups, and the statistics would have been compromised. Group size also should be consistent. If the groups had been 18–20 (a 3-year span), 21–25 (a 4-year span), and over 25 (a 3-year span), then inaccurate analysis of data would occur. While grouping data might make it easier

TABLE 12-3 Example of Frequency and Percentage Distributions of Ages

Raw Data
18 18 18 19 19 19 20 21 21 21 21 21 22 22 22 23 23 25 27 28

	Ungrouped Data				Grouped Data		
Age	Tally	Frequency	Percent	Age	Tally	Frequency	Percent
18	|||	3	15	18–19	++++		6	30
19	|||	3	15	20–21	++++		6	30
20			1	5	22–23	++++	5	25
21	++++	5	25	24–25			1	5
22	|||	3	15	>25	||	2	10
23	||	2	10	**Total**		**20**	**100**
25			1	5				
27			1	5				
28			1	5				
Total		**20**	**100**				

to understand, it also results in some loss of information. The grouped data presented in Table 12-3 indicate that 30% of the subjects were between 20 and 21 years of age; however, there is no way of knowing that most subjects (five of the six) were 21, and only one subject was 20 years of age.

In addition to frequency distributions, *percentage distributions* are often used to present descriptive statistics. A percentage distribution is calculated by dividing the frequency of an event by the total number of events. For example, in Table 12-3 the three 18-year-old subjects in the study represent 15% of the total number of subjects reported. Providing information about percentages is another way to group data to make results more comprehensible and allow for easier comparisons with other studies.

After data are tallied and a frequency distribution is determined, data may be converted to graphic form. Graphs provide a visual representation of data and often make it easier to discern trends. The most common types of graphs are line charts, bar graphs, pie charts, histograms, and scattergrams (or scatterplots). **Figure 12-1** depicts two different ways to present the age data from Table 12-3.

KEY TERM

Percentage distributions: Descriptive statistic used to group data to make results more comprehensible

FIGURE 12-1 **Frequency Polygon and Histogram of Age Data**

Frequency Polygon for Grouped Age Data

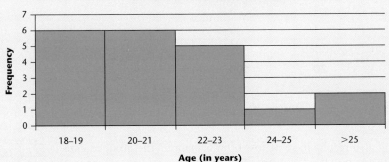

Histogram for Grouped Age Data

TEST YOUR KNOWLEDGE 12-2

True/False

1. Frequency distributions are an effective way to present inferential statistics.

2. Categories in grouped data must be mutually exclusive.

3. Percentages are often used to describe characteristics of samples.

4. The total number of subjects in a sample is represented by the symbol n.

How did you do? 1. F; 2. T; 3. T; 4. F

12.3 Measures of Central Tendency

At the end of this section, you will be able to:

< Describe measures of central tendency and their uses

Another method used to describe raw data is the *measures of central tendency*. These measures provide information about the "typical" case to be found in the data. The mean, median, and mode are the three terms most commonly used to describe the tendency of data to cluster around the middle of the data set (i.e., "averages" for the data). The mean and median are used to describe continuous level data, while the mode is used to describe both continuous and nominal level data. Because the mean and median may be calculated values, they can be rounded to the nearest number; however, the mode is never rounded because it is an actual data point.

Mode

The *mode* is the easiest measure of central tendency to determine because it is the most frequently occurring value in a data set. It is the highest tally when counting and is the highest frequency in a distribution table. *Modality* refers to the number of modes found in a data distribution. Data can be *amodal* (without a mode), *unimodal* (with one mode), or *bimodal* (with two modes). There is no specific term to indicate when data have more than two modes. The mode does not mean that a data value occurs more than once in a frequency distribution because the mode is an actual data point. The mode is not affected by the existence of any extreme values in the data. **Table 12-4** demonstrates

KEY TERMS

Measures of central tendency: Measures (e.g., mean, median, mode) that provide information about the typical case

Mode: The most frequently occurring value in a data set

Modality: The number of modes found in a data distribution

Amodal: A data set that does not have a mode

Unimodal: A data set with one mode such as a normal distribution

Bimodal: A data set with two modes

TABLE 12-4 **Mode**

Data Points	Type of Mode	Location of Mode
{0, 1, 2, 3}	amodal	N/A
{0, 1, 2, 2}	unimodal	2
{1, 1, 2, 2}	bimodal	1 and 2
{1, 1, 1, 2, 2}	unimodal	1
{1, 1, 1, 2, 596}	unimodal	1

how the change in just one data point affects the modality of the data. Using the age data presented in Table 12-3, note that the ungrouped data are unimodal with the mode being 21. However, when the data are grouped, they become bimodal with modes at 18–19 years as well as 20–21 years of age (**Table 12-5**). It is easy to see the modes on the frequency polygon and histogram in Figure 12-1 because the modes have the highest peaks and tallest bars. The mode is considered to be an unstable measure of central tendency because it tends to vary widely from one sample to the next. Given its instability, the mode is rarely presented as the sole measure of central tendency.

Median

The *median* is the center of the data set. Just as the median of the road divides the highway into two halves, the median of a data set divides data in half. If there are an odd number of data points, the median is the middle value or the score where exactly 50% of the data lie above the median and 50% of the data lie below it. If there is an even number of values in the data set, the median is the average of the two middle-most values and as such may be a number not actually found in the data set. The median actually refers to the average position in the data, and it is minimally affected by the existence of an outlier.

The *position of the median* is calculated by using the formula $(n + 1)/2$, where *n* is the number of data values in the set. It is important to remember

TABLE 12-5 Mode of Age Data for 20 Subjects

Ungrouped Data			Grouped Data		
Age	Tally	Frequency	Age	Tally	Percent
18	|||	3	18–19	⸗⸗		6
19	|||	3	20–21	⸗⸗		6
20			1	22–23	⸗⸗	5
21	⸗⸗	5	24–25			1
22	|||	3	>25	||	2
23	||	2	**Total**		**20**
25			1			
27			1			
28			1			
Total		**20**			

that this formula only gives the position, and not the actual value, of the median. For example, in a study describing the number of hours that five ($n = 5$) sedentary subjects spent watching television last week, the following data were collected: {5, 7, 3, 38, 7} hours. To determine the median, the researcher would perform a number of easy steps.

1. Sort the data. 3 5 7 7 38
2. Determine the median's location. The median is at the $(5 + 1)/2$, or third, position from either end.
3. Count over three places to find that the median is 7. In this example, 7 is also the mode.

If the data set is changed to {3, 5, 7, 7}, then the position of the median would be 2.5 or halfway between the second and third sorted data points. In this example, the median is 6, and 7 is the mode. If the data set is changed again to include {3, 5, 7, 100}, the position of the median still will be 2.5 or halfway between the second and third sorted data points, and the median remains 6. This example demonstrates that the outlier value of 100 did not affect the median value. For this reason, the median is generally used to describe average when there is an extreme value in the data.

When data are grouped, the median is determined using cumulative frequencies. In **Table 12-6** age data are reported for 20 subjects. The median is

FYI

The three most commonly used measures of central tendency are the mean, median, and mode. The mean and median are used to describe continuous level data, while the mode is used to describe both continuous and nominal level data.

TABLE 12-6 Median of Age Data for 20 Subjects

Ungrouped Data				Grouped Data			
Age	Tally	Frequency	Cumulative Frequency	Age	Tally	Frequency	Cumulative Frequency
18	|	3	3	18–19	⊢⊣⊣⊣ |	6	6
19	|||	3	6	20–21	⊢⊣⊣⊣ |	6	12
20	|	1	7	22–23	⊢⊣⊣⊣	5	17
21	⊢⊣⊣⊣	5	12	24–25	|	1	18
22	|||	3	15	>25	||	2	20
23	||	2	17	**Total**		**20**	
25	|	1	18				
27	|	1	19				
28	|	1	20				
Total		**20**					

located at $(20 + 1)/2$, the 11.5th position, and it is the average of the 11th and 12th data values. Using the ungrouped data, the median would be 21 years old, while the grouped median would be 20–21 years.

Mean

When people refer to an average, what they are really referring to is the *mean*. The mean is calculated by adding all of the data values and then dividing by the total number of values. The mean is the most commonly used measure of central tendency. It is greatly affected by the existence of outliers because every value in the data set is included in the calculation. The larger the sample size, the less an outlier will affect the mean. For example, using the previous data example about number of hours spent watching television, subjects reported watching 5, 7, 3, 38, and 7 hours of television per week. Using these data, the mean is calculated to be 12 hours ($60 / 5 = 12$). However, 12 hours does not present a clear picture of the amount of television watched by most subjects because the one extreme value of 38 hours skews the data. Because the mean is the measure of central tendency used in many tests of statistical significance, it is imperative for researchers to evaluate data for outliers before performing statistical analyses. When reading articles in which averages are used, nurses must carefully examine the conclusions drawn. For example, suppose a nursing unit employs five staff nurses and a nursing manager. Annual salaries of these employees are $26,500, $26,500, $27,000, $28,000, and $29,000. The nursing manager earns $123,000. During contract negotiations, nurses indicate that they need a raise. One individual claims the "average" salary is $27,000 per year (median), while another says the "average" salary is $26,500 (the mode). When confronted by the administration, the nurse manager responds by saying the "average" salary is actually $43,333.33 (mean). So who is correct? In fact, they are all correct. They are just using different meanings of "average." This example demonstrates how easy it is to manipulate statistics and why careful attention must be given to the interpretation of data being presented. When appraising evidence, it is helpful to remember that the mean is the best measure of central tendency if there are no extreme values, and the median is best if there are extreme values. Because they are calculated, the mean and median are not necessarily actual data values, although the mode must be an exact data point. The mean and median are unique values (again, because they are calculated), but the mode might be unique, might not exist at all, or there might be multiple modes. The mean is greatly affected by extreme values, the median is marginally affected, and the mode is not affected. The mean and median use continuous level data values for their calculations, while the mode can use either continuous or nominal data values. The mean is the most stable in that if repeated samples were drawn from the same population, the mean would vary less than either the median or the mode from sample to sample.

TEST YOUR KNOWLEDGE 12-3

1. The most frequent data value in a set of data is the
   a. mean.
   b. median.
   c. mode.
   d. average.

2. When data have no outliers, researchers prefer to report the
   a. mean.
   b. median.
   c. mode.
   d. magnitude.

How did you do? 1. c; 2. a

Because it is the most stable, the mean is most often used when computing other statistics. The median is used when the center of a data set is desired, and the mode is used to determine the most typical case.

12.4   Distribution Patterns

At the end of this section, you will be able to:

< Name patterns of data distribution correctly

Normal Distributions: Symmetrical Shapes

Measures of central tendencies are used to define distribution patterns. When the distribution of the data is symmetrical (that is, when the two halves of the distribution are folded over, they would be superimposed on each other and therefore be unimodal), then the mean, median, and mode are equal. In this situation, the data are considered to be normally distributed. A *normal distribution* has a distinctive bell-shaped curve and is symmetric about the

KEY TERM

Normal distribution: Data representation with a distinctive bell-shaped curve, symmetric about the mean

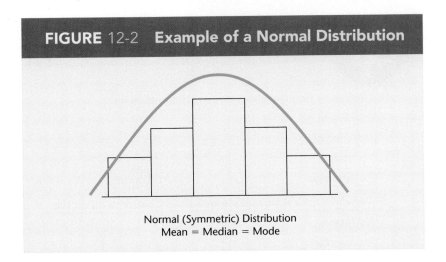

FIGURE 12-2 **Example of a Normal Distribution**

Normal (Symmetric) Distribution
Mean = Median = Mode

mean. In **Figure 12-2**, note that the decreasing bars, or area under the curve, indicate that the data cluster at the center and taper away from the mean. A number of human traits, such as intelligence and height, are considered to be normally distributed in the population.

When Data Are Not Normally Distributed

Often data do not fit a normal distribution and are considered to be asymmetric or *skewed*. In asymmetric distributions, the peak of the data is not at the center of the distribution, and one tail is longer than the other. Skewed distributions are usually discussed in terms of their direction. If the longer tail is pointing to the left, the data are considered to be *negatively skewed* (**Figure 12-3**). In this situation, the mean is less than the median and mode. For example, a group of students take a test for which all but one student studied. The one student, who did not study, scores very low. This low score, because it is an outlier, affects the mean because the scores of students who studied are high. This outlier contributes to a negatively skewed distribution. The low score pulls down the mean and pulls with it the tail of the distribution to the left. If the mean is greater than the median and mode, then the data are *positively skewed*, pulling the tail to the right. For example, an instructor gives a difficult test. Only one or two students scored high on the test. The rest of the students' scores were low. Most students' scores are lower than the mean because the outliers affect the mean. The distribution of these scores is positively skewed. The extremely high scores pull up the mean and pull the tail in a positive direction (**Figure 12-4**).

KEY TERMS

Skewed: An asymmetrical distribution of data

Negatively skewed: A distribution when the mean is less than the median and the mode

Positively skewed: Distribution when the mean is greater than the median and the mode

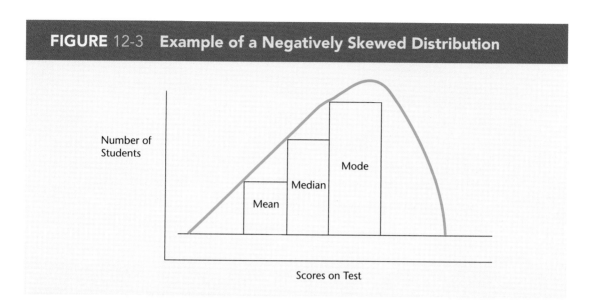

FIGURE 12-3 **Example of a Negatively Skewed Distribution**

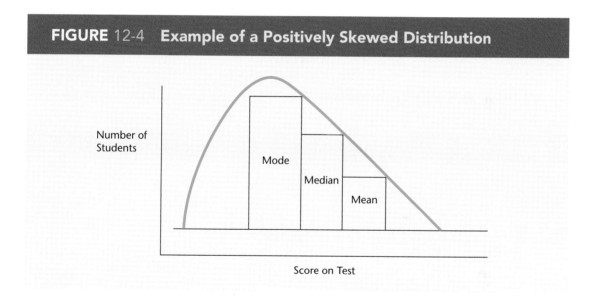

FIGURE 12-4 **Example of a Positively Skewed Distribution**

Attention should be given to how the data are spread, or dispersed, around the mean. Just as school children or military personnel wear uniforms to be like each other, uniform data have very little spread and look like each other. When there is greater variation in data, a wider spread results. When looking at graphic representations of data (see **Figure 12-5**), highly uniform data have a high peak and highly variable data have a low peak. *Kurtosis* is the term used to describe the peakedness or flatness of a data set.

KEY TERM

Kurtosis: The peakedness or flatness of a distribution of data

FIGURE 12-5 **Example of Kurtosis**

High Uniformity   Moderate Uniformity   Low Uniformity

TEST YOUR KNOWLEDGE 12-4

True/False

1. If the tail of a distribution is skewed to the left, the data are negatively skewed.

2. In a normal distribution, the mean, median, and mode are the same value.

3. If data are highly uniform, a low peak will be observed in a graphic representation of the data.

How did you do? 1. T; 2. T; 3. F

12.5 Measures of Variability

At the end of this section, you will be able to:

‹ Describe measures of variability and their use

KEY TERM

Measures of variability: Measures providing information about differences among data within a set

Measures of variability provide information regarding how different the data are within a set. These can also be known as measures of dispersion because they provide information about how data are dispersed around the mean. If the data are very similar, there is little variability, and the data are considered to be *homogeneous*. If there is wide variation, the data are considered to be *heterogeneous*. Common measures of variation include range, semiquartile

TABLE 12-7 Example of Ranges of Income		
	Control	**Experimental**
	$30,000	$15,000
	$38,000	$23,000
	$42,000	$42,000
	$57,000	$57,000
	$73,000	$103,000
Range	$43,000	$88,000

range, percentile, and standard deviation. Z scores and variance are used to compare the variability among data using different units of measure.

Range

A statistical *range* is the difference between the maximum and minimum values in a data set. Because the range is very sample specific, it is considered to be an unstable measure of variability. **Table 12-7** shows the income reported for subjects in the experimental and control groups of a study designed to evaluate health literacy. The mean for both data sets is $48,000, and the medians are each $42,000. However, the data are quite different because the data for the experimental group are more heterogeneous than for the control group. The experimental group's income varies from a minimum of $15,000 to a maximum of $103,000, with a range of $88,000. The control group's income has a minimum of $30,000 and a maximum of $73,000. While salaries are still quite variable, they are more uniform than the experimental group's salaries because their range is $43,000. When comparing like data, the smaller the range, the more uniform the data, and the greater the range, the more variable the data will be.

Semiquartile Range

Just as the median divides data into two halves, there are other values that divide these halves in half, meaning into quarters. The *semiquartile range* is the range of the middle 50% of the data. **Figure 12-6** illustrates the semiquartile range of the age data from a previous example. The semiquartile range lies between the lower (first) and upper (third) quartile of ages. The first quartile value is the median of the lower half of the data set; one fourth of the data lie below the first quartile and three fourths of the data lie above it. The third

FYI

The most commonly reported measure of variability, the standard deviation, is the measure of the average deviations of a value from the mean in a given data set. Because standard deviations are based on the mean of the data set, information collected using different measurement scales cannot be directly compared.

FIGURE 12-6   **Semiquartile Range of Age Data**

18 18 18 19 19 | 19 20 21 21 21 | 21 21 22 22 22 | 23 23 25 27 28

$Q_1=19$ Median=21 $Q_3=22.5$

---

quartile value is the median of the upper half of the data; three fourths of the data lie below the third quartile and one fourth of the data lie above it. The semiquartile range is the difference between the third and first quartile values and describes the middle half of a data distribution. In Figure 12-6, note that 50% of the data lie between 19 and 22.5, and the range is 3.5.

Percentile

A *percentile* is a measure or rank. Each percentile represents the percentage of cases that a given value exceeds. The median is the 50th percentile, the first quartile is the 25th percentile, and the third quartile is the 75th percentile score in a given data set. For example, if a newborn baby boy's weight is in the 39th percentile, he would weigh more than 39% of babies tested but less than 61% of the other babies.

Standard Deviation

The most commonly reported measure of variability is *standard deviation,* which is based on deviations from the mean of the data. While the mean is the expectation value (the expected "average" of the data set), the standard deviation is the measure of the average deviations of a value from the mean in a given data set. Because it is a measure of deviation from the mean, a standard deviation should always be reported with a mean. Standard deviation is based on the normal curve and is used to determine the number of data values that fall within a specific interval in a normal distribution. Understanding the stan-

---

CRITICAL THINKING EXERCISE 12-1

Consider how your ACT or SAT scores were reported. What was your raw score? What was your percentile? What do these data indicate about your performance on these tests?

TABLE 12-8 Standard Deviations of Income

	Control	Experimental
	$30,000	$15,000
	$38,000	$23,000
	$42,000	$42,000
	$57,000	$57,000
	$73,000	$103,000
SD	$17,073.37	$34,842.50

dard deviation allows you to interpret an individual score in comparison with all other scores in the data set. Recall the salary example presented earlier. The data were variable because of the extreme ranges of salary values. Calculating a standard deviation provides different information about variability. It is now apparent that the average deviation from the mean for the experimental group is $34,842.50, which is more than double that of the control group's $17,073.37 deviation (see **Table 12-8**).

Comparing Variability When Units of Measure Are Different

Because standard deviations are based on the mean of the data set, information collected using different measurement scales cannot be directly compared. For example, the mean of a sample's age is reported in years while the mean of a sample's weight is reported in pounds. To make comparisons among unlike data requires that all the data means be converted to standardized units called standardized or *z scores*. Z scores are then used to describe the distance a score is away from the mean per standard deviation. A z score of 1.25 means that a data value is 1.25 standard deviations above the mean. A z score of 2.53 means that a data value is 2.53 standard deviations below the mean. Using the z score allows researchers to compare results of age and weight.

The *coefficient of variation* is a percentage used to compare standard deviations when the units of measure are different or when the means of the distributions being compared are far apart. The coefficient of variation is computed by dividing the standard deviation by the mean and recording the result as a percentage. For example, if you were to compare age and income of a sample of nurses, you could not use range or standard deviations to discuss their com-

CRITICAL THINKING EXERCISE 12-2

Do you have a professor who uses means and standard deviations, known as norm referencing, for grading exams? What are the advantages to using this approach as opposed to straight scales for grading? What are some disadvantages? Why would it be false to assume that having more questions on exams would be advantageous to students when norm referencing is used?

KEY TERMS

Tailedness: Degree to which a tail in a distribution is pulled to the left or to the right

Rule of 68-95-99.7: 68% of the data fall within one standard deviation of the mean; 95% fall within two standard deviations; 99.7% of the data fall within three standard deviations

parative spread because they are measured with different units. If the mean salary for nurses is $44,000, with a standard deviation of $4,000 and the mean age is 32 years, with a standard deviation of 4 years, the coefficient of variation for the salary is 9.1%, and the coefficient of variation for age is 12.5%. Using the coefficient of variation shows that age is more variable than salaries among this group of nurses.

Tailedness: The Rule of 68-95-99.7

The concept of *tailedness* is important to understand when reading statistical reports. Recall that a normal distribution is one in which the mean, median, and mode are all equal and that the data are symmetrical. In discussing tailedness, the graph of a normal distribution is depicted as a bell-shaped curve, centered about the mean ($\bar{x}$), with three standard deviations marked to the right (positive) and also to the left (negative) (see **Figure 12-7**). Normal distributions are not shown beyond three standard deviations in either direction because approximately 99.7% of the data will lie within this range. Approximately 68% of all data in a normal curve lie within one standard deviation of the mean, and 95% of the data lie within two standard deviations of the mean. Thus, the *Rule of 68-95-99.7* tells us that for every sample, 99.7% of the data will fall within three standard deviations of the mean. In **Figure 12-8**, note the symmetry about the mean for the standard deviations as they are divided in half for each distribution percentage. For example, one standard deviation contains 34% of the scores above and 34% of the scores below the mean to total 68%; two standard deviations contain 34% 13.5% above and below the mean to equal 95% of the scores. On a standard deviation graph, the mean has a z score of zero. Other z score percentages may be determined by using a table showing the area under the curve data.

Figure 12-9 shows that normal distributions may also be used to approximate percentile ranks. Actual percentile values must always be determined by using a normal distribution table to look up a given z score.

FIGURE 12-7   **Normal Distribution With Standard Deviations**

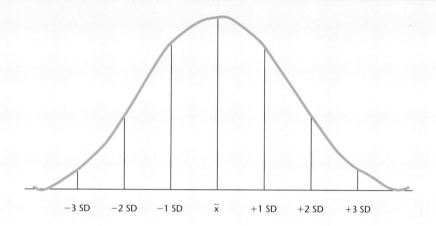

FIGURE 12-8   **Standard Deviations and Percentage Distribution**

FIGURE 12-9 **Percentile Rank Based on Normal Distribution**

The age data from previous examples do not approximate a normal distribution because the mean, median, and mode are not equal. If, however, we used data that were standardized with a mean of 23 and a standard deviation of 1.5 years, the normal curve for these data would look like the graph in **Figure 12-10**. Sixty-eight percent of these people would be between 21.5 and 24.5 years of age, and someone 26 years old would be in the 95th percentile.

FIGURE 12-10 **Standard Deviations of Age Data**

Half of the people would be 23 or older, while half would be younger than 23 years old.

Correlation Coefficients

Bivariate analyses are performed to calculate *correlation coefficients*, which are used to describe the relationship between two variables. Correlational coefficients provide information regarding the degree to which variables are related. Correlations are evaluated in terms of magnitude direction and sometimes significance. Scatterplots of data can provide hints about direction and magnitude of the correlation (**Figure 12-11**). *Direction* refers to the way the two variables covary. A positive correlation occurs when an increase in one variable is associated with an increase in another or when a decrease in one variable is associated with a decrease in the other. For example, if a researcher found that as weight increased so did systolic blood pressure, or if weight decreased so did systolic blood pressure, a "positive" relationship between weight and blood pressure exists. A negative correlation occurs when two variables covary inversely; that is, when one decreases, the other increases.

Magnitude refers to the strength of the relationship found to exist between two variables. A correlation can range from a perfect positive correlation of 1.00 to a perfect negative correlation of 1.00. A correlation of zero means that there is no relationship between the two variables. It is generally accepted that correlations ranging between 0.10 and 0.30 are considered to be weak, 0.30 to

FIGURE 12-11   **Scatterplots of Correlational Relationships**

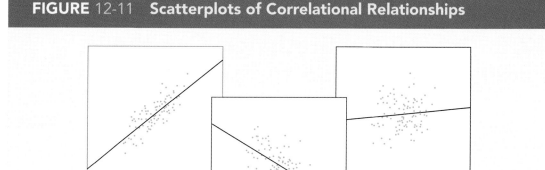

Large Magnitude, Positive Correlation

Large Magnitude, Negative Correlation

No Correlation

TEST YOUR KNOWLEDGE 12-5

Match the following terms:

1. Range
2. Semiquartile range
3. Percentile
4. Standard Deviation
5. Z score
6. Coefficient of variation

a. rank
b. difference between maximum and minimum value
c. measure of the average deviations of a value from the mean
d. percentage comparing standard deviations when units of measure are different
e. range of the middle 50% of data
f. converted standard deviation to a standardized unit

How did you do? 1. b; 2. e; 3. a; 4. c; 5. f; 6. d

0.50 moderate, and greater than 0.50 strong; however, the final determination is based on the variables being examined. It is important to remember that magnitude is not dependent on or related to the direction of the correlation.

12.6   Inferential Statistics: Can the Findings Be Applied to the Population?

At the end of this section, you will be able to:

‹ Discuss the purpose of inferential statistical tests
‹ Explain how statistical testing is related to chance

www

When to Use Inferential Statistics

First, samples are analyzed using descriptive statistics. Then, if appropriate, inferential statistical tests can be conducted to: a) make decisions about whether findings can be inferred to the population, and b) test hypotheses. For some studies, the use of inferential statistics is not appropriate, and their use depends on the research questions being asked. Research questions that are descriptive would not require inferential statistics. For example, the research question "How often do nurses assess the use of herbal remedies by patients?" would best be answered by using descriptive statistics, such as frequencies, means, and standard deviations.

Using parameter estimation to determine inferences to the population is less common in nursing research; however, this approach is becoming more popular with the emphasis on evidence-based practice (EBP) in nursing and medicine (Borenstein, 1997; Straus, Richardson, Glasziou, & Haynes, 2005). Most frequently, these estimates are reported as *confidence intervals* (CI). CI are ranges established around means that estimate the probability of being correct (American College of Physicians—American Society of Internal Medicine, 2001; Polit & Beck, 2004). In other words, CI estimate the degree of confidence one can have about the inferences. Researchers typically report confidence levels of 95% or 99%.

When using inferential statistics to test hypotheses, they are best suited to research questions or hypotheses asking one of two broad questions:

1. Is there a difference among the groups?
2. Is there a relationship among the variables?

Most experimental and quasi-experimental designs involve questions asking if there is a difference among the groups. For example, the use of inferential statistics to test the hypothesis, "Patients who have uninterrupted sleep cycles have better wound healing than patients who awaken throughout the night" would be appropriate. Research questions or hypotheses that ask about relationships among variables, such as "Is there a relationship between the number of hours of sleep and a score on a memory exam?" can also be tested using inferential statistics.

When deciding which statistical tests to use to analyze data, researchers must take into account many factors (Hayes, 1994). After considering whether the research questions or hypotheses involve groups or variables, the next most important factor to be considered is the level of measurement. Whether variables are nominal, ordinal, interval, or ratio is important because some tests are appropriate for interval and ratio data but not for other levels of measurement. Other factors that can influence selection of inferential statistical tests include whether: a) a probability sampling method was used, b) the data are normally distributed, and c) there is potential confounding of the variables. Nurses should keep in mind that the strongest inferences can be made when the level of measurement is interval or ratio, a probability sampling method was used, the sample size is adequate, and the data are normally distributed.

FYI

Regardless of the type of question being asked, the major unanswered question is: Are the findings a result of the treatment, or did the findings happen by chance? Statistics enable nursing researchers to determine the probability that results are a result of treatment or chance.

KEY TERM

Confidence intervals: Ranges established around means that estimate the probability of being correct

KEY TERMS

Probability:
Likelihood or chance
that an event will
occur in a situation

Sampling error:
Error resulting
when elements in
the sample do not
adequately represent
the population

**Statistically
significant:** When
findings did not
happen by chance

Nonsignificant: When
critical values fall
within three standard
deviations of the
mean

It's All About Chance

Regardless of the type of question being asked, the major unanswered question is: Are the findings a result of the treatment, or did the findings happen by chance? For example, suppose that you toss a coin 10 times, and each time it lands heads up. Could that happen by chance? Absolutely. Now suppose you flip it another 10 times and it lands heads up every time. While it is possible that a coin could land heads up 20 times in a row, this would be a rare occurrence. Would you begin to wonder if this were happening by chance or would you suspect that the coin is not fair? How many times would you want to toss the coin before you conclude that the coin is not fair?

Researchers are asking the same types of questions when they analyze data using inferential statistics. They are asking, "What is the probability that the findings were a result of chance?" *Probability* is the likelihood of the frequency of an event in repeated trials under similar conditions. Probability is based on the concept of sampling error, that is, how probable it is that results were obtained by chance. *Sampling error* is the tendency for statistics to fluctuate from one sample to another. There is always a possibility of errors in sampling, even when the samples are randomly selected. The characteristics of any given sample are usually different from those of the population. For example, suppose a fair coin was tossed 10 times for 10 different trials. A tally of the results in **Table 12-9** shows that the trials varied; but as expected, more of the trials were nearer 50% heads than 100% heads.

Researchers determine whether the results were obtained by chance using inferential statistical tests, sometimes known as tests of significance. Mathematical calculations are performed, usually by computers, to obtain critical values. These values are plotted on a normal distribution, and determinations of whether findings are *statistically significant* or *nonsignificant* are made. Statistically significant critical values fall in the tails of the normal distributions, usually three standard deviations from the mean or where about only 0.3% of the data occur. Thus, when critical values are in that area, researchers believe it is appropriate to claim that the findings did not happen by chance.

CRITICAL THINKING EXERCISE 12-3

When is there enough testing to make a decision?

TABLE 12-9 Coin Toss Example

	Trial 1	Trial 2	Trial 3	Trial 4	Trial 5	Trial 6	Trial 7	Trial 8	Trial 9	Trial 10
0 Heads 10 Tails										
1 Head 9 Tails										
2 Heads 8 Tails						X				
3 Heads 7 Tails										
4 Heads 6 Tails		X					X			
5 Heads 5 Tails	X				X					X
6 Heads 4 Tails				X					X	
7 Heads 3 Tails								X		
8 Heads 2 Tails			X							
9 Heads 1 Tail										
10 Heads 0 Tails										

TEST YOUR KNOWLEDGE 12-6

1. Inferential statistical tests are used to
   a. make decisions about the population.
   b. describe the sample with means and standard deviations.
   c. test hypotheses asking if there is a difference among the groups.
   d. select a sample.
   e. determine if results occurred by chance.

How did you do? 1. a, c, e

12.7 Reducing Error When Deciding About Hypotheses

At the end of this section, you will be able to:

< Distinguish between type I and type II errors
< Describe alpha levels commonly used in nursing research

FYI

Researchers attempt to reduce error so that nurses can have confidence in findings. Methods for reducing error include selecting designs that fit with research questions, controlling the independent variable, carefully measuring variables, and reducing threats to internal and external validity.

Researchers do many things to reduce error so that nurses can have confidence in findings. They reduce error by selecting designs that fit with research questions, controlling the independent variable, carefully measuring variables, and reducing threats to internal and external validity. They also do things to reduce error when deciding whether a research hypothesis is supported or not supported.

When making decisions about hypotheses, it is helpful to keep several principles in mind (Hayes, 1994). First, hypotheses are claims about the world. Second, decisions are made about null hypotheses, not research hypotheses. The purpose of inferential statistical tests is to determine if the null hypothesis should be accepted or rejected. Third, it is important to remember that no matter how well errors are reduced or how powerful the findings are, nothing is ever proven. The most that can be claimed is that a research hypothesis is either supported or unsupported. Lastly, it is wise to understand that an empirical view is adopted and an assumption is made that there is a single reality in the physical world and that science can be used to discover the truth about reality.

For example, suppose a researcher is testing a new way to assess risk for skin breakdown over the sacrum. The researcher hypothesizes that prior to the presentation of redness, skin temperature will be increased. From an empirical viewpoint, it is assumed that skin temperature, redness, and sacrum are real entities and, that in the real world, one of four situations is true. Prior to the appearance of redness over the sacrum, either the skin temperature will be increased, unchanged, decreased, or varied. Now suppose that in the real world, the unknown truth is that skin temperature does increase before redness appears over the sacrum. After collecting and analyzing data, statistically significant results were obtained. The researcher decides to reject the null hypothesis, that there will be no difference in skin temperature before the appearance of redness, and the research hypothesis is supported. In this instance, unbeknown to the researcher, an error was not made. The claim of the original hypothesis, that skin temperature would be increased prior to the appearance of sacral redness, matches what actually happens in the world. The researcher rejected the null hypothesis, and it was indeed false. If nurses accumulated additional supporting evidence, findings would make their way into practice, and patients at risk for skin breakdown could be identified earlier.

Errors are avoided when researchers accept the null hypothesis when it is true. Consider this variation of the preceding example. The researcher hypothesizes that prior to the presentation of redness over the sacrum, skin temperature will be increased; however, in the real world there is no change in skin temperature over the sacrum prior to the appearance of redness. After collecting and analyzing data, the researcher finds that calculations from inferential statistical tests are nonsignificant and therefore the null hypothesis is supported. Although disappointed, the researcher accepts the null hypothesis and unwittingly avoids error because there is no temperature change in the real world. The goal of hypothesis testing is to accept true claims and reject false ones.

Type I and Type II Errors

The goal is to avoid the two kinds of errors that can be made when making decisions about null hypotheses. These errors are known as type I and type II errors. A *type I error* occurs when the researcher rejects the null hypothesis when it should have been accepted. In nursing, when the null hypothesis is wrongly rejected, the usual result is that the researcher is making false claims about the research hypothesis. Usually this means that the researcher is claiming that some treatment works or some relationship exists, when in actuality that is not the case. For example, in the previous examples, the researcher hypothesized that skin temperatures over the sacrum would be increased prior to the appearance of redness. Now suppose that in the real world, there is no change in the temperature; however, analysis of the data collected indicates that there is an increase of temperature. In other words, the researcher has obtained statistically significant results. This false finding could be the result of any number of errors, such as sampling bias and measurement error. The false finding could have happened by chance, just as it would be possible by chance to get 20 heads in a row when tossing a fair coin. The researcher, unaware about what is true in the world, rejects the null hypothesis based on the statistical analysis and claims that the research hypothesis is supported. This is a type I error. If nurses adopt this finding into practice, they will unnecessarily spend time measuring skin temperature because it would provide no indication of risk. If the practice of measuring skin temperature continued without evaluation of patient outcomes, it is possible that this type I error would never be discovered. A *type II error* occurs when researchers accept the null hypothesis when it should have been rejected. In nursing, this type of error usually means that practice does

CRITICAL THINKING EXERCISE 12-4

Individuals make decisions every day. They make decisions based on their assumptions about the world, only to find out later that the assumptions were incorrect. Can you think of times when you have made a type I error? What about a situation when a type II error was made?

not change when it should have. The opportunity to implement an effective treatment or claim the discovery of a relationship has been missed. Consider this variation of the previous example. The researcher still hypothesizes that sacral skin temperature is increased prior to the appearance of redness, and in the real world this is true. The researcher completes the analysis, which has statistically nonsignificant results. These nonsignificant results can be due to error or chance. Based on the statistical analysis, the researcher is forced to accept the null hypothesis, unaware that the research hypothesis is true in the real world. A type II error has occurred, and nurses miss an opportunity to predict which patients are at risk for skin breakdown.

There are a few strategies for remembering type I and type II errors. One way is through the graphic representation in **Table 12-10**. One axis of the table represents whether the null hypothesis is true or false in the real world. The other axis represents the two decisions that can be made by researchers about the null hypothesis: to accept or to reject. The center boxes are then filled in as appropriate. No errors are made when a decision to accept a null hypothesis is made when it is true in the real world. Likewise, there is no error when a false null hypothesis is rejected. A type I error is made when researchers, obtaining statistically significant results, reject the null hypothesis when in fact it was true. A type II error occurs when researchers fail to obtain statistically significant results, and thus they accept the null hypothesis despite the fact that it is false. Another way to remember type I and type II errors is to think of the ac-

TABLE 12-10 Type I and Type II Errors

	The Null Hypothesis Is True in "Real World"	The Null Hypothesis Is False in "Real World"
Researcher accepts the Null Hypothesis	No Error	Type II Error
Reseacher rejects the Null Hypothesis	Type I Error	No Error

ronym "RAAR" (Gillis & Jackson, 2002). RAAR stands for the phrase: "Reject the null hypothesis when you should accept it, and accept the null hypothesis when you should reject it." The first two letters, RA, stand for type I error. The second two letters, AR, stand for type II error.

Level of Significance: Adjusting the Risk of Making Type I and Type II Errors

In nursing, type I errors are considered to be more serious than type II errors (Munro, 2004). It seems much more risky to claim that a treatment works, when in reality it does not, than to miss the opportunity to claim that a treatment works. For example, a researcher invents and tests a new device for measuring blood sugar. If a type I error is made, the researcher will claim that the new device works, when in reality it does not. Patients begin using the device, which inaccurately measures blood sugar. Because nurses evaluate the implementation of this new device, they eventually realize that the device is not effective as the researcher claimed. The type I error could result in accusations of harming diabetics with a fraudulent measuring device. Because patients who used the device might have been harmed, they might want to sue the researcher. However, if a type II error is made, the researcher throws away the device for measuring blood sugar even though in reality it is superior to other devices. In this situation, the researcher misses the opportunity to market the device and earn money, and diabetics miss the opportunity to benefit from the measuring device. While neither scenario is desirable, most researchers would choose to miss the opportunity to make money rather than to harm patients and risk the legal implications.

Researchers must make decisions about how much risk they are willing to tolerate. When interventions are complex, expensive, invasive, or have many side effects, such as a new procedure for cardiac surgery, researchers are usually less willing to make type I errors. When interventions are simple, inexpensive, or noninvasive, such as a new teaching method, the tolerance for a type I error is increased.

Researchers use statistics to adjust the amount of risk involved in making type I and II errors. It is helpful to remember that type I and type II errors have an inverse relationship. When type I error is increased, type II error is decreased. Risks for these errors are adjusted by selecting the *alpha level*, which is the probability of making a type I error. Alpha level is designated at the end of the tail in a distribution (see **Figure 12-12**). In nursing research, the alpha levels are usually either 0.05 or 0.01. In the figure, the placement of the alpha level shows how type I and type II errors can be adjusted. In this example of a one-tailed test, the area under the curve to the left of the alpha level represents

KEY TERM

Alpha level:
Probability of making a type I error

FIGURE 12-12 **Placement of Alpha Level on Normal Distribution**

the amount of type II error. The area under the curve to the right of the line is the amount of type I error. Notice that when the alpha level is larger, there is more space to the right of the line than when the alpha level is smaller.

What are the implications of these alpha levels? When the alpha level is set at 0.05, it is likely that 5 times out of 100, the researcher would make a type I error by wrongly rejecting the null hypothesis. When 0.01 is used for the alpha level, a researcher would make a type I error only 1 time out of 100. Thus, alpha levels of 0.05 increase type I errors while reducing type II errors. While alpha levels of 0.01 reduce type I errors, the likelihood of making a type II error increases. In nursing, 0.05 is used more commonly than 0.01; however, when multiple statistical tests are being conducted, researchers should use an alpha level of 0.01.

While the mathematical difference between these alphas is miniscule, the implications for decision making are great. **Figure 12-13** provides an illustration of how the acceptance or rejection of the null hypothesis is affected by the alpha level selected. When conducting statistical tests to test hypotheses, suppose there is a chance for three possible critical values. Note in Figure 12-13 that critical value "A" falls to the left of both alpha levels. Regardless of the alpha level chosen, the results will be statistically nonsignificant, and the null hypothesis will be accepted. Critical value "B" falls to the right of both alpha levels. The results will be statistically significant regardless of the alpha level selected. Now consider the position of critical value "C." How would the decision about the null hypothesis be affected by either of these two alphas? If the alpha level is set at 0.05, the critical point would be significant and the null hypothesis would be rejected. However, if an alpha level of 0.01 is selected,

FIGURE 12-13   **Relationship of Alpha Levels and Critical Values**

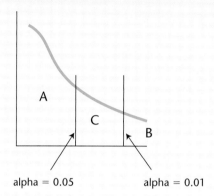

the critical point would be nonsignificant, and the researcher would accept the null hypothesis. To avoid any temptation to select alpha levels that bias decision making, researchers must always state their selected alpha levels in the initial research proposal. Strong rationales for the one selected must also be provided.

TEST YOUR KNOWLEDGE 12-7

1. When a researcher accepts the null hypothesis when it really should have been rejected, the researcher:
   a. committed a type I error
   b. committed a type II error
   c. obtained significant results
   d. obtained nonsignificant results

2. The most commonly used alpha level in nursing research is
   a. 0.001
   b. 0.0001
   c. 0.005
   d. 0.05

How did you do? 1. b, d; 2. d

12.8   Using Statistical Tests to Infer to Populations

At the end of this section, you will be able to:

‹ Match common notations with associated statistical tests

‹ Identify common statistical tests as parametric or nonparametric

‹ Describe tests used to determine statistically significant differences among groups

‹ Discuss tests used to determine statistically significant differences among variables

‹ Assign commonly used statistical tests to examples based on type of research question and level of measurement

The Language of Inferential Statistics

A unique language is used by statisticians to communicate statistical data. There is a variety of terms and statistical symbols (**Table 12-11**) associated with inferential statistics. Statistical tests are frequently named after the individuals who devised them, which can sometimes make the names seem arbitrary and hard to remember. The following fundamental terms are ones with which nurses should become familiar. *Parametric* tests are used to infer to the population when specific conditions have been met (Hayes, 1994; Munro, 2004). These conditions include: a) use of probability sampling, b) normal distribution of data, c) measurement of variables at the interval or ratio level, and d) reduction of error. For example, data collected using a visual analog scale would be analyzed using parametric tests. These important conditions make parametric tests especially powerful. When parametric tests are used, nurses can have high levels of confidence about the conclusions made. When all four conditions are not met, researchers must use less powerful tests known as *nonparametric* tests. In nursing research, nonparametric tests are frequently used because many variables are measured at nominal and ordinal levels. For example, data collected using Likert scales would be analyzed using nonparametric tests. Because these tests are considered to be less powerful, the level of confidence nurses have about inferring to the population is not as strong as when parametric tests are used. Another term used when talking about statistics is *degrees of freedom*. Degrees of freedom, based on the number of elements in a sample, are used to correct for possible underestimation of population parameters when performing mathematical equations (Munro, 2004). For example, suppose a data set consists of four scores: 1, 4, 4, and 7. Before any of these scores were collected, the researcher did not know what these scores would be. Each score was free to vary. This means that each score

KEY TERMS

Parametric:
Inferential statistical tests involving interval or ratio level data to infer to the population

Nonparametric:
Inferential statistics involving nominal or ordinal level data to infer to the population

Degrees of freedom:
Refers to the number of sample values that are free to vary; n–1

Symbol/Abbreviation	Definition
ANOVA	Analysis of variance
df	Degrees of freedom
F	Fisher's *F* ratio
ns	Nonsignificant
p	Probability
r	Pearson product-moment correlation
R	Multiple correlation
R^2	Multiple correlation squared
t	Computed value of *t* test
α	Alpha; probability of type I error
β	Beta; probability of type II error
Δ	Delta; amount of change
Σ	Sigma; sum or summation
χ^2	Chi square

TABLE 12-11 **Statistical Symbols for Inferential Statistics**

was independent from the other scores. Because there are four scores, there are four degrees of freedom. However, when the mean is calculated, one degree of freedom is lost. This is because after the mean is known, along with three of the scores, the fourth score is no longer free to vary. The fourth score can be calculated, and only one value will be correct. Therefore, the data set of four scores has three degrees of freedom, $n - 1$, because one degree of freedom is lost. Many inferential statistics include degrees of freedom in their calculations. Another concept important in the language of inferential statistics is *sampling distribution* (Munro, 2004; Nieswiadomy, 2008). In theory, an infinite number of samples can be drawn from a population. Some samples are more likely to be drawn than others. For example, when sampling coin tosses, getting half heads and half tails when tossing a coin 20 times is far more likely than tossing heads 20 times in a row. For many inferential tests, statisticians have calculated the likelihood of obtaining different samples and reported them in tables. When researchers perform certain inferential tests, they refer to these tables to find out if their results are likely or unlikely. Results that are unlikely to occur as a result of chance are then considered to be statistically significant.

KEY TERM

Sampling distribution: Theoretical distribution representing an infinite number of samples that can be drawn from a population

There are a number of inferential tests that nurses will commonly see in the literature. While the study of statistical tests can seem overwhelming to some individuals, it might not be necessary to fully understand why each test is conducted and how the calculations are performed to appraise evidence. Nurses should be able to discern that the correct tests were used to analyze data. This can be determined by focusing on two broad questions: 1) "What type of question is being asked by the researcher?" and, 2) "What is the level of measurement being used to measure the variables?" Some inferential statistical tests that are commonly used in nursing research are listed in **Table 12-12**. While it is beyond the scope of this textbook to elaborate on all the tests listed in the table, information about some of the most common tests is worth remembering. When answering questions about statistically significant differences among groups, nurses should be familiar with Chi square, *t* tests, and analysis of variance (ANOVA). They should also be familiar with Pearson's *r* and multiple regression, which are tests used to determine if there is a statistically significant correlation among the variables.

Testing for Differences Among Groups

As shown in Table 12-12, a variety of tests are used to analyze data for the purpose of determining if there is a statistically significant difference among the groups. When deciding which test to use, researchers must consider the number of groups to be included in the analysis and at what level variables were measured. Pilots frequently involve one group, while classic experiments and quasi-experiments can include two or more groups. Before analyzing data, researchers need to consider whether the groups are dependent or independent to select the correct tests to perform. For example, suppose a researcher is studying perceptions of health in married couples before and after a class about stress reduction. The researcher tests both men and women who are married to one another. Because individuals in a marriage will have many characteristics in common, the data collected should be analyzed using inferential tests for dependent groups. Data from designs using subjects as their own controls, for example, measuring blood pressures before and after exercise, are also treated as data from dependent groups. More likely than not, researchers collect data from independent groups, for example, test scores from two groups of diabetic patients.

The Chi Square Statistic

Chi square is a very commonly used statistic (Hayes, 1994; Munro, 2004). Calculated when analyzing nominal and ordinal data, it is a nonparametric

---

KEY TERM

Chi square: Statistic used to analyze nominal and ordinal data to find differences between groups

TABLE 12-12 Inferential Tests Commonly Used in Nursing

		What is the hypothesis asking?			Is there a relationship among the variables?	
		Is there a difference among the groups?				
	1 Group	2 Groups		>2 Groups	2 Variables	>2 Variables
		Related	Independent			
Nonparametric — Nominal	Chi Square	Chi Square Fisher's Exact Probability Test	Chi Square	Chi Square	Phi Coefficient Point Biserial	Contingency Coefficient
Nonparametric — Ordinal	Kolmogorov-Smirnov	Sign Test Wilcoxon Matched Pairs Signed Rank	Chi Square Median Test Mann-Whitney U	Chi Square	Kendall's Tau Spearman Rho	
Parametric — Interval or Ratio	Correlated t (Paired t)	Correlated t	Independent t	ANOVA ANCOVA MANOVA	Pearson's r	Multiple Regression Path Analysis Canonical Correlation

What is the level of measurement?

KEY TERMS

t statistic: Inferential statistical test to determine if a statistically significant difference between groups exists

Correlated t test: *t* test variant used for only one group or when groups are related

Independent t test: *t* test variant used when data values vary independently from one another

test. One reason Chi square is used so often is because it is very useful for finding differences between the groups on demographic variables. For example, suppose that a researcher is studying the effect of aromatherapy on blood pressure and randomly assigns 200 individuals to one of two groups. The experimental group contains 54 women and 46 men, while the control group has 46 women and 54 men. By performing a Chi square test, the researcher can determine if the groups are alike on the extraneous variable of gender. If the groups are not significantly different on gender, it can be assumed that changes in blood pressure are more likely as a result of the intervention than gender. When Chi square statistics are used, the frequencies that are observed during the study are compared to the frequencies that would be expected to occur if the null hypothesis were true. Observed and expected frequencies are entered into contingency tables, and a Chi square statistic is calculated. Using the calculated Chi square statistic, the degrees of freedom, and the alpha level, researchers consult Chi square tables to determine the critical value and judge whether the critical value is statistically significant. In the literature, notations for Chi square, such as $X^2 = 1.89$, $df = 1$, $p < 0.05$, appear reported with degrees of freedom and significance. Another reason Chi squares are frequently used is that they can be calculated without the use of computers. However, the sample size must be adequate because there must be at least six observed frequencies in each cell of the table. If this minimum is not met, then a variation of the Chi square, known as Fisher's exact probability test, is used.

The t Statistic

The *t statistic* is another inferential statistical test commonly reported in nursing research to determine if there is a statistically significant difference between two groups. It is commonly known as the *t* test, or Student's *t* test, and is a parametric measure (Hayes, 1994; Munro, 2004). There are two variations of the *t* test. One variation, known as the *correlated t test* or paired *t* test, is used when there is only one group or when the groups are related. The other variation is known as an *independent t test* and is used when data values vary independently from one another. In experimental and quasi-experimental designs, the *t* test is used to determine whether the means of two groups are statistically different. Suppose a researcher is measuring pain following the application of ice to a new cast applied for fracture of the tibia. The mean pain intensity rating for the experimental group is 5.6, while for the control group it is 6.0. As with a Chi square test, researchers calculate the *t* statistic and consult tables using the statistic, degrees of freedom, and alpha levels to find the critical value. The critical value is obtained and a decision about its statistical significance is made. In reports, *t* tests are reported in the following manner: $t = 2.54, p < 0.01$.

Analysis of Variance

Analysis of variance (ANOVA) is used when the level of measurement is interval or ratio and there are more than two groups (Hayes, 1994; Munro, 2004). The broad question being answered is whether group means significantly differ from one another. Using ANOVA allows researchers to compare a combination of pairs of means while reducing the odds for a type I error. For example, suppose that a researcher is testing three different styles of education with adolescent asthmatics: peer, text messaging, and Web-based. There would be three different pairs of means to compare: peer to text messaging, peer to Web-based, and text messaging to Web-based. If *t* tests were conducted for each pair, the same null hypothesis would be tested three times, increasing the risk of a type I error. By using an ANOVA, researchers can compare the variations among the groups using one statistical test, thereby reducing the chances of making a type I error. ANOVA and *t* tests are very closely related. When testing two groups, the same mathematical answer would result whether an ANOVA or a *t* test were used. Using ANOVA, researchers calculate the *F* statistic, which is based on the *F*-distribution using degrees of freedom. The greater the *F* statistic, the greater the variation among the means of the groups. Tables of the *F*-distributions and degrees of freedom are also used. $F = 4.65, df = 2, 50, p < 0.05$ is an example of the notation that would be used to report an ANOVA. Two variations of ANOVA, analysis of covariance (ANCOVA) and multiple analysis of variance (MANOVA), are also used in nursing research. ANCOVA is used to statistically control for known extraneous variables. For example, if a researcher believes that level of education affects the amount learned by the adolescent asthmatics, the researcher may use ANCOVA to control for grade in school. When researchers have more than one dependent variable, they used MANOVA instead of ANOVA to analyze data.

Other Tests of Significance

It can be noted in Table 12-12 that there is a number of other inferential statistics that can be used to determine if there are statistically significant differences among groups. These include Kolmogorov-Smirnov test, sign test, Wilcoxin matched pairs test, signed rank test, median test, and Mann-Whitney U test (Hayes, 1994; Munro, 2004). These tests are used when ordinal level data are involved; thus they are categorized as nonparametric tests. Tests are selected based on considerations such as the number of groups being compared, the distribution pattern of the data (normal or skewed), and other nuances that can be found in the data.

Testing for Relationships Among Variables

To determine if there are relationships among variables, a variety of statistical tests is used to determine the significance of correlations (see Table 12-2). Decisions about which statistical tests to use are based on whether there are two variables or more than two variables. Consideration is also given to the level of measurement used. Understanding how decisions are made allows nurses to ascertain the quality of the findings.

Pearson's r

When researchers pose hypotheses about the relationships among variables, they are testing for the significance of the correlation coefficient. When two variables are measured at the interval or ratio level, they calculate the *Pearson's r* statistic, also known as the Pearson product-moment correlation (Hayes, 1994; Munro, 2004). The degrees of freedom for this test are always $N - 2$, which means that the correlation coefficient can be affected by the sample size. It is possible for a small correlation coefficient to be statistically significant when there is a large sample. In the literature, the notation $r = 0.62$, $p < 0.01$ is used. For example, suppose a researcher hypothesized that in adolescent anorexics attending an inpatient clinic, a positive relationship exists between self-esteem and weight gain. The null hypothesis would be that there is no relationship between self-esteem and weight gain. If the researcher obtained a correlation coefficient of 0.83, it is very likely that self-esteem and weight gain are related. However, if the correlation coefficient was 0.23, it would be a guess as to whether self-esteem and weight gain are related or whether the value resulted by chance. To test if 0.23 was significant, a Pearson's r statistic would be used.

Small correlations can be statistically significant because it does not take much variation to be significantly different from a correlation of zero (Nieswiadomy, 2008). Therefore, researchers can use a variation of Pearson's r that determines the percentage of variance shared by two variables, which provides more meaningful information. By squaring the coefficient (r^2), the overlap, or shared variance, is computed. A helpful way to think about variance is to think of a pie chart. The entire pie chart represents all the variables that can contribute to changes in the dependent variable. Each r^2 indicates how large a section of the pie chart that variable earns. With this information, knowledge of one variable can be used to predict the value of the other variable. For example, suppose that a correlation coefficient of 0.23 was obtained for the variables self-esteem and weight gain. Squaring 0.23 equals 0.0529. This is interpreted to mean that self-esteem accounts for about 5% of weight gain. Thus, the researcher would know that other variables must also contribute to weight gain.

Multiple Regression

A change in one variable is usually the result of many factors. Thus, when researchers want to study the relationship of many independent variables on a dependent variable, they use *multiple regression* (Hayes, 1994; Munro, 2004). Calculations such as these have become much more sophisticated with the use of computers because they are able to perform simultaneous calculations. Like Pearson's *r*, multiple regression is used when variables are measured at the interval or ratio level. For example, suppose a researcher wants to determine which factors best predict an anorexic adolescent's success at maintaining a weight in the normal range. Independent variables might include self-esteem, social support, anxiety, and locus of control. Nurses will often see variations of multiple regression reported in the literature. One variation is known as step-wise. This approach is used to find the smallest number of independent variables that account for the greatest proportion of variance (Pedhazur, 1982). For example, in a study of anorexic adolescents, a researcher might find that self-esteem, anxiety, and locus of control account for 24% of the variance and that social support does not make any significant difference in weight gain. Another variation of multiple regression used by researchers is hierarchical regression. This approach is typically used when the importance of variables has been specified in theories. For example, suppose it is proposed in a theory about anorexic adolescents that locus of control is the most important factor, followed by self-esteem and then anxiety. Based on this theory, the researcher would be able to specify the order the independent variables are to be entered into the equations. As in step-wise multiple regression, the amount of variance that is significant is reported.

Other Tests of Significance

Because all variables are not measured at interval and ratio levels, there are other tests of significance that can determine if changes in variables are significant (Hayes, 1994; Munro, 2004). When nominal data are involved, statistics such as Phi coefficients, point biserials, and contingency coefficients are reported. Researchers use Kendall's Tau, Spearman Rho, and discriminate function analysis to analyze ordinal level data. There are also very sophisticated methods for testing and predicting the strength and direction of relationships among multiple variables. These analytical methods, such as linear structural relationships or structural equation modeling, are useful ways to use data to generate theories.

KEY TERM

Multiple regression: Inferential statistical test that describes the relationship of three or more variables

TEST YOUR KNOWLEDGE 12-8

Match the following

1. Chi square

2. *t* test

3. ANOVA

4. Pearson's *r*

5. Multiple regression

a. Uses the *F* statistic

b. tests for the significance of a correlation between two variables

c. has independent and correlated variations

d. tests the significance of relationships among three or more variables

e. tests for differences among groups using nonparametric data

6. A researcher is studying the relationship between the amount of time intensive care unit patients spend lying on their backs to urine output. Which test would the researcher use to analyze the data?
   a. Chi square
   b. Pearson's *r*
   c. Phi coefficient
   d. Multiple regression

How did you do? 1. e; 2. c; 3. a; 4. b; 5. d; 6. b

12.9   What Does All This Mean for EBP?

At the end of this section, you will be able to:

‹ Interpret data reported in statistical tables
‹ Differentiate between statistical significance and clinical significance
‹ Appraise data analysis sections of an article

When reading research articles, nurses must assume that mathematical calculations were done accurately because raw data are not included. What nurses should appraise is that the correct tests were performed. Table 12-12 is a helpful tool for appraising the analysis sections of articles.

Nurses should also appraise data presented in tables to determine if conclusions drawn by researchers are supported by the findings. While many readers frequently skip over the tables when reading research articles, this is not a good practice. The tables contain evidence on which practice changes can be made, and for this reason they may be one of the most important components of the report. Nurses need to acquire skill at reading and interpreting tables. Some hints for doing so are presented in **Table 12-13**.

It is also important to differentiate between statistical significance and clinical significance. For example, suppose a drug lowered cholesterol levels on average from 135 to 118. Analysis indicated that this decrease was statistically significant; however, because any cholesterol value below 200 is considered

FYI

While many readers frequently skip over the tables when reading research articles, this is not a good practice. Data presented in tables may contain evidence on which practice changes can be made, and thus may be one of the most important components of a report.

TABLE 12-13 Tips for Reading Statistical Tables

Be familiar with symbols used.
Read the title of the table first.
Pay attention to the labels of each axis.
Observe when headings for subsamples and subscales are indented in axis.
Follow columns carefully both horizontally and vertically.
Attend to significant findings.
Alpha levels are either reported with a notation or under the table with an asterisk (*).
Pay attention to superscript or footnote markings.
Do not skip tables, because information can be clearer after studying a table.
Put the table with the text because the table tends to explain or amplify text.
Recognize that there can be typos and math errors.
Remember that subsamples can be omitted from table (i.e., sample indicates total subjects and number of women, leaving reader to calculate number of men).

to be within normal range, there is no clinical significance to this finding. In another example, consider an experimental study involving guided imagery. Children in the guided imagery group had average pain ratings of 4.2, while children in the control group had average pain ratings of 5.2. While the difference between these means is not statistically significant, it may be clinically significant to have pain ratings a whole point lower. Furthermore, because guided imagery was noninvasive, inexpensive, and children reportedly enjoyed it, it might be worth incorporating as a practice intervention. When appraising evidence, it is wise for nurses to keep in mind that statistical significance and clinical significance are different.

Appraising the results section of research reports can be challenging. An understanding of the material presented in this chapter can assist you in meeting this challenge. **Table 12-14** lists questions that should be considered when evaluating data analysis.

TABLE 12-14 Questions for Appraising Analysis of Data

1. What statistics were used to describe the characteristics of the sample and the results of the instruments used? Were the statistics appropriate for the level of measurement?

2. Were measures of central tendency provided? If so, which ones were used? Are they the most appropriate? How sensitive to outliers is the measure reported?

3. Were measures of variation/dispersion provided? Were standard deviations reported for each mean that was reported?

4. What was the distribution of the data? Were data normally distributed? Was skewness or kurtosis discussed?

5. What statistics were used to determine differences among the groups? Were the results significant?

6. What statistics were used to express relationships among variables of interest? What was the magnitude and direction of the relationship? Was it significant?

7. Are all the hypotheses addressed in the analysis section of the report?

8. Is the level of significance selected appropriate for the purpose of the study and the types of analyses being conducted?

9. Do the tables and graphs agree with the text? Are they precise and do they offer economy of information?

10. Are the results understandable and presented objectively?

TEST YOUR KNOWLEDGE 12-9

True/False

1. Nurses should determine that researchers are using the correct statistical tests to analyze data.

2. Data contained in tables are an important source of evidence for practice.

3. All statistically significant findings have clinical significance.

4. Reading the table after the text is a helpful strategy that can improve comprehension of ideas.

How did you do? 1. T; 2. T; 3. F; 4. T

12.10   Keeping It Ethical

At the end of this section, you will be able to:

< Discuss ethical considerations when conducting statistical analyses

All researchers hope that their hypotheses will be supported. Researchers develop a passion for their topics that keeps them invested in their research. However, researchers must use care when analyzing data and selecting alpha levels. It is best if decisions about which statistical tests to conduct and which alpha levels to use are made prior to implementing the study. These decisions

CRITICAL THINKING EXERCISE 12-5

Imagine that manuscripts for 10 different studies conducted about the effect of massage on the oxygen saturation of infants in the neonatal intensive care unit are sent to a variety of journals. Only one study had significant findings, and it was accepted for publication. If none of the other nine studies were accepted for publication, what evidence would be available to nurses for EBP? How might practice be affected if all 10 studies are published?

TEST YOUR KNOWLEDGE 12-10

Which of the following are unethical?

1. Selecting an alpha of 0.05 so that the research hypothesis is supported when it would not be if the alpha were set at 0.01.

2. Publishing articles about studies with nonsignificant findings.

3. Including information about incidental findings, especially when they involve side effects or risks.

How did you do? 1. unethical; 2. ethical; 3. ethical

are usually presented, with strong rationales for the decisions, in the proposal for the study. While there are situations when it is appropriate to conduct additional statistical tests, it is unethical for researchers to "go fishing" for evidence to support their hypotheses.

Editors and research conference planners who review studies are faced with making decisions about which studies warrant dissemination. Studies with significant findings are much more likely to be accepted for presentation or publication. Because nonsignificant findings have an important role in making decisions about practice, decision makers, such as conference planners and journal publishers, need to give more consideration to studies with nonsignificant findings.

Ignoring incidental findings that are pertinent to decision making is also unethical. Incidental findings are findings that were not purposefully sought. A dilemma can occur when an intervention is found to be effective, but incidental findings, such as side effects or risks, are found to be associated with the intervention. It is possible for researchers to report additional analyses comparing risks and benefits. Reporting adverse effects is necessary so that professionals and patients can make informed choices. Researchers should also report incidental findings when findings have clinical significance or are interesting and indicate a need for further research.

RAPID REVIEW

Statistics are used to describe numerical outcomes and the probabilities derived from calculations on raw data.

There are two types of statistics: descriptive and inferential. Descriptive statistics explain characteristics of variables found in a sample. Inferential statistics are the basis for predictions about the phenomenon.

Univariate analysis involves only one variable at a time and includes frequency distributions, measures of central tendency, shape of the distribution, and measures of variability.

Bivariate analysis is conducted to describe relationships between two variables.

Frequencies may be grouped or ungrouped data describing how often a variable is found to occur. Line charts, bar graphs, pie charts, histograms, and scattergrams are ways frequencies can be depicted.

The mode, median, and mean are measures of central tendency. In a normal distribution, they are all the same value.

A normal distribution is a bell-shaped curve that is symmetric around the mean. Asymmetric distributions are known as skewed and have either positive or negative directions.

Data with little variability are considered to be homogeneous, while data with wide variations are considered to be heterogeneous.

Measures of variability include the range, semiquartile range, percentile, standard deviation, z scores, and coefficient of variation.

The Rule of 68-95-99.7 is a way of describing the percentage of scores falling within specific standard deviations of the mean.

Correlation coefficients are used to describe the relationship between two variables.

Inferential statistics are used to estimate population parameters and test hypotheses.

Confidence intervals describe the probability of being correct.

When selecting which statistical tests to use, the type of question being asked and the level of measurement must be considered. The null hypothesis is statistically tested and is rejected when significant findings occur. Research hypotheses are supported but never proven.

Probability is the likelihood of a frequency of an event in similar trials under similar conditions and indicates how probable it is that the results were obtained by chance. Sampling error is the tendency for statistics to fluctuate from one sample to another and forms the basis for probability.

APPLY WHAT YOU HAVE LEARNED

The committee is nearly done analyzing the evidence. Complete the last column of the grid found on the companion website for the various articles using quantitative designs that you have read by indicating what strategies were most effective in reducing medication errors. In some cases, it may be helpful to include some important statistics. The other quantitative articles that the committee has been reading are already completed.

- Type I errors occur when researchers reject the null hypothesis when it should have been accepted. Type II errors occur when researchers accept the null hypothesis when it should have been rejected.

- Alpha levels of either 0.05 or 0.01 are typically used in nursing research. Alpha levels affect the amount of risk involved for making type I and type II errors.

- Parametric tests are more powerful than nonparametric tests because they are used with interval or ratio level data.

- To test for differences among groups, researchers can use Chi square, *t* test, and ANOVA.

- To test for relationships among variables, Pearson's *r* and multiple regression can be used.

- To apply findings to EBP, nurses must be able to interpret statistical tables, differentiate between clinical and statistical significance, and appraise data analysis.

- To maintain ethical integrity, researchers should select statistical tests and alpha levels in advance and report incidental findings. It is as important to disseminate nonsignificant findings as it is to disseminate significant findings.

REFERENCES

American College of Physicians—American Society of Internal Medicine (2001). Primer on 95% confidence intervals. *Effective Clinical Practice, 4,* 229–231. Retrieved September 13, 2010, from http://www.acponline.org/journals/ecp/sepoct01/primerci.htm

Borenstein, M. (1997). Hypothesis testing and effect size estimation in clinical trials. *Annals of Allergy, Asthma, and Immunology, 78,* 5–11.

Gillis, A., & Jackson, W. (2002). *Research for nurses: Methods and interpretation*. Philadelphia: Davis.

Hayes, W. L. (1994). *Statistics*. Boston: Wadsworth.

Munro, B. H. (2004). *Statistical methods for health care research* (5th ed.). Philadelphia: Lippincott Williams and Wilkins.

Nieswiadomy, R. M. (2008). *Foundations of nursing research* (5th ed.). Upper Saddle River, NJ: Prentice Hall.

Pedhazur, E. J. (1982). *Multiple regression in behavioral research: Explanation and prediction* (2nd ed.). Philadelphia: Harcourt Brace.

Polit, D. E., & Beck, C. T. (2004). *Nursing research: Principles and methods* (7th ed.). Philadelphia: Lippincott Williams & Wilkins.

Straus, S. E., Richardson, W. S., Glasziou, P., & Haynes, R. B. (2005). *Evidence-based medicine: How to practice and teach EBM* (3rd ed.). Edinburgh, Scotland: Churchill Livingstone.

Wikitionary. (2007). *Statistics*. Retrieved September 13, 2010, from http://en.wiktionary.org/wiki/Statistics

At the end of this chapter, you will be able to:

< Compare and contrast ways that qualitative data are analyzed

< Discuss two types of software that may assist with managing qualitative data

< Describe how researchers draw and verify conclusions from the data

< Recognize the common ways data are presented in reports

< State why qualitative research is evaluated differently than quantitative research

< Define trustworthiness in terms of credibility, transferability, dependability, and confirmability

< Describe strategies for evaluating qualitative research

< Describe key ethical issues in qualitative research

auditability
axial coding
coding
confessionist tales
confirmability
credibility
data reduction

data saturation
dependability
impressionist tales
member checks
negative case analysis
open coding
peer debriefing

personal narrative
qualitative data analysis
realist tales
replicated
representativeness
transferability
trustworthiness

CHAPTER 13

What Do the Qualitative Data Mean?

Kristen L. Mauk

13.1 Qualitative Data Analysis

At the end of this section, you will be able to:

‹ Compare and contrast ways that qualitative data are analyzed

‹ Discuss two types of software that may assist with managing qualitative data

What Is Qualitative Data Analysis?

Qualitative data analysis is a much less straightforward process than quantitative data analysis. Using words versus numbers to explain phenomena is both more subjective and more labor intensive. Qualitative data analysis has been described as "guided by few standardized rules" (Polit & Beck, 2006, p. 419), and there are many acceptable methods to analyze the data. Sandelowski (1995) pointed out that although data analysis and interpretation often occur simultaneously in qualitative research, they should be considered distinct processes. "Qualitative analysis is a means to knowledge production" (Sandelowski, p. 373) that involves the breakdown, categorization, and prioritization of data into a useful system. She described data analysis as having two major parts: getting a sense of the whole and developing a system. According to Strauss and Corbin (1998), data analysis is "the process of breaking down, examining, comparing, conceptualizing, and categorizing data" (p. 57). Bogdan and Biklen (2003) described data analysis in two stages: analysis (systematically arranging the data) and interpretation.

Miles and Huberman (1994) defined qualitative analysis as having three "concurrent flows of activity: data reduction, data display, and conclusion drawing/verification" (p. 10). Although each of these definitions differs somewhat, there is agreement that data analysis involves some type of process in which data are managed, organized, arranged, or prioritized.

Managing the Data

Researchers begin analysis by examining data. Remember that qualitative researchers may have mounds of data from numerous pages of transcribed interviews and field notes. This large amount of data must be reduced or broken into manageable units (Jacelon & O'Dell, 2005). Because the nature of qualitative research is thick description, "the purpose of analysis is to organize the description so that it is manageable" (Patton, 1990, p. 430).

Coding and Data Reduction

Line-by-line *coding* was historically a common way to begin data analysis and one by which many new researchers learned about this process. It involves reading transcripts line-by-line and attaching labels to each line. Coding is done to categorize the data into groups. Line-by-line coding done by hand, as many novice researchers do to gain practice, is tedious and frustrating work and not always as fruitful as one would like. Stepping back and taking in the whole data set by thorough reading and rereading prior to considering the grouping of data into meaningful and manageable units should precede any type of systematic coding. There are many ways to approach coding, or labeling. Some researchers use a note card system with labels, filing key quotes under the basic codes, while others handwrite codes into the margins in a complicated hierarchy according to a codebook they have developed. Color coding is another option, as well as the use of computer software, but ultimately researchers come up with their own systems by which to organize the data into manageable units. Tesch (1990) believed that traditional hand coding resulted in more data instead of less, and that *data reduction* is a better alternative. Miles and Huberman (1994) stated that "data reduction refers to the process of selecting, focusing, simplifying, abstracting, and transforming the data that appear in written-up field notes or transcriptions" (p. 10). Data reduction is part of analysis, and the researcher must make decisions about which data are most representative of the entire story being told. As researchers choose which patterns or categories best present the most essential chunks of the data, they become the tool for data analysis and interpretation. There is no perfect process for coding data, and there is no wrong process either. Jacelon and O'Dell (2005) maintained that "through the process of coding, the researcher fractures that data and organizes it by the ideas contained within . . . it is the knowledge and perceptions of the researcher that are used to identify the ideas in the data" (p. 218). This is why the knowledge and skill of the qualitative researcher takes on such great significance and importance in qualitative research.

Traditional *opening coding* (Corbin & Strauss, 1990) is one way to describe the first step in grouping the data into categories that seem logical. Researchers should always leave an audit trail by keeping a log of their ongoing thoughts and ideas about the naming and assigning of categories to the data so that they can later examine why certain labels were chosen and others discarded. *Axial coding* (Corbin & Strauss) takes the analysis process further and requires researchers to compare the categories and labels, defining and exploring relationships among them.

After the data have been organized by basic coding, Marshall and Rossman (1995) suggest that the next step is to generate categories, themes, and patterns. Researchers must search for categories of meaning that best express "salient themes, recurring ideas or language, and patterns of belief that link people and settings together" (Marshall & Rossman, p. 114). Codes might be connected through a common theme. There might be patterns across and within the themes. Researchers look at how codes overlap and how themes and patterns emerge in relationship to each other. The analysis process is done with the end result in mind: to stay true to the data and best represent the story or phenomenon being studied.

After the data are categorized and themes emerge, researchers need to pull everything together to paint a picture of the underlying truths revealed by the data. This pulling together of the evidence into a meaningful report that can be communicated to others is another challenge. As Sandelowski (1995) stated, "qualitative analysis also has artistic dimensions that are often inchoate and incommunicable, involving playfulness, imaginativeness, and creativity" (p. 375).

The examples below were taken from interviews with stroke survivors (Easton, 2001). The examples provide some raw data from which you can derive some ideas or common threads. In the first example, what do you perceive? Are there any important concepts, ideas, or themes expressed? What was the participant trying to convey?

> Well I know one of the therapists, physical therapists here at the campus uh, I talked to her about it and then she says, oh she says, it may never get all right. It was sorta a jolt for me. (p. 148)

Compare the next example with the previous and see if you notice any similarities or differences. If so, what are they? Are the different participants in these

KEY TERMS

Open coding:
Grouping of qualitative data into categories that seem logical

Axial coding:
Analysis of categories and labels after completion of open coding

interviews saying anything that might lead you to believe they had similar experiences?

> That uh, you know, just get up and go do what you were gonna do. But that was just a flashing—and then we realized that uh, we can't do that no more. (p. 148)

Look at one more quote from yet another stroke survivor. Are there any similarities between this participant's ideas and those of the other two cited above? If so, what are they?

> I was home probably, oh, I had been to the SOS meeting, and after listening and watching some of the people there, I realized I may never get back everything. (p. 148)

In the previous examples, one might observe some common threads such as: *a sense of loss* or *realizing that things may not be the same as before the stroke.* These snippets of data are examples of those that researchers might identify as containing codes or ideas. Using the ideas found within the data as codes, researchers compile lists of codes and then return to the data again and again to categorize data into organized units. Remember that analysis is occurring while data collection is still in progress. When common ideas begin to emerge, the analysis should be used to adapt future interviews and direct and focus the data collection process. This entire process of data analysis and interpretation can be compared to discovering and putting together the pieces of a puzzle to form a meaningful picture that best represents the essence of the story told by the participants.

Sandelowski (1995) recommended some alternative strategies to traditional coding for developing a system to manage the data. She suggested extracting the facts and looking for story lines, topics, and content in addition to reduction of the data. Facts are those items of data that are not subject to debate, that are "givens," and later may be important for establishing the context of the research. When trying to capture the data in a systematic way, this avoids line-by-line coding. The aim is to think of the data as telling a story. Researchers approach the data by trying to identify the main points of the story or the major idea. Sandelowski suggested making a list that captures all the topics present in the data, much like the major plot points in each scene of a play.

When formulating labels for codes, themes, or patterns, it is always best to try to use the language of the participants. Qualitative researchers, in efforts to remain true to the data, will select words that reflect the participants' language and ideas, even often using those native terms as key labels for the data. For example, in Easton's (2001) stroke survivor study, a major subconcept early in the stroke recovery process was labeled the *mirage of recovery*, using a term coined by Veith (1988), an author of one of the books used in the theoretical

TABLE 13-1 **Quotes from Stroke Survivors**

"I always expected it to go away."
"I didn't think it was going to be very bad. I thought it was just going to be a mild stroke . . . I thought I'd be recovered before I went home."
"Even after 3 years, I can't help but believe that, eh, your, that's always a little progress . . . and I can't help but believe that it's all gonna go away."
"I always thought I would [recover]. I had a feeling that if I tried hard enough I could beat it."
"I had a neurologist told me, he said 6 weeks . . . but then . . . he [another doctor] said 9 months."
"He [the doctor] said that this was all on the left side, and I should have complete recovery, that's what he said."
Source: Easton, 2001, p. 148; used with permission of author

development for the framework of the study. Veith used this term in reference to the optimistic and unrealistic assurances given to her by physicians that she would recover from her stroke with no residual effects. The quotations in **Table 13-1** are direct quotes from face-to-face interviews with stroke survivors whose average time at the interview since their stroke was 5 years. Do these quotes illustrate any similar ideas that may have supported Easton's label of the mirage of recovery?

Computer Software

Software can assist researchers in managing qualitative data. Just as statistical software helps to manage and manipulate numbers, software for qualitative data helps to manage multitudes of words. The software available today falls into several categories that include word processing, text, analysis, grouping and linking, and displaying relationships. The type of software researchers choose will be determined by what they intend to do with the data and how they will be displayed or managed. Although software can be extremely helpful in managing large amounts of data, it does not do the work of coding for the researcher. Qualitative researchers are still responsible for analyzing and labeling the data. Software programs can help with the sorting and grouping of data so that researchers can view similar statements or categories in a systematic way. This is often referred to as computer-assisted qualitative data or qualitative data analysis software (Jacelon & O'Dell, 2005). A basic word processor, such as Microsoft Word, generally serves as the initial data entry software. That is, the interviews or field notes will be transcribed from audiotapes into a word processing document. Such software itself is a useful tool and works well for simple data analysis. However, if the study is large and will result in copious amounts of data, it is wise to investigate the benefits of a software program such as QRS NUD*IST, which stands for qualitative research and solutions nonnumerical unstructured data indexing searching and theorizing. This program is one of the most widely used for qualitative data analysis and helps to group and link concepts within the data.

This software assists researchers to label statements within the transcriptions, group them into categories, and then make interpretations or inferences. QRS NUD*IST has enormous searching capabilities to help researchers look through hundreds of pages of text to find items of specific data.

Likewise, Ethnograph (Seidel, Friese, & Leonard, 1995) is a software program for the analysis of text-based data that is highly regarded by qualitative researchers, particularly those doing ethnography. Ethnograph was first introduced in 1985 and has continued to be developed in various forms. The major categories in Ethnograph include creating and managing data files, coding data files, the code book, master list, family tree, and analytic writing. Ethnograph

TEST YOUR KNOWLEDGE 13-1

1. Put the following in the correct order:
   a. Pull together evidence into a meaningful report
   b. Code line by line
   c. Transcribe interviews
   d. Group coded data to generate categories, themes, and patterns

True/False

2. Computer software programs used to analyze qualitative data automatically generate themes based on participants' words.

3. There are many different strategies for coding data.

4. Analysis of data in qualitative research is done simultaneously with data collection.

How did you do? 1. c, b, d, a; 2. F; 3. T; 4. T

is not an easy system to learn and has few resources for technology support in the event of questions or problems.

While software can be helpful, qualitative packages are generally cumbersome to learn and require a commitment on the part of researchers to master the software to maximize its usefulness. Data entry and coding are still time consuming and tedious. The greatest benefit to such software is the ability to group, compare, and contrast data more efficiently because of easier accessibility after all data are entered. Software is also helpful when preparing written reports of the data and selecting quotations or collapsing data for presentations, although some researchers find that basic word processing software is sufficient for these purposes.

13.2   Qualitative Data Interpretation

At the end of this section, you will be able to:

< Describe how researchers draw and verify conclusions from the data
< Recognize the common ways data are presented in reports

Sandelowski (1995) distinguished between analysis and interpretation of data by stating, "In contrast, qualitative interpretation is the knowledge produced: the end-product of analysis where the researcher construes or renders the analyzed data in such a way that something new is created that is different from, yet faithful to, that data in its original form" (p. 372). In other words, data analysis is the means to an end, with the final outcome being a useful piece of research that can be applied in practice. Thus, one could say that the interpretation of qualitative data provides evidence for practice. This is the evidence of words.

Drawing and Verifying Conclusions

As the data are being analyzed, researchers are also drawing some conclusions that are continually tested and either modified, discarded, or verified. So how does one figure out what all the data and codes mean? How do researchers know that codes they have chosen to use are correct? **Table 13-2** lists five levels of qualitative data (Jacelon & O'Dell, 2005; Kearney, 2001) that range from simple to most complex. To address this question of what the data mean, one could start with the simplest level of research analysis and merely describe the phenomenon. As the levels progress to more complex, researchers become increasingly engaged in exploration, explanation, and synthesis. Qualitative

TABLE 13-2 Five Levels of Qualitative Data

Level of Data	Summary
1) A priori framework	Data analyzed according to a preexisting framework; lowest level of data; provides no new knowledge
2) Descriptive	Researcher develops labels for data categories but does not explicate relationships among the categories; useful for devising lists of descriptors on a topic
3) Developing a synthesis	Researcher explains and explores relationships among themes with logical integration
4) Increased complexity and case variance	Researcher explains variations and negative case examples of the research; a step beyond developing a synthesis
5) A product that comprehensively explains a complex human phenomenon	The level of research that is considered to be the gold standard; provides an explanation of a phenomenon with depth and breadth as to increase others' understanding and advance the science

Source: Adapted from Jacelon & O'Dell, 2005; Kearney, 2001.

researchers should strive for a product that meets level five in Table 13-2 and provides the most useful level of information aimed at positively influencing nursing practice.

For practical purposes, Miles and Huberman (1994) suggested 13 tactics for generating meaning from data. These are summarized in **Table 13-3**. Using strategies such as these, qualitative researchers extract the most important points from large amounts of data to form a logical conclusion.

To verify the conclusions drawn, Miles and Huberman (1994) suggested several other strategies. These included checking for researcher effects or bias that might have been introduced by the researcher's presence among the participants. Researchers must ask themselves if their presence may have influenced the participants to act any differently, and if so, how? Researchers should also check for *representativeness*. This means that researchers should challenge their assumption that the participants included in a study indeed represent the group. In addition, all cases that do not fit the typical profile that emerged from the data should be examined. These extreme or negative cases should be analyzed to see why they are not represented by the researchers' findings. Such exceptional cases should be few and able to be logically explained.

KEY TERM

Representativeness: Degree to which participants are like the population

TABLE 13-3 Strategies for Generating Meaning

Strategy	Summary
Noting patterns, themes	Items that "jump out" at you; commonalities
Seeing plausibility	When categories make sense, feel right, fit
Clustering	Clumping or grouping data into categories
Making metaphors	Making comparisons with things that people identify with
Counting	Looking at number of times, recurrence
Making contrasts/ comparisons	Comparing cases with practical significance
Partitioning variables	Unbundling variables as needed; separating variables that should not be clumped together
Subsuming particulars into the general	Ask if a specific thing really stands alone, or does it belong in a more general category
Factoring	Identifying general themes to see which go together
Noting relations between variables	Describing the effects of one variable on another and any relationships between concepts
Finding intervening variables	Identifying the variables that go together only with the help of an additional variable to facilitate
Building a logical chain of evidence	Defining causal links that make logical sense when viewed as a whole
Making conceptual/ theoretical coherence	Moving from constructs and interrelationships to theories and can be predictive

Source: Adapted from Miles & Huberman, 1994, pp. 245–262.

FYI

The interpretation of qualitative data should provide evidence for practice; the results of the study must be reported with sufficient rigor and details about the methods used to establish trustworthiness of the findings so that readers can have confidence that the results represent suggestions for best practice. There are three common approaches to reporting qualitative data: realist tales, confessionist tales, and impressionist tales.

Confirmation of a study's findings is enhanced if they can be *replicated*. This means that if another researcher can essentially do the same study with similar results, this helps to validate the original researcher's findings. Another strategy is to get feedback from the study participants about how well the results represent what they actually experienced. Having the participants themselves confirm the findings of the study lends credibility to the results.

Writing Reports

Another challenge of qualitative research is reporting the results. Traditional formats for reporting quantitative research do not fit well with most qualitative studies, and many authorities have suggested that qualitative reports focus much more on detailed description and integration of the discussion of methods (Burnard, 2004; Dickie, 2003). A typical report of qualitative research would follow a format similar to that presented in **Table 13-4**. Traditional reports contain an introduction, explanation of the significance of the project, a review of the relevant literature, description of methods, findings, discussion, and conclusions. However, there are several ways in which qualitative research may be presented, and researchers should carefully choose the strategy for presentation that best represents what they are trying to convey. Thought should be given to creatively reporting findings if it would enhance the ability

TABLE 13-4 **Example of Standard Components of a Qualitative Research Report**

Title page
Abstract
Introduction
Aim or purpose of the study
Review of literature
Methods
    Sample
    Setting
    Data collection methods
    Data analysis methods
Findings or results
Discussion
    Nursing implications
    Limitations of study
Conclusions

KEY TERMS

Replicated: When another researcher has findings similar to a previous study of nurses to better apply the research in practice. That said, the results of the study must be reported with sufficient rigor and details about the methods used to establish trustworthiness of the findings so that readers can have confidence that the results represent suggestions for best practice.

While there are several ways to approach the reporting of qualitative data, Van Manen (1988) identified three that are often referred to when considering how to write the report: *realist tales, confessionist tales*, and *impressionist tales*. Realist tales are the most common and were used by ethnographers such as Margaret Mead (Marshall & Rossman, 1995). When using this approach, researchers write a real-life account of the culture being studied and present it by using a third-person voice, clearly separating researchers from the participants in the study. The focus is on the many details about the group while there is very little description of methods. The researcher is almost invisible (Miles & Huberman, 1994). Peer-reviewed articles in scholarly journals or monographs are common places to publish this type of writing. These are standard and respected types of articles, but they have been criticized for being dull and boring.

Confessional tales are more personalized accounts in which the writer gives more insight into the process of data collection and shows the scientific rigor of the field methods. The confessional voice is written from the researcher's viewpoint with personal authority and thick description (Van Manen, 1988).

Impressionist tales allow researchers to chronicle their experiences in a "sort of auto-ethnography" (Marshall & Rossman, 1995, p. 118). Researchers speak more personally about the experiences of conducting the study, and they are participant observers versus disconnected realists. These reports are often more like storytelling and help the reader relive the experience.

Whichever voice researchers choose to use when reporting the results of the study, the decision should be made with the goal of communicating results in the most useful manner. Reports should be written with the audience in mind. If the audience is nursing students, the focus will be different than a focus for registered nurses who are working on their master's degrees and different still if the readers are interdisciplinary team members outside of nursing.

Patton (1990) stated that the most important aspect of reporting is focus. When writing qualitative research reports, researchers must take care to include enough detail but not too much so as to preclude the major purpose of communicating useful, evidence-based information that impacts practice. "Sufficient description and direct quotations should be included to allow the reader to enter into the situation and thoughts of the people represented in the report. Description should stop short, however, of becoming trivial and mundane" (p. 430). Sandelowski summarized her view by saying, "I think one

KEY TERMS

Realist tales: Account of culture presented in a third person voice clearly separating researchers from participants

Confessionist tales: Qualitative researchers' personal accounts that provide insight about data collection and scientific rigor

Impressionist tales: Qualitative researchers' storytelling and personal descriptions about conducting studies

KEY TERM

Personal narrative:
Conveying the
meaning of
experiences through
storytelling

of the hallmarks of a good qualitative researcher is someone who writes in a very accessible way for particular audiences" (Morse, 1994, p. 280).

Some differences in reporting formats between the four major types of qualitative research should also be noted. In phenomenological research, researchers can use realist tales, confessionist tales, or impressionist tales when writing. The choice depends on the audience and certainly on the sample size. If the sample is small, perhaps a storytelling approach would best convey the participants' experiences. The *personal narrative*, as a way of conveying the meaning of experiences, has recently received increased attention. Gaydos (2005) suggested that nurses can use their intuition to assist key informants who are ready to tell their stories in a type of cocreation of a personal narrative by using memories and metaphors. "The experience of creating a self story with a nurse can be healing, as the self story is heard by a caring person, memories are understood in new ways, and the self story is both confirmed and recreated" (p. 254). This may represent yet another way to report information about lived experience.

Grounded theory, conversely, is often presented more traditionally because it seeks to communicate a process that the researcher has discovered, lending itself to a more detached, analytical mode of reporting. So, while one could use a variety of voices in reporting qualitative data, it is key to focus the report to the audiences and choose the best approach to communicate with that audience.

With ethnography, researchers often choose the realist voice, but perhaps the impressionist tale would be better to describe information about a certain concept with a different culture. For example, if a researcher was studying death and burial practices of an unknown tribe in the jungle, perhaps a storytelling approach would be the most effective way to communicate the message

CRITICAL THINKING EXERCISE 13-1

You have just finished helping with a qualitative research study on homeless people in the rural Midwest, in which you assisted with data collection. The research team has discovered some essential health-related information about the homeless living in the vicinity of your university. The lead researcher asks your opinion about how the research should be presented for publication. She wants the information to be targeted to nurses and nursing students. How should the article be written for the target audience? What suggestions would you make about the best way to present this information to students? How could information be disseminated to promote evidence-based practice (EBP) or to improve the community outreach efforts of your university?

TEST YOUR KNOWLEDGE 13-2

1. Which of the following are strategies for drawing and verifying conclusions?
    a. checking for representativeness
    b. ignoring negative cases
    c. being sensitive to bias
    d. confirming findings through replication

2. Match the following:

    a. real life account using-third person voice   1. realist tales

    b. speaking as a participant observer about the experience   2. confessionist tales

    c. emphasizing scientific rigor in the method   3. impressionist tales

How did you do? 1. a, c, d; 2. a. 1 b. 3 c. 2

learned from the research. Henderson (2005) suggested that dramaturgy (a description of the scene or social situation that is similar to a play) be included in field notes and reported in conjunction with ethnography to better explain the societal context of social activity.

In historical research, the typical voice is the realist because the data are usually obtained from documents. Miller and Alvarado (2005) suggested that documents could be used as commentary and as actors in qualitative research. Reports using documents would include more talk and observation. Certainly with this approach, one might choose a different voice to present the results or at least take a more creative approach to reporting.

13.3   Qualitative Data Evaluation

At the end of this section, you will be able to:

‹   State why qualitative research is evaluated differently than quantitative research
‹   Define trustworthiness in terms of credibility, transferability, dependability, and confirmability
‹   Describe strategies for evaluating qualitative research

Standards for Evaluating Qualitative Data

As with quantitative research, there are certain standard criteria that are accepted for evaluating qualitative studies. These were developed because quantitative criteria such as internal validity, external validity, generalizability, reliability, and objectivity were for evaluating numbers and did not fit well when evaluating words. It is expected that qualitative studies be conducted with extreme rigor because of the potential for subjectivity that is inherent in this type of research. In addition to addressing ethical issues, such as informed consent and use of data, qualitative researchers are guided by the requirements for establishing *trustworthiness* of the study. This is a more difficult task when dealing with words and people than numbers and statistics. Lincoln and Guba (1985) proposed a different set of criteria with unique terminology that is appropriate for evaluation of qualitative research. These criteria are considered to be a gold standard to establish trustworthiness of a study.

Establishing Trustworthiness

Trustworthiness refers to the quality, the authenticity, and the truthfulness of findings in qualitative research. It relates to the degree of trust, or confidence, readers have in the results. Trustworthiness can be established by meeting four criteria (Lincoln & Guba, 1985): *credibility*, *transferability*, *dependability*, and *confirmability*. **Table 13-5** provides a summary of strategies for meeting these criteria.

Credibility

Credibility in qualitative research is akin to internal validity in quantitative research. To meet the criterion of credibility, the research must be shown to be authentic and truthful. The results should make sense and be believable. There are many strategies to help establish and evaluate credibility. Researchers should use well-established research methods and describe them with sufficient detail so the study can be replicated. If a similar study can show similar results using another method, credibility is supported.

Good interviewing skills help to establish credibility of the data. Shenton (2004) suggested that specific questions be asked of participants to ensure that they are giving the truth and not misleading researchers during interviews. *Data saturation*, when no new information is being provided by participants, should be achieved. When evaluating qualitative research for credibility, readers should be able to see that researchers used *peer debriefing* to ensure that truth emerged from the data. Peer debriefing provides researchers with another

TABLE 13-5 Strategies to Establish Trustworthiness of a Study

Credibility

Use of well-established research methods
Use of random sampling methods when possible
Triangulation
Thick description
Detailed interviews
Questioning to prevent deliberate deception by informants
Data saturation
Peer debriefing
Peer critique
Member checks
Constant comparison
Negative case analysis
Reflective commentary in journals
Established expertise and appropriate experience of the researcher
Ability to relate previous research findings to the current study

Confirmability

Audit trail
Peer debriefing
Member checks
Acknowledgment of potential sources of bias
Self-reflection of the researcher evidenced by journals
Accurate record keeping of methods and procedures
Credibility and authenticity of the data

Dependability

Audit trail
Peer debriefing
Stability of observations over time
Multiple interviews
Data saturation
Coding checks that show agreement
Uniformity of responses across subjects

Transferability

Clear explanation of the boundaries/limitations of the study
Description of the context of the study
Thick description
Deliberately trying to find negative case examples
Checking for representativeness of the data

Auditability

Fittingness
Congruent findings with other research or theories
Suggestions of other settings to test findings
Replication of the study

Sources: Adapted from Lincoln & Guba, 1985; Miles & Huberman, 1994; Sandelowski, 1986; and Shenton, 2004.

FYI

The standard criteria accepted for evaluating quantitative data (internal validity, external validity, generalizability, reliability, and objectivity) fit well for evaluating numbers, but not words, the basic unit of qualitative data. Establishing the trustworthiness of qualitative data is particularly challenging because of the potential for subjectivity that is inherent in this type of research; however it can be achieved by meeting four criteria: credibility, transferability, dependability, and confirmability.

professional's opinion and views of the data. A peer debriefing should be at the same educational and positional level as the researcher and be considered a colleague but not a supervisor or boss.

Using the constant comparison method, researchers may choose to do *member checks* in which participants are asked to confirm the results as data collection progresses. Another strategy, *negative case analysis*, includes analyzing cases that do not seem to fit the patterns or categories that are emerging and exploring the reasons for this. Other strategies involve keeping a reflective journal that details thoughts and ideas as they emerge and relating the research findings of others' studies to one's own. In addition, researchers should have appropriate expertise, skills, and established credentials to carry out the study. All of these strategies are used to both establish and evaluate credibility.

Transferability

Transferability relates to external validity, generalizability, or fittingness of the data (Miles & Huberman, 1994). Although the purpose of qualitative research is not specifically to generalize, it is necessary to note the significance of the study with relation to its importance in helping understand a phenomenon in different contexts or situations. For example, a qualitative study uncovers themes about the lived experience of waiting for a heart transplant. Nurses working with transplant patients would need to consider if these findings are transferable to individuals waiting for another type of organ transplant. Certainly if the findings of a study are congruent with existing research or theoretical frameworks, this supports transferability. Other strategies used to meet this criterion include providing a clear explanation of the limitations of the study, giving thick descriptions of the study context and setting, leaving a paper trail that can be followed, checking that the data are representative in most cases, and making suggestions for other settings to test the findings. In addition, if the study is sufficiently described so that it can be replicated, transferability is supported.

Dependability

Reliability in quantitative research is similar to dependability or *auditability* in qualitative research. This means that the study should be consistent over time and that enough observations were made that showed this consistency. Dependability is supported when coding checks show that there is agreement within and among the concepts and themes. When existing theories can be tied to new findings, dependability is enhanced. Review by peers or colleagues, as with peer debriefing, also supports dependability. There should be a logical consistency between responses of participants that carries over into the coding and analysis procedures. The audit trail should show rigor of research method with multiple journals being used to record thoughts, decisions, and reflections about the data and coding procedures.

Confirmability

Confirmability in qualitative research is most like objectivity in quantitative research. Neutrality refers to the findings of the research, versus the researcher (Sandelowski, 1986). Some subjectivity is inherent in qualitative methods because the researcher is the instrument for data gathering as well as analysis and interpretation. It is when any potential biases are not recognized or accounted for that confirmability may be in question. Member checks and peer debriefing may help researchers to remain true to the data. Methods of the study should be described completely with an audit trail clearly detailing all aspects of the study. The self-reflections of researchers should be recorded in journals. Record keeping must be accurate. Data should make sense and appear to be real and authentic.

In summary, qualitative researchers should consciously address the four criteria that are the standard for establishing trustworthiness. Nurse researchers should review the strategies for meeting these criteria and build them into the research plan. Journaling, good record keeping, recording detailed field notes

KEY TERMS

Member checks: When the researcher shares the results with participants to ensure the findings reflect what they said

Negative case analysis: Qualitative strategy involving the analysis of cases that do not fit patterns

Auditability: Degree to which qualitative data can be shown to be consistent over time and support findings

CRITICAL THINKING EXERCISE 13-2

Compare and contrast each of the four criteria of trustworthiness of a qualitative study with what you have learned about the criteria for evaluating quantitative studies. How are they alike? How are they different? What is your understanding of the reasons behind using different measures to evaluate qualitative versus quantitative research?

TEST YOUR KNOWLEDGE 13-3

1. Which of the following are criteria for establishing trustworthiness?
   a. credibility
   b. reliability
   c. confirmability
   d. inferability

2. Which of the following are techniques used by qualitative researchers?
   a. peer review
   b. member checks
   c. data saturation
   d. audit trails

How did you do? 1. a, c; 2. b, c, d

with thick descriptions, and recognizing sources of bias are essential to meet these criteria. In addition, scientific and ethical standards for rigor in qualitative research must be maintained to provide the best possible believability and trustworthiness for the study.

13.4   Keeping It Ethical

At the end of this section, you will be able to:

‹ Describe key ethical issues in qualitative research

There are numerous ethical issues inherent in qualitative research. Some issues arise during the initial phases of planning a research study, and others arise during implementation. Certain ethical issues are of note during data analysis, interpretation, and evaluation. Miles and Huberman (1994), long considered a standard resource for qualitative data analysis, recommended that specific ethical issues be given particular attention. They are summarized in **Table 13-6**.

Many of the ethical issues posed in Table 13-6 can be addressed by establishing trustworthiness of the research project. Researchers should be able to defend and explain why a study is significant and describe what it adds to EBP.

TABLE 13-6 Ethical Issues to Consider in Qualitative Research

Issue	Ask Yourself (Implications for Nursing)
Worthiness of the project	Is this a worthwhile project to pursue? Does it have value? What will it add to nursing knowledge?
Competence boundaries	Am I adequately prepared to conduct this study? If not, what would I need to become so, or who can I get to assist me?
Informed consent	Have I obtained informed consent from participants? Did I explain the purpose, risks, and benefits of the study and allow time for questions?
Benefits, costs, and reciprocity	Does the cost/benefit ratio make sense? Is it fiscally responsible?
Harm and risk	Is there minimal harm or risk to participants? Have any potential effects been explained to participants?
Honesty and trust	Have I established trust and been honest with participants?
Privacy, confidentiality, and anonymity	Have I received institutional review board approval? How have I assured privacy, confidentiality of responses, and anonymity of participants?
Intervention and advocacy	Do I advocate for the right when I observe wrong behavior of other researchers? Can my subjects count on me to put their interests above my own?
Research integrity and quality	Do I adhere to accepted standards of practice and embrace scientific integrity? Am I absolutely true to the data to avoid fraud and deception in analysis?
Ownership of data and conclusions	Have I clarified who owns my work and the results of it? Who has access to the data, and have I protected the data, and thus my subjects, sufficiently?
Use and misuse of results	Have I taken adequate care to avoid interventions and persuasion instead of remaining in the role of the researcher? Have my findings been sufficiently described so as not to be misinterpreted or misused by others for their own purposes?
Conflicts, dilemmas, and trade-offs	Have I examined all of the possible ethical dilemmas that could arise, or have arisen, from my data collection and analysis? Have I thought of my position related to these possible dilemmas and how I would handle them?

Source: Adapted from Miles & Huberman, 1994.

Potential risks to participants should be carefully weighed against benefits, and justifications for decisions should be made. Researchers should be competent to carry out proposed studies and have the necessary skills and expertise to interpret findings and to convey them for use in practice.

Because qualitative research deals with unique human situations that are largely interpreted by researchers, issues related to scientific rigor seem to be always present. It is essential, then, that qualitative researchers take every care to ensure anonymity and confidentiality of study participants. In sharing people's words and thoughts, the potential for inappropriate disclosure of personal information is greater than in studies where numbers and statistics form the descriptions. Careful explanations of how data will be used and how participants' identities will be protected must be given to participants. Researchers must make certain to honor these obligations. Participants must be able to trust that if they share their innermost thoughts with researchers, researchers will do what has been promised with regard to protecting privacy and safeguarding personal data. Details of the study must be carefully planned in advance so that even the smallest matter is not left to chance.

Qualitative researchers have an inherent obligation and contract with participants to use data in the way that has been specified, to analyze data with an open mind, and to be true to the data when reporting findings. For example, when using ethnography as a method, researchers must address challenges such as avoiding bias when studying cultural groups different from their own and finding how best to ensure informed consent among these groups (Lipson, 1994).

When the research findings further nursing science and translate into better care and outcomes for study participants, or those like them, then researchers

TEST YOUR KNOWLEDGE 13-4

True/False

1. Qualitative researchers do not need to obtain informed consent because they participate in the process.

2. Qualitative researchers often assign code names to participants to protect their privacy.

3. There is no harm or risk associated with participation in qualitative research because data are typically collected through interviews.

How did you do? 1. F; 2. T; 3. F

can be assured that an important task has been accomplished. If this goal is kept in mind while maintaining the expected rigor of this type of research, researchers are much less likely to violate ethical standards.

RAPID **REVIEW**

- In qualitative research, data collection, data analysis, and data interpretation often occur simultaneously.

- Data analysis involves coding data into manageable units. This can involve data reduction, open coding, or axial coding.

- Coded data are used to generate categories, themes, and patterns.

- Themes, using the language of the participants, paint a meaningful picture of the phenomenon.

- Computer software, such as QRS NUD*IST and The Ethnograph, can assist researchers in organizing and managing data.

- Interpretations of qualitative data strive to produce a description of complex phenomena.

- Qualitative research reports have a format different from quantitative reports. Authors use one of three approaches: realist tales, confessionist tales, or impressionist tales.

- Criteria used to evaluate quantitative studies cannot be applied when evaluating qualitative studies. Qualitative studies are trustworthy when strategies have been used to meet credibility, transferability, dependability, and confirmability.

- Maintaining confidentiality and protecting anonymity are especially important when conducting qualitative studies. Researchers have an obligation to remain true to the data during analysis and interpretation.

APPLY WHAT YOU HAVE LEARNED

www

The committee has almost completed entering information into the grid on the companion website. Conclude the analysis by reporting the findings from the Schwappach, Hochreutener, and Wernli (2010) article. Because this is a qualitative study, it is appropriate to indicate the themes in the findings column.

REFERENCES

Bogdan, R. C., & Biklen, S. K. (2003). *Qualitative research for education: An introduction to theory and methods* (4th ed.). Boston: Allyn & Bacon.

Burnard, P. (2004). Writing a qualitative research report. *Accident & Emergency Nursing, 12*(3), 176–181.

Corbin, J., & Strauss, A. L. (1990). Grounded theory research: Procedures, canons, and evaluative criteria. *Qualitative Sociology, 13*(1), 3–21.

Dickie, V. A. (2003). Data analysis in qualitative research: A plea for sharing the magic and the effort. *American Journal of Occupational Therapy, 57*(1), 49–56.

Easton, K. L. (2001). *The post-stroke journey: From agonizing to owning.* Unpublished doctoral dissertation, Wayne State University, Detroit, MI.

Gaydos, H. L. (2005). Understanding personal narratives: An approach to practice. *Journal of Advanced Nursing, 49*(3), 254–259.

Henderson, A. (2005). The value of integrating interpretive research approaches in the exposition of healthcare context. *Journal of Advanced Nursing, 52,* 554–560.

Jacelon, C. S., & O'Dell, K. K. (2005). Analyzing qualitative data. *Urologic Nursing, 25,* 217–220.

Kearney, M. (2001). Focus on research methods: Levels and applications of qualitative research evidence. *Research in Nursing & Health, 24,* 145–153.

Lincoln, Y. S., & Guba, E. G. (1985). *Naturalistic inquiry.* Newbury Park, CA: Sage.

Lipson, J. G. (1994). Ethical issues in ethnography. In J. M. Morse (Ed.), *Critical issues in qualitative research methods* (pp. 333–356). Newbury Park, CA: Sage.

Marshall, C., & Rossman, G. B. (1995). *Designing qualitative research.* Thousand Oaks, CA: Sage.

Miles, M. B., & Huberman, A. M. (1994). *Qualitative data analysis.* Thousand Oaks, CA: Sage.

Miller, F. A., & Alvarado, K. (2005). Incorporating documents into qualitative nursing research. *Journal of Nursing Scholarship, 37,* 348–353.

Morse, J. M. (1994). *Critical issues in qualitative research methods.* Newbury Park, CA: Sage.

Patton, M. Q. (1990). *Qualitative evaluations and research methods.* Newbury Park, CA: Sage.

Polit, D., & Beck, C. T. (2006). *Essentials of nursing research: Methods, appraisal, and utilization* (6th ed.). Philadelphia: Lippincott Williams & Wilkins.

Sandelowski, M. (1986). The problem of rigor in qualitative research. *Advances in Nursing Science, 8*(3), 27–37.

Sandelowski, M. (1995). Qualitative analysis: What it is and how to begin. *Research in Nursing & Health, 18,* 371–375.

Schwappach, D. L. B., Hochreutener, M. A., & Wernli, M. (2010). Oncology nurses' perceptions about involving patients in the prevention of chemotherapy administration errors. *Oncology Nursing Forum, 37,* E84–E91.

Seidel, J., Friese, S., & Leonard, D. C. (1995). *The Ethnograph V4.0: A users guide.* Unpublished manuscript.

Shenton, A. K. (2004). Strategies for ensuring trustworthiness in qualitative research projects. *Education for Information, 22,* 63–75.

Strauss, A., & Corbin, J. (1998). *Basics of qualitative research: Techniques and procedures for developing grounded theory.* Thousand Oaks, CA: Sage.

Tesch, R. (1990). *Qualitative research: Analysis types and software tools.* New York: Falmer Press.

Van Manen, M. (1988). *Tales of the field: On writing ethnography.* Chicago: University of Chicago Press.

Veith, I. (1988). *Can you hear the clapping of one hand?: Learning to live with a stroke.* Berkeley, CA: University of California Press.

At the end of this chapter, you will be able to:

< Describe strategies that individuals use to reduce uncertainty when making decisions

< Explain how findings from quantitative designs contribute to evidence

< Discuss characteristics that should be appraised when evaluating qualitative and quantitative designs

< Rank pieces of evidence using a rating system

< Explain the development and use of clinical practice guidelines

< Discuss reasons why nurses should follow agency policies even when they conflict with evidence

active rejection
adoption
AGREE II
case control studies
clinical practice guidelines
cohort studies

descriptive studies
evidence hierarchies
GRADE
levels of evidence
meta-analyses
passive rejection

pilot
randomized controlled
    trial
rejection
uncertainty

CHAPTER 14

Weighing In on the Evidence

Carol O. Long

14.1 Deciding What to Do

At the end of this section, you will be able to:

< Describe strategies that individuals use to reduce uncertainty when making decisions

Evidence-based nursing is the process whereby nurses make clinical decisions that integrate the best available research with clinical relevance and incorporate the patient's preferences, values, and circumstances (University of Minnesota, 2001). This assumes that sufficient evidence or research that is clinically relevant, methodologically sound, and of scientific merit exists (Sackett, Straus, Richardson, Rosenberg, & Haynes, 2000). Some practice decisions will be made by a committee responsible for overseeing policies and procedures. Other decisions can be made when circumstances warrant a timely decision. For example, a patient may have an unusual complication where the current protocol has not been successful. Healthcare providers may collaborate after securing evidence about an innovative treatment, and after consulting with the patient, they decide to implement it.

How do clinicians make decisions? There are really only two options: *adoption* or *rejection* of the innovation. Individuals aim to select the option about which they are the least uncertain. "*Uncertainty* is the degree to which a number of alternatives are perceived with respect to the occurrence of an event and the relative probability of these alternatives" (Rogers, 2003, p. 6). Individuals typically select to adopt an innovation when uncertainty is reduced. When there is a significant amount of uncertainty about a new innovation, individuals generally reject adopting the innovation.

KEY TERMS

Adoption: Applying an innovation to practice

Rejection: Decision not to adopt an innovation

There are different strategies that individuals use to reduce uncertainty during the decision-making process (Rogers, 2003). Sometimes individuals may decide to try a portion of the innovation or adopt the innovation on a trial basis, which is called a *pilot*. For example, a new infusion pump may be piloted on one unit to determine its efficiency before implementing the new model throughout the facility. In some cases, a trial of a new idea by peers and their recommendations are sufficient to affect a decision about adoption. Respected individuals are often asked to endorse innovations as a marketing strategy. Offering free samples, a frequent practice among pharmaceutical companies, is another strategy that can facilitate the adoption of an innovation. Demonstrations can also be effective in furthering the adoption of innovations.

There are two kinds of rejection: active and passive (Rogers, 2003). Just because an innovation is adopted for a period of time, there are no guarantees that rejection will not occur. *Active rejection* involves active decision making after a pilot and purposefully deciding not to adopt the innovation. For example, in the pilot testing of the new infusion pump, nurses reported that alarms sounded for no reason, requiring more time to monitor infusions. Therefore, it was decided not to adopt the new infusion pumps in the facility. *Passive rejection* is when there is no consideration given to adopting the innovation. In essence, no decision is ever made and old practices are continued.

Culture plays an important role in the decision-making process. In some cultures, it is common for decisions to be made collectively. For example, married women in an Asian village attended a presentation by a government change agent about intrauterine devices (IUD). At the conclusion of the presentation, 18 women voted to adopt this method of birth control. They immediately went to a nearby clinic to have an IUD inserted (Rogers, 2003). In some cultures, such as mainstream America, individual goals supersede the goals of the group and a vote described above would be rare.

TEST YOUR KNOWLEDGE 14-1

1. Which of the following strategies reduce uncertainty during decision making?
   a. pilot testing
   b. reviewing samples
   c. listening to the opinions of peers
   d. relying on intuition

How did you do? 1. a, b, c

TABLE 14-1 Five-Step Approach for Evidence-Based Nursing Practice	
Ask	Identify the research question. Determine if the question is well constructed to elicit a response or solution.
Acquire	Search the literature for preappraised evidence or research. Secure the best evidence that is available.
Appraise	Conduct a critical appraisal of the literature and studies. Evaluate for validity and determine the applicability in practice.
Apply	Institute recommendations and findings and apply them to nursing practice.
Assess	Evaluate the application of the findings, outcomes, and relevance to nursing practice.

Source: Adapted from Straus, 2005.

KEY TERMS

Uncertainty: Degree to which alternatives are preceived as potentially successful

Pilot: Adopting an innovation on a trial basis

Active rejection: Purposefully deciding not to adopt an innovation

Passive rejection: Lack of consideration given to adopting an innovation, hence old practices are continued

14.2   Appraising the Evidence

At the end of this chapter, you will be able to:

< Explain how findings from quantitative designs contribute to evidence
< Discuss characteristics that should be appraised when evaluating qualitative and quantitative designs
< Rank pieces of evidence using a rating system

Does the Study Provide Good Evidence?

Determining the relevance of the evidence requires skill in analyzing research studies. These skills include techniques used for determining the strength, significance, and relevance of the evidence. There are five steps for evaluating and implementing evidence-based practice (EBP), which are listed and briefly described in **Table 14-1** (Straus, 2005). While each step requires solid analytical skills and application of good research methods, these are especially important for weighing the evidence. When appraising, nurses need to ensure that the first two steps, ask and acquire, were thoroughly executed.

After specific literature about the research question has been collected, a rigorous evaluation is conducted. The mere fact that an individual study has been published in a peer-reviewed journal does not ensure that the findings are sound (Steinberg & Luce, 2005). During appraisal, the study design, how the research was conducted, and the data analysis are all scrutinized to ensure that the study was sound. **Table 14-2** presents questions that should be considered when examining individual studies.

Quantitative Designs

By this point, you are familiar with quantitative methods and are ready to learn to apply your knowledge about research principles to make decisions about the evidence. A critical appraisal of quantitative studies is necessary for nurses to determine the validity, reliability, statistical significance, clinical importance, and applicability of the findings (University of Alberta, 2003a).

TABLE 14-2 **Questions to Consider When Appraising Nursing Studies**

Introduction

(1) Does the introduction demonstrate the need for the study?
(2) Is the problem clearly and concisely identified?
(3) Is the problem presented with enough background material to acquaint the reader with the importance of the problem?
(4) Is the purpose of the study clearly stated?
(5) Are the terms and variables relevant to the study clearly defined?
(6) Are the assumptions clearly and simply stated?
(7) If appropriate to the design, are hypotheses stated?
(8) Does the study use a theoretical framework to guide its design?

Review of the Literature

(1) Is the review of the literature (ROL) relevant to the problem?
(2) Is the ROL adequate in terms of the range and scope of ideas, opinions, and points of view relevant to the problem?
(3) Is the ROL well organized and synthesized?
(4) Does the ROL provide for critical appraisal of the contribution of each of the major references?
(5) Does the ROL conclude with a summary of the literature with implications for the study?
(6) Is the ROL adequately and correctly documented?

Methods

(1) Is the research approach appropriate?

(2) Was the protection of human subjects considered?

(3) Are the details of data collection clearly and logically presented?

(4) Are the instrument(s) appropriate for the study both in terms of the problem and the approach?

(5) Are the instrument(s) described sufficiently in terms of content, structure, validity, and reliability?

(6) Is the population and the method for selecting the sample adequately described?

(7) Is the method for selection of the sample appropriate?

(8) Is the sample size sufficient?

(9) Is attrition of sample reported and explained?

(10) Does the design have controls at an acceptable level for the threats to internal validity?

(11) What are the limits to generalizability in terms of external validity?

Results

(1) Is the presentation of data clear?

(9) Are the characteristics of the sample described?

(2) Was the best method(s) of analysis selected?

(3) Are the tables, charts, and graphs pertinent?

Discussion

(1) Are the results based on the data presented?

(2) Is the evidence sufficient to draw conclusions?

(3) Are the results interpreted in the context of the problem/purpose, hypothesis, and theoretical framework/literature reviewed?

(4) Are the conclusions and generalizations clearly stated?

(5) Are the limitations of the findings clearly delineated?

(6) Are the generalizations within the scope of the findings or beyond the findings?

(7) Does the study contribute to nursing knowledge?

When appraising *meta-analyses*, nurses should establish if well-designed studies that fit with the research question are included. Both published and unpublished studies should be included. One must be confident that the literature was systematically searched to obtain an adequate sample size. There should be evidence that statistical findings from the studies were merged to identify incongruencies and similarities of findings among the studies.

Other kinds of studies that nurses are likely to appraise are *randomized controlled trials* (RCT). RCT sometimes also stands for randomized clinical trials. Studies of this type can be found in the nursing literature and are especially important to the advancement of EBP. Studies showing that a treatment has a

FYI

There are five steps for evaluating and implementing EBP: ask, acquire, appraise, apply, and assess. Nurses need to examine all the evidence to make recommendations about practice changes.

greater effect, rather than studies showing a small effect, weigh more heavily in the appraisal. Sample sizes are typically large, and often patients are recruited from multiple sites. Studies are strengthened by using strategies such as blinded designs, ensuring that interventions are controlled, and by showing that patient groups were similar at the beginning of the trial (University of Alberta, 2003b). Reviewers should determine if there is bias by using the five Cs approach for evaluation: contamination, crossover, compliance, cointervention, and count, that is, attrition (Attia & Page, 2001). Results should be readily applicable to patients with similar clinical and demographic backgrounds.

Cohort studies, sometimes known as quasi-experimental studies, examine a large sample of the population and observe changes in characteristics over time. Like RCT, there are two groups: one that receives the treatment and one that does not. Then both groups are followed for a period of time related to the outcome of interest. Cohort studies are considered to be less rigorous than RCT because subjects are not randomly assigned to groups; therefore the two groups may vary on other characteristics and the controls may be difficult to identify. Cohort studies may be retrospective or prospective.

Case control studies compare two groups: those who have a specific condition and those who do not have the condition. This type of research usually focuses on rare disorders or disorders where there is considerable time between exposure or treatment and the onset or change in outcome. In case control studies, fewer subjects are needed than in cross-sectional studies. The disadvantages of case control studies include the potential for confounding variables, bias (recall and selection), and difficulty in selecting the control group.

Descriptive studies aim to provide information about a phenomenon. They are nonexperimental in design and most often lack an independent variable. They are often used when little is known about the phenomenon. Correlational and survey designs fall into this category of research. These types of studies may have large or small samples, be cross-sectional or longitudinal, and typically report means, standard deviations, and frequencies. Correlations are reported if the purpose of the study is to determine relationships.

Qualitative Designs

Qualitative nursing research provides a valuable contribution to building nursing theory and understanding the practice of nursing. Qualitative studies have not been highly regarded in the growing field of EBP. Traditionally, it has been difficult for many individuals to accept qualitative findings because the criteria to determine scientific rigor are so different from quantitative methods. However, the contributions of qualitative research should not be underestimated because findings provide the patient perspective, which is an important component of EBP.

KEY TERMS

Cohort studies: Quasi-experimental studies using two or more groups

Case control studies: Studies that compare two groups, those with and without a specific condition

Descriptive studies: Nonexperimental studies used to provide information about a phenomenon

When nurses appraise qualitative studies there are several characteristics that should be evaluated. The qualitative method selected should be appropriate for the research question. Unlike quantitative research, samples tend to be small, and nurses should determine that researchers report reaching saturation. Scientific rigor should be maintained through orderly and detailed data collection. Strong evidence is generated when analyses are systematic, rigorous, and auditable (Thorne, 2001). Conclusions should be grounded in the data.

Ranking the Evidence

Decisions should not be based on one piece of evidence. Nurses need to examine all the evidence to make recommendations about practice changes. You may think that this will be difficult to do; however, it is usually easier than appraising an individual study. There are predetermined scales, known as *evidence hierarchies*, that guide decisions for ranking studies. Because authors are typically very clear in their descriptions of their studies, it is usually easy to rank the evidence correctly. In EBP, there are a variety of ways to rate evidence. These rating systems have been designed by professional organizations or expert panels. **Figure 14-1** provides a rating system that

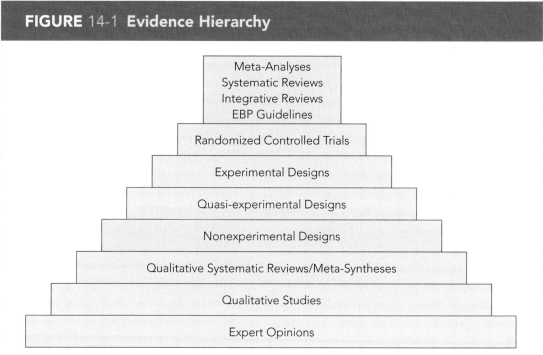

FIGURE 14-1 **Evidence Hierarchy**

Meta-Analyses
Systematic Reviews
Integrative Reviews
EBP Guidelines

Randomized Controlled Trials

Experimental Designs

Quasi-experimental Designs

Nonexperimental Designs

Qualitative Systematic Reviews/Meta-Syntheses

Qualitative Studies

Expert Opinions

Source: Adapted from Melnyk & Fineout-Overholt, 2005, p. 10.

KEY TERMS

Evidence hierarchies:
Predetermined scales
that guide decisions
for ranking evidence

Levels of evidence:
Predetermined scales
that guide decisions
for ranking evidence

is commonly used in nursing to make decisions about evidence (Melnyk & Fineout-Overholt, 2005).

While the rating system in Figure 14-1 provides a commonly encountered method for rating evidence, you will likely come across other useful rating scales. Regardless of the scale selected, they all have in common ranking/rating systems to stratify the evidence by quality. Several notable rating scales are presented so that you can become familiar with alternative approaches.

Members of the Canadian Task Force on Preventive Health Care were one of the first to generate *levels of evidence* (Centre for Evidence-Based Medicine, 2001). The recommendations that typically accompany clinical practice guidelines are graded by examining the risk versus the benefit and the quality or strength of the evidence on which the information is derived. Reviewers determine if the results are transferable to the clinical setting with qualifications for the uncertainty of risk for the population at large (Swinglehurst, 2005).

First convened by the U.S. Public Health Service in 1984, the U.S. Preventive Services Task Force (USPSTF) is currently sponsored by the Agency for Healthcare Research and Quality (AHRQ). As a federally funded agency, AHRQ's mission is to support quality of care and EBP most notably through its Evidence-based Practice Centers (EPCs) throughout the United States. USPSTF is supported by an EPC. It is the "leading independent panel of private-sector experts in prevention and primary care" (USPSTF, 2006. p. 1). The USPSTF evaluates scientific studies related to clinical preventive services and makes recommendations based on explicit criteria, generally intended for use in the primary care setting. Recommendations provide information about the evidence, allowing clinicians to make informed practice decisions. The task force grades the strength of the evidence from "A" (strongly recommends), "B" (recommends), "C" (no recommendation for or against), "D" (recommends against), or "I" (insufficient evidence to recommend for or against).

CRITICAL THINKING EXERCISE 14-1   [www]

Read the following description and determine how you would rank this study using the rating system in Figure 14.1.

The purpose of this experimental study was to test the efficacy of two interventions for mothers and their adolescents in delaying initiation of sexual intercourse for youth who are not sexually active and encouraging the use of condoms among sexually active youth. Adolescents (N-582) and their mothers were randomly assigned to one of two groups (Dilorio et al., 2006).

Recognizing the diversity of rating systems, they identified three relevant domains and elements for systems to grade the strength of the evidence: Grade definitions can be accessed at http://www.uspreventiveservicestaskforce.org/uspstf/grades.htm.

1. Quality: The aggregate of quality rating for individual studies, predicted on the extent to which bias was minimized
2. Quantity: The magnitude of effect, numbers of studies, and sample size or power
3. Consistency: For any given topic, the extent to which similar findings are reported using similar and different study designs (AHRQ, 2002, p. 4)

The Cochrane Collaboration, founded in 1993, is an international not-for-profit organization that is dedicated to disseminating information about the effects of health care worldwide. The Cochrane Collaboration has several resources at the disposal of evidence-based practitioners, one of them being the Cochrane Database of Systematic Reviews, published quarterly from The Cochrane Library (The Cochrane Collaboration, 2006). They are best known for their comprehensive evidence-based summaries written in an easy-to-read style.

The Joanna Briggs Institute (2006), a formidable institution whose central mission is to evaluate health outcomes for the client and community from an economic and clinical perspective, also focuses on the evaluation of research. The institute identifies topics for systematic review, plans the review, and uses expert panels and reviewers to publish systematic reviews. Steps identified by The Cochrane Collaboration and levels of evidence are used in the reviews. Levels of evidence, ranked one through four, are based on the following factors: feasibility, appropriateness, meaningfulness, effectiveness, and economic evidence. The Joanna Briggs Institute uses the criteria of feasibility, appropriateness, meaningfulness, and effectiveness to grade recommendations used in clinical practice guidelines and gives them letter grades of A through E.

Clearly there are many evidence rating and grading schemes. There is controversy about which scheme provides the best evaluation. Yet deciding on one universal rating scheme may not be feasible. Grades of Recommendations, Assessment, Development, and Evaluation, known as *GRADE*, has been an international effort to develop a universal system of evaluation. The mission has been to consolidate the forces of many reputable organizations and agencies, such as AHRQ, the U.K. National Institute for Health and Clinical Excellence, and the World Health Organization (Guyatt et al., 2006). GRADE is closely aligned with The Cochrane Collaboration. The GRADE system ranks the strength and quality of evidence into four levels: (1) high, (2) moderate, (3) low, and (4) very low. The recommendation is either (1) strong or (2) weak. Plans are underway for the United States to consider the adoption of GRADE

(Falck-Ytter, 2006). Criteria of the GRADE system can be accessed at http://www.gradeworkinggroup.org/FAQ/index.htm.

When weighing evidence, nurses may be involved in discussions that involve determining the clinical significance of the findings (Straus, Richardson, Glasziou, & Haynes, 2005). Questions about diagnosis, therapy, prognosis, causation, harm, and etiology can be discussed. Examples are provided in **Table 14-3**. It would not be unusual for the discussion to include concepts such as relative risk, relative risk reduction, absolute risk reduction, numbers needed to treat, and odds ratio. Definitions of these terms are provided in **Table 14-4**. This content is included so that you can become familiar with the terminology, not so that you become adept at performing calculations.

It should be noted that not all the rating systems discussed include a way to rank qualitative studies. Melnyk (2004) notes that EBP must consider their inclusion when reviewing studies of merit, and those qualitative studies should assume a step on the hierarchy ladder. The research findings that emerge from qualitative research are valued because they incorporate the "patients' voice into evidence based process" (p. 142). As such, qualitative research deserves a place in the hierarchy of evidence although it may not be considered to have a "high" rating (Swinglehurst, 2005).

TABLE 14-3 Common Clinical Questions

Diagnosis	Queries the selection and interpretation of diagnostic tests
Therapy	Examines therapeutic treatment(s) for healthcare problems and their efficacy, cost, and potential harm
Prognosis	Evaluates the course of treatment over time, any complications, and overall prognosis
Causation/Harm/Etiology	Looks at the causes of disease, including iatrogenic causes, potential harm, and benefits
Other	Questions may be written related to prevention, clinical examinations, cost, point of contact, or patient/client data

Source: Adapted from Straus et al., 2005.

TABLE 14-4 Definitions of Clinically Significant Statistics

Relative risk (*RR*) is the risk of the outcome in the treated group (*Y*) compared to the risk in the control group (*X*). $RR = Y / X$

Relative risk reduction (*RRR*) is the percentage reduction in risk in the treated group (*Y*) compared to the control group (*X*). $RRR = 1 - Y / X \times 100\%$

Absolute risk reduction (ARR) is the difference in risk between the control group (*X*) and the treatment group (*Y*). $ARR = X - Y$

Numbers needed to treat (*NNT*) is the number of patients that must be treated over a given period of time to prevent one adverse outcome. $NNT = 1 / (X - Y)$

Odds ratio (*OR*) is the odds of an experimental patient suffering an event compared to a patient in the control group or the odds of risk.

Source: Adapted from Straus et al., 2005.

TEST YOUR KNOWLEDGE 14-2

1. Which of the following would be considered when appraising quantitative studies?
   a. representativeness of the sample
   b. trustworthiness
   c. sample size
   d. control over extraneous variables

2. Which of the following would be considered when appraising qualitative studies?
   a. validity and reliability
   b. audit trail
   c. thick description
   d. participants are experienced in the phenomenon

3. Place the following kinds of evidence in order from highest to lowest.
   a. meta-analysis
   b. case studies
   c. RCT
   d. cohort studies
   e. expert opinion

How did you do? 1. a, c, d; 2. b, c, d; 3. a, c, d, b, e

14.3   Clinical Practice Guidelines: Moving Ratings and Recommendations Into Practice

At the end of this section, you will be able to:

‹ Explain the development and use of clinical practice guidelines

---

KEY TERM

Clinical practice guidelines:
Recommendations based on evidence that serve as useful tools to direct clinical practice

Various professional associations and other clinical entities have developed *clinical practice guidelines* to be used in practice settings. The National Guideline Clearinghouse, under the auspices of the AHRQ and the U.S. Department of Health and Human Services (http://www.guidelines.gov), hosts a myriad of these documents. Nurses can purchase other guidelines through professional associations.

Most guidelines have a standard format and therefore provide similar information. Most often they identify the names of the reviewers or development team or a listing of the background of experts who served on the panel. The method of review is generally presented, such as the number of citations, databases searched, and other means to capture relevant research and secondary sources of interest. Panel members typically review findings and reach consensus about best practice. Usually limitations of the review are listed, which may include exclusions of certain topics tangential to the guidelines or issues that were beyond the scope of the review, such as issues related to legal matters, economics, or healthcare system issues. Recommendations by the panel members form the basis of clinical practice guidelines. Appendixes often contain the rating scales used to evaluate the evidence, tables, and figures. Often a disclaimer is included that notes that recommendations serve as guides and are not to be used in lieu of "critical thinking, sound judgment, and clinical experience" (American Geriatrics Society, 2002, p. S207).

Clinical practice guidelines are just that: guidelines. A guideline is a "unit of knowledge devised on the basis of a review of the current state of scientific evidence" (Heath, 2005, p. 269). As such, they serve as useful tools to direct clinical practice. They typically include all relevant process and outcome measures that would be indicated for the average patient with a specific diagnosis or treatment problem. Guidelines provide an easy-to-read consolidation of research findings. Algorithms or decision trees are used in some guidelines to demonstrate a stepwise process for resolving a specific clinical problem. Although evidence-based clinical practice guidelines specify good clinical practice, healthcare providers may not be using them to their maximum potential. Clinicians, patients, and healthcare systems stand to benefit when guidelines are easy to follow and widely used (Bazian Ltd., 2005).

While guidelines may appear to be comprehensive, they do not include all of the variables that clinicians encounter when managing patient conditions or treatments. Guidelines are unable to address unique patient characteristics. Social, psychological, emotional, spiritual, environmental, and biomedical factors are not considered in the guidelines. Using guidelines can result in making generalizations that can be problematic. Guidelines provide a general approach to clinical management based on scientific evidence, but caution must be exercised when applying them to individual patients.

Heath (2005) warns about the use of clinical practice guidelines as an "instrument of surveillance" (p. 269), whether it is for financial reward, measures of quality, punitive action, or ethical or legal considerations. Manipulation of guidelines for such purposes should be considered carefully because their primary intent is to describe best practice for the typical patient. Nurses must be aware that guidelines may also contain bias and therefore must critically evaluate them.

To remedy some of the concerns about bias, the Appraisal of Guidelines Research and Evaluation (*AGREE II*) instrument was developed as part of an international collaborative of researchers and policy makers. The instrument provides a standard framework for the development and implementation of clinical practice guidelines. A checklist of 23 items across six different quality domains provides a useful tool for the generation and evaluation of guidelines (AGREE Collaboration, 2009: **Table 14-5**). The AGREE II instrument is generic and can be applied to all types of clinical practice guidelines. The instrument can be accessed at http://www.agreecollaboration.org/pdf/agree-instrumentfinal.pdf.

Clinical practice guidelines will continue evolving because of the momentum generated by EBP. Evidence is more available because of the increased

FYI

CRITICAL THINKING EXERCISE 14-2

Think about your last clinical experience. What practice guidelines would have been helpful? Where might you find these guidelines? Do you think the staff would be receptive to your using clinical guidelines on the unit?

TABLE 14-5 Domains of Quality in the AGREE II Instrument

Domain 1	Scope and purpose of the guidelines
	Purpose, aims, clinical questions, and target population are evaluated
Domain 2	Stakeholder involvement
	Identifies the congruence of meeting the needs of the intended users
Domain 3	Rigour of development
	Evaluates the process of gathering and synthesizing the evidence and how it was examined
Domain 4	Clarity and presentation
	Evaluates the format and clearness of the guideline
Domain 5	Applicability
	Addresses the behavioral, cost, and organizational consequences of applying the guideline
Domain 6	Editorial independence
	Specification of possible conflicts of interest are enumerated and the independence of the recommendations

Source: AGREE Collaboration, 2009.

capacity to search the literature. Computerization capabilities are allowing information from guidelines, such as algorithms or decision tools, to be loaded into the PDAs of practicing nurses. Others, such as insurers, attorneys, and ethicists will be interested in guideline development.

TEST YOUR KNOWLEDGE 14-3

True or False

1. Patient care must follow clinical guidelines exactly.

2. A panel of experts synthesizes evidence to make recommendations for clinical guidelines.

3. Nurses should evaluate clinical guidelines because they may be biased.

How did you do? 1. F; 2. T; 3. T

14.4   Keeping It Ethical

At the end of this section, you will be able to:

< Discuss reasons why nurses should follow agency policies even when they conflict with evidence.

When weighing evidence, nurses need to remember that there are no perfect studies; therefore, there are always limitations of the evidence. Even though systematic reviews are highly regarded, they may not provide all the answers a researcher would like to have or that the clinician might want to know. Evidence might support a certain treatment or intervention, but one must remember that the literature might not report all aspects that were tested. For example, the use of case reports might reveal harm from a pharmaceutical agent, such as an adverse drug reaction. A systematic review might ensue to appraise harmful consequences of the pharmaceutical agent. However, because negative trials typically never make it to publication, the information would not be uncovered during a systematic review. Similarly, the evidence derived from research might be perceived to be ironclad, without exception or deviation. This cannot be further from the truth. Clinicians must examine the evidence within the context of the question, and consequently, the answer that is revealed. Nurses must incorporate several sources of evidence at the bedside: the individual patient experience, the clinical experience, and policy or cost considerations (Rycroft-Malone, 2003). Questions that nurses can ask are (Straus et al., 2005):

< Are our patients enough like those in the study so that results can apply?
< Is the treatment feasible in our setting?
< What are the potential benefits and harms from the treatment for our patients?
< What are our patients' values and expectations about the treatment and the outcomes?

Generalizability is always a concern when deciding how to apply evidence to practice. Application of evidence to practice relies on findings and recommendations generated from samples. Individual patients may not have the same characteristics as study subjects, and this raises concern for nurses when considering the adoption and application of the evidence to the point of care.

Gray (2005) suggests that the path from the evidence to utilization in practice can be value laden and raise ethical concerns. For example, recommendations for specific diagnostic screenings, such as routine cancer testing for

FYI

Nurses who engage in activities that promote EBP, such as journal clubs and policy committees, may find that even after diligently reviewing the evidence, practice changes are not implemented. Nurses need to follow agency policy and act as change agents to effectively bring the evidence to the point of care.

TEST YOUR KNOWLEDGE 14-4

True or False

1. Decisions about clinical practice are based solely on evidence.

2. If a conflict exists between evidence and facility policy, the nurse should implement procedures based on the evidence.

How did you do? 1. F; 2. F

specific age groups or genders, may be scientifically justified based on incidence and prevalence rates and other population characteristics. In a perfect world of unlimited resources, a full battery of cancer screening tests could begin at age 21 and be done annually thereafter. However, in the real world with limited resources and potential harm from repeated screening, it would be difficult to justify this standard of screening. Using resources for routine, comprehensive cancer screening at age 21 would be considered foolish and wasteful. Clinical decisions are ultimately derived from choices that are impacted by the needs and values of the population. Even when practice is based on evidence, other factors might impact clinical decision making.

An ethical dilemma may arise if agency policy conflicts with evidence. Nurses who engage in activities that promote EBP, such as journal clubs and policy committees, may find that even after diligently reviewing the evidence, practice changes are not implemented. But for legal reasons, nurses need to follow agency policy and act as change agents to effectively bring the evidence to the point of care.

RAPID REVIEW

 When weighing the evidence, clinicians can either adopt or reject an innovation. Innovations are adopted when uncertainty is reduced.

 There are two kinds of rejection: active and passive.

 Appraisal involves reviewing the design, sampling methods, and data analysis.

 Quantitative designs must be appraised to ensure that appropriate conclusions are drawn.

APPLY WHAT YOU HAVE LEARNED

The committee has been meeting regularly to analyze evidence and is now able to make recommendations for best practice. Of course, if you were on an actual EBP committee, there would be much more evidence about medication errors that you would need to consider. We have provided only a sample of evidence for you in this exercise. When making a policy decision in clinical practice, you would need to consider all the evidence. First, examine each study to determine if the study is valid by considering the questions presented in Table 14-2. Then use the rating system described in Figure 14-1 to assign each piece of evidence a ranking. Make a decision about the evidence and write a nursing policy that you think will reduce medication errors. Be sure to consider the feasibility (organizational and individual barriers) of your policy. A template is included on the companion website that serves as an example of a format that can be used to standardize the way policies are written in a healthcare facility. Use this template to record your policy.

 Qualitative research is appraised for scientific rigor, systematic analysis, and conclusions that are grounded in data.

 Evidence hierarchies provide a meaningful way to rank research studies based on scientific rigor and the levels of evidence: clinical practice guidelines, meta-analyses, systematic reviews, RCTs, cohort studies, case control studies, descriptive studies, qualitative studies, expert opinions, and case studies.

 A variety of professional organizations and clinical entities have developed rating systems that provide a systematic way to rate risks, benefits, quality, and strengths of the evidence. An international collaboration proposes to use the GRADE system as a single standard.

 Clinical practice guidelines provide recommendations for practice based on a thorough review of evidence conducted by expert panel members. Because clinical practice guidelines might have bias, the AGREE instrument assists nurses in evaluating guidelines.

 Nurses must consider other factors aside from evidence that impact clinical decision making.

REFERENCES

Agency for Healthcare Research and Quality. (2002). *Systems to rate the strength of scientific evidence.* Evidence Report/Technology Assessment. No 47. AHRQ Pub. No. 02-E015. Retrieved May 26, 2005, from http://www.ahrq.gov

AGREE Collaboration. (2009). *Appraisal of guidelines for research and evaluation (AGREE) instrument.* Retrieved October 9, 2010, from http://www.agreecollaboration.org/pdf/agreeinstrumentfinal.pdf

American Geriatrics Society. (2002). The management of persistent pain in older persons. AGS panel on persistent pain in older persons. *Journal of the American Geriatrics Society, 50,* S205–S224.

Attia, J., & Page, J. (2001). A graphic framework for teaching critical appraisal of randomized controlled trials. *Evidence Based Medicine, 6,* 68–69.

Bazian Ltd. (2005). Do evidence-based guidelines improve the quality of care? *Evidence-Based Healthcare and Public Health, 9,* 270–275.

Centre for Evidence-Based Medicine. (2001). *Oxford Centre for Evidence-based Medicine Levels of Evidence.* Retrieved October 8, 2010, from http://www.cebm.net/index.aspx?o=1025

Dilorio, C., Resnicow, K., McCarty, F., De, A. K., Dudley, W. N., Wang, D. T., & Denzmore, P. (2006). Keepin' it R. E. A. L.! Results of a mother-adolescent HIV prevention program. *Nursing Research, 55*(1), 43–51.

Falck-Ytter, Y. (2006). *GRADE–Moving towards a consensus on a consistent approach to grading evidence and recommendations.* Small conference grant abstract. Retrieved October 9, 2010, from http://www.gradeworkinggroup.org/publications/AHRQ-grant_2006.pdf

Gray, J. A. (2005). Evidence-based and value-based healthcare. *Evidence-based Healthcare and Public Health, 9,* 317–318.

Guyatt, G., Vist, G., Falck-Ytter, Y., Kunz, R., Magrini, N., & Schünemann, H. (2006). An emerging consensus on grading recommendations? *Evidence Based Medicine, 11,* 2–4.

Heath, I. (2005). The use and abuse of guidelines. *Evidence-based Healthcare and Public Health, 9,* 268–269.

Joanna Briggs Institute. (2006). *Levels of evidence.* Retrieved October 9, 2010, from http://www.joannabriggs.edu.au/pubs/approach.php

Melnyk, B. M. (2004, Second Quarter). Evidence digest. *Worldviews on Evidence-based Nursing,* 142–145.

Melnyk, B. M., & Fineout-Overholt, E. (2005). *Evidence-based practice in nursing and healthcare: A guide to best practice.* Philadelphia: Lippincott Williams & Wilkins.

Rogers, E. M. (2003). *Diffusion of innovations* (5th ed.). New York: Free Press.

Rycroft-Malone, J. (2003). Consider the evidence. *Nursing Standard, 17*(45), 21.

Sackett, D. L., Straus, S. E., Richardson, W. S., Rosenberg, W., & Haynes, R. B. (2000). *Evidence-based medicine: How to practice and teach EBM* (2nd ed.). Edinburgh, Scotland: Churchill Livingstone.

Steinberg, E. P., & Luce, B. R. (2005). Evidence based? Caveat emptor! *Health Affairs, 24*(1), 80–92.

Straus, S. E. (2005). *Introduction to teaching evidence-based health care.* University of Toronto Knowledge Translation Program. PowerPoint Presentation. Retrieved September 25, 2006, from http://www.cebm.net/?o=1021

Straus, S. E., Richardson, W. S., Glasziou, P., & Haynes, R. B. (2005). *Evidencebased medicine: How to practice and teach EBM* (3rd ed.). Edinburgh, Scotland: Elsevier.

Swinglehurst, D. (2005). Evidence-based guidelines: The theory and the practice. *Evidence-based Healthcare and Public Health, 9,* 308–314.

The Cochrane Collaboration. (2006). *What Is The Cochrane Collaboration?* Retrieved January 10, 2007, from http://www.cochrane.org/docs/descrip.htm

Thorne, S. (2001). Data analysis in qualitative research. *Evidence Based Nursing, 3,* 68–70.

University of Alberta. (2003a). *Introduction to evidence based medicine.* Retrieved November 12, 2010, from http://www.ebm.med.ualberta.ca/EbmIntro.html

University of Alberta. (2003b). *Therapy/Prevention Article Appraisal Guide.* Retrieved November 12, 2010, from http://www.ebm.med.ualberta.ca/Therapy.html

University of Minnesota. (2001). *Evidence based nursing.* Retrieved October 9, 2010, from http://evidence.ahc.umn.edu/ebn.htm

U.S. Preventive Services Task Force. Agency for Healthcare Research and Quality. (2006). *About USPSTF.* Retrieved October 9, 2010, from http://www.uspreventiveservicestaskforce.org/about.htm

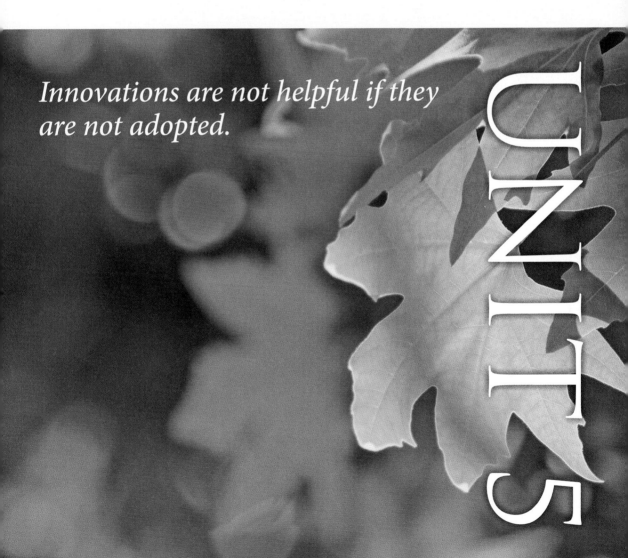

Implementation

Innovations are not helpful if they are not adopted.

UNIT 5

CHAPTER OBJECTIVES

www.

At the end of this chapter, you will be able to:

< Identify evidence-based practice (EBP) models

< Discuss barriers to application of evidence to practice

< Discuss strategies for creating change to support EBP

< Describe strategies for engaging others in change

< List Kotter's eight phases of change

< Discuss dilemmas that can be encountered during change

KEY TERMS

barriers
change
change phases model
conduct and utilization of research in nursing (CURN)

cost-benefit ratio
disciplined clinical inquiry model
Iowa model for EBP to promote quality care
journal club

Nursing Quality Indicators
Stetler model

CHAPTER 15

Transitioning Evidence to Practice

Maria Young

15.1 Evidence-Based Practice Models to Overcome Barriers

At the end of this section, you will be able to:

< Identify EBP models
< Discuss barriers to application of evidence to practice

By now you should have an understanding of EBP. As you recall from Chapter 1, trial and error, educated guesses, or intuition are all useful in contributing to a nurse's experience that guides practice, but these processes or behaviors do little to provide the stronger evidence needed to achieve positive patient outcomes. In today's rapidly changing, highly complex healthcare environment, patient outcomes based upon evidence provide the foundation for safe, quality patient care. So how do we take the evidence and apply it to the point of care? What EBP models have the potential to increase our use of research to guide care? What are the barriers to applying evidence to practice? What elements are necessary if nurses are to create a practice culture that is committed to and supports evidence-based processes, policies, and actions? Answers to these questions will be examined in this chapter as well as exploring some strategies to create an EBP setting.

Evidence-Based Practice Models

EBP is nothing new to nurses. Florence Nightingale, through her use of meticulous record keeping and data analysis, was able to demonstrate that mortality rates decreased when sanitary methods were improved (Riddle, 2006). By using the data she had gathered, Nightingale was able to develop interventions that, when applied to medical and surgical patients, reduced mortality rates caused by unsanitary conditions. In general, the term "EBP" describes a model of care whereby nurses, using current evidence or research knowledge, make decisions using clinical expertise and patient preferences to guide patient care (Melnyk & Fineout-Overholt, 2005). The University of Minnesota (2001) has on its website the following definition of evidence-based care: "Evidence Based Nursing is the process by which nurses make clinical decisions using the best available research evidence, their clinical expertise and patient preferences" (p. 1). Clinical practice based on evidence would seem to be an important goal for nurses, yet many nurses acknowledge that they do not incorporate research findings into their practices (Fink, Thompson, & Bonnes, 2005). Why this is so has been explored by many researchers (Hommelstad & Ruland, 2004; Pettengill, Gillies, & Clark, 1994; Retsas, 2000; Rutledge, Greene, Mooney, Nail, & Ropka, 1998; Sitzia, 2001) and is a topic that remains under continued examination (French, 2002).

Several models have emerged and serve as the foundation for evidence-based nursing practice. Some models are the *conduct and utilization of research in nursing (CURN)* project, the *Stetler model*, and the *Iowa model for EBP to promote quality care*.

CURN

The CURN project was one of the earliest attempts to increase the use of research in practice by registered nurses (RNs). It was a 5-year project awarded to the Michigan Nurses' Association by the Division of Nursing in the 1970s and focused on helping nurses transition research findings into their practice settings (Polit & Beck, 2004). An outcome of the CURN project was a realization that practicing nurses would use research only if it had been widely disseminated and was relevant to their practice (Horsely, Crane, & Bingle, 1978). The CURN project moved nursing practice from customs, opinions, and authority to searching for the best research available and integrating the evidence with a nurse's clinical expertise, patient preferences, and existing resources (Polit & Beck). To appreciate the importance of the CURN project, consider that in the 1970s nurses engaged in practice behaviors solely because "we've always done it this way." For example, consider the practice of restraining patients by tying them to their beds or chairs to prevent falls. It has only been through research studies examining this practice that nurses now know that while tying patients to beds or chairs may have prevented falls, it also predisposed patients to other injuries, such as strangling, as they tried to get out of the restraints. Because 70% of accidents among hospitalized patients are related to falls, the need to conduct research and disseminate the findings about the prevention of patient falls remains a priority (Agency for Healthcare Research and Quality, 2005). Without the work of the CURN project, an understanding of how nurses embrace and use research in their clinical practice might not have occurred.

The Stetler Model

While the CURN project has given nurses insight about how and why nurses embrace research in clinical practice, the Stetler model (Stetler, 2001) focuses upon how individual practitioners adopt research findings at the bedside. Originally developed in 1976 as the Stetler/Merram model for research utilization, this model can be used to systematically integrate research into practice. The model was updated to facilitate examination of both the product and process of research. Products of research are things such as research findings. An example of this would be that 9 out of 10 dentists recommend a certain chewing gum for their patients who chew gum. The process of research tells how to go about solving a problem. For example, nurses on a busy medical surgical unit want to explore why they have noticed an increase in patient falls. They begin by examining the problem by conducting a chart audit of all the patients who have fallen in the past year. Next they determine if there are any common factors. When the common factors are identified, a list of risk factors is developed that can guide interventions to reduce the number of falls. These nurses are engaging in a process of research. As evidenced in these examples, both product and process are important to facilitate EBP.

Because Stetler's model (2001) is prescriptively designed, it provides practitioners with step-by-step instructions for integrating research into practice and is useful to help nurses deliver safe patient care. In the updated version of the model (see **Figure 15-1**), Stetler provides a traditional graphic accompanied by a narrative of the five phases of the model.

In the first phase of the model, known as the preparation phase, Stetler (2001) encourages nurses to be very clear about the purpose, the context, and the sources of any research evidence. Questions to be answered include what are the issues, who are the stakeholders, and how will we define our outcomes? Questions such as these assist nurses to be very purposeful in their thinking when making decisions about EBP.

The second phase of the model is the validation phase. In this phase, nurses analyze the evidence to determine if it is sufficient and credible to use in the practice setting. You should be familiar with techniques, such as creating a grid to summarize and weigh research articles, that are important for successfully progressing through this phase.

FYI

In today's rapidly changing, highly complex healthcare environment, patient outcomes based upon evidence provide the foundation for safe, quality patient care. Several models have emerged and serve as the foundation for evidence-based nursing practice, including the CURN project, the Stetler model, and the Iowa model for EBP to promote quality care.

FYI

By understanding barriers to creating EBP, nurses are better able to anticipate potential problems when initiating research activities in clinical practice. Barriers to applying research to practice include organizational culture, nurses' belief systems related to practice, and research-related barriers.

The third phase, also called the comparative evaluation/decision making phase, is when nurses engage in labeling, condensing, organizing, and attributing meaning to all the assembled evidence. Questions that could be considered during this phase are do you have all the data needed to make a good decision and is the evidence that you have uncovered reliable? For example, you would not want to make a practice change if the only evidence came from a nonpeer-reviewed journal because this would not be very strong evidence. By the end of this phase a decision is made about whether to use the research to guide practice.

In the fourth phase, the challenge is to translate or apply the research in the practice setting (Stetler, 2001). For many organizations this may be easier said than done. For example, consider the difficulties encountered when integrating knowledge related to smoking cessation into practice. Based on various studies, researchers project that smoking rates can be reduced by 50% over the next decade if patients receive smoking cessation advice before they leave the hospital (USDHHS, 2006). Thus, while cessation advice would seem to be a necessary component for quality patient care, many organizations struggle to integrate smoking cessation advice into a patient's plan of care as is apparent from the dismal results on the government website www.hospitalcompare.hhs.gov. This illustrates how difficult it can be to adopt innovations in a social system. When applying research to practice, it is important for nurses to think carefully about how the evidence will be communicated, disseminated, and applied. In this example, relevant questions to consider include who will be responsible for implementing smoking cessation guidelines into practice, what resources (time, money, personnel) are available to operate the program, and how will the success of the program be measured? Change is at the heart of this phase.

In the fifth and final phase of the Stetler model (2001), nurses evaluate the outcomes of the change in practice. Continuing with the example of smoking cessation, questions from the fourth phase provide a means for evaluating how well research is applied to practice. In the fourth phase it was decided that practice should be based on the knowledge that patients respond best to smoking cessation advice when they are hospitalized because of symptoms related to smoking and indicate they are ready to quit. Practice was changed to have nurses assess patient readiness to quit and immediately provide written and verbal smoking cessation information. The success of this practice change can be evaluated by comparing how often patients are given smoking cessation advice with how many of them actually quit smoking.

The Iowa Model

The Iowa model for EBP to promote quality care is a systematic method that explains how organizations change practice (see **Figure 15-2**). Originally

FIGURE 15-1   Stetler Model of Research Utilization to Facilitate EBP

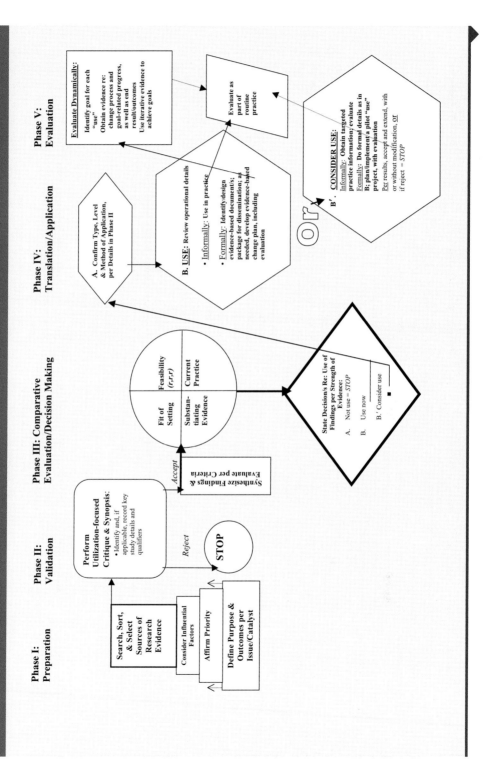

(continued)

Phase I: Preparation	Phase II: Validation	Phase III: Comparative Evaluation/Decision Making	Phase IV: Translation/Application	Phase V: Evaluation
Purpose, Context, & Sources of Research Evidence:	Credibility of Findings & Potential for/Detailed Qualifiers of Application:	Synthesis & Decisions/Recommendations per Criteria of Applicability:	Operational Definition of Use/Actions for Change:	Alternative Types of Evaluation:
• **Potential Issues/Catalysts** = *a problem, including unexplained variations or less-than-best practice; or routine update of knowledge; or validation/ routine revision of procedure, policy, etc; or innovative program goal*	• **Critique & synopsize essential components, operational details, and other qualifying factors, per source**	• **Synthesize the cumulative findings:** o *Logically organize & display the similarities and differences across multiple findings, per common aspects or sub-elements of the topic under review*	• **Types** = *cognitive, symbolic &/or instrumental* • **Methods** = *informal or formal; direct or indirect* • **Levels** = *individual, group, or department/organization* • **Direct instrumental use:** *change individual behavior (vis-à-vis assessment; plan/intervention options); implementation details; &/or evaluation), or change policy, procedure, protocol, algorithm, program components, etc.*	• **Evaluation can be formal or informal, individual or institutional** • **Consider cost-benefit of various evaluation efforts** • **Use RU as a process to enhance credibility of evaluation data** • **For both dynamic & pilot evaluations, include two types of evaluative information:** o *formative, regarding actual implementation & goal progress* o *summative, regarding Phase I outcomes and goal results*
• **Affirm perceived problems with internal evidence**		o *See instructions for use of utilization-focused review tables to facilitate this task; fill in the tables for group decision making or potential future synthesis*		
• **Focus on high priority issues**	• **Critique systematic reviews**	o *Evaluate degree of substantiation of each aspect/subelement; reference any qualifying conditions* • **Evaluate degree & nature of other criteria:** *feasibility (r,r,r = risk, resources, readiness); pragmatic fit; & current practice*	• **Cognitive use:** *validate current practice; change personal way of thinking; increase awareness; better understand or appreciate condition/s or experience/s* • **Symbolic use:** *develop position paper or proposal for change; persuade others regarding a way of thinking*	
• **Decide if need to form a team or involve formal "structures"/key stake-holders**	• **Reassess fit of individual sources** • **Rate the level & quality of each evidence source per a "table of evidence"**	• **Make a decision whether/what to use:** o *Can be a personal practitioner-level decision or a recommendation to others* o *Judge the strength of this decision; indicate if primarily "research-based" or, "evidence-based"; qualify the related level*	**CAUTION: Assess whether translation/product or use goes beyond actual findings/evidence:** o *Research evidence may or may not provide various details for a complete policy, procedure, etc.; indicate this fact to users, and note differential levels of evidence therein*	
• **Consider other influential internal and external factors, such as beliefs, resources, or timelines**	• **Differentiate statistical and clinical significance** • **Eliminate noncredible sources**	*of strength of decision/recommendations per related table* o *For formal recommendations, determine degree of stakeholder consensus*	• **Formal dissemination & change strategies should be planned per relevant research** *(Include Dx analysis):* o *Simple, passive education is rarely effective as an isolated strategy. Consider multiple strategies; e.g., interactive education, opinion leaders, educational outreach, audit, etc.*	
• **Define desired, measurable outcome/s**	• **End the process if there is no evidence or if there is clearly insufficient credible research evidence that meets your need**	• **If decision = "Not use" research findings:** o *May conduct own research or delay use until additional research is done by others* o *If still decide to act now; e.g., on evidence of consensus or another basis for practice,*	o *Consider implementation models (e.g., Kitson or PRECEDE)* • **Consider need for appropriate, reasoned variation** • **WITH B, where a decision to use in the setting:** o *With formal use, may need a dynamic evaluation to effectively implement & continuously improve/refine use of best available evidence*	
• **Seek out systematic reviews** • **Determine need for an explicit type of research evidence, if relevant** **Select research sources with conceptual fit**	See Stetler et al. (1998) for noted tables, reviews, & synthesis process.	*STOP use of model but consider need for planned change and evaluation* • **If decision = "Use/Consider Use," can mean a recommendation for or against a specific practice**	• **WITH B', where made a decision to consider use & thus obtain additional, pragmatic information before a final decision** o *With formal consideration, need a pilot project* o *With a pilot project, must assess if need IRB review, per relevant institutional criteria*	NOTE: Model applies to all forms of practice, i.e., educational, clinical, managerial, or other

Source: Stetler, C. (2001). Evidence-based practice and the use of research: A synopsis of basic concepts and strategies to improve care. Washington, DC: NOVA Foundation.

FIGURE 15-2 The Iowa Model of Evidence-Based Practice to Promote Quality Care

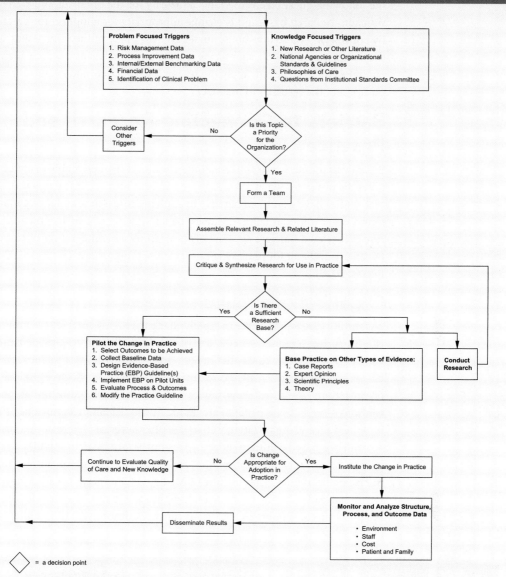

Reference
Titler, M.G., Kleiber, C., Steelman, V., Rakel, B., Budreau, G., Everett, L.Q., Buckwalter, K.C., Tripp-Reimer, T., & Goode C. (2001). The Iowa model of evidence-based practice to promote quality care. *Critical Care Nursing Clinics of North America, 13*(4), 497-509.

Source: Used/reproduced with permission from Marita G. Titler, PhD, RN, FAAN, University of Iowa Hospitals and Clinics. Copyright 1998.

KEY TERM

Barriers: Factors
that limit or prevent
change

a research utilization model, it has been updated recently to include more
emphasis on EBP and renamed the Iowa model of evidence-based practice
to promote quality care (Titler et al., 2001). In this model nurses consider
the following questions: is the topic a priority for the organization, is there a
sufficient research base, and is change appropriate for adoption for practice?
By considering these questions, nurses address many of the same issues as in
the Stetler model (2001), such as the need to gather relevant research, identify
outcomes to be achieved, apply the research to practice, and evaluate the application of the research to practice.

Barriers to Connecting Research and Practice

By understanding *barriers* to creating EBP, nurses are better able to anticipate
potential problems when initiating research activities in clinical practice. Several studies have examined barriers to applying research to practice and have
found organizational culture, nurses' belief systems related to practice, and
research-related barriers as some of the reasons why integration of research
findings is difficult for practicing nurses at the point of care (Fink et al., 2005;
Retsas, 2000).

Organizational Culture

That health care is practiced in a rapidly changing, highly complex environment
is no surprise to nurses. Nurses are constantly challenged to provide patients
with high quality, safe care with limited resources. How successful nurses are at
delivering high quality patient care can depend upon how effective professional
organizations are in fostering nurses' abilities to develop and initiate interventions aimed at safe patient care. Funk, Tornquist, and Champagne (1995)
identified several organizational characteristics necessary to create and sustain
an evidence-based culture: a) adequate resources for research activities, b) support and encouragement for inquiry, and c) an expectation for staff to engage
in research activities. The Institute of Medicine (2004) report called for organizational leaders to "incorporate multiple academic and other research-based
organizations to support HCOs [healthcare organizations] in the identification

CRITICAL THINKING EXERCISE 15-1

Why do nurses seem reluctant to incorporate research findings into their
practice? The next time you are on a clinical unit, ask the staff how they
apply research findings in their practice.

and adoption of evidence-based management systems" (p. 155). This is good news to nurses who have often practiced in environments that seldom recognized the need for, nor appreciated, the evidence needed for best practice.

Within the nursing profession there is evidence of changing expectations as noted by the American Nurses Association's (ANA) development of ***Nursing Quality Indicators*** (ANA, 1998). These indicators show the outcomes of nursing care and are meant to address patient safety and quality of care. Organizations committed to quality assurance collect data on the following initiatives:

KEY TERM

Nursing quality indicators: Outcomes of nursing care that address patient safety and quality of care

- ‹ Patient satisfaction with pain management
- ‹ Patient satisfaction with educational information
- ‹ Patient satisfaction with overall care
- ‹ Patient satisfaction with nursing care
- ‹ Mix of RNs, licensed practical nurses (LPNs), and unlicensed staff caring for patients in acute care settings
- ‹ Total nursing care hours provided per patient day
- ‹ Pressure ulcers
- ‹ Patient falls
- ‹ Nosocomial infection rate
- ‹ Nursing staff satisfaction

Nurses are expected to use the best evidence available to achieve the best patient outcomes possible (Krugman, 2003). Many organizations have come to appreciate the link between EBP and positive patient outcomes as a result of changing reimbursement policies. Third party payers are demanding the implementation of policies, processes, and practices that have the greatest potential to contribute to the best outcomes. When organizations support EBP, the potential exists to balance costs as well as benefits to patients (Hill, 1999). The reason this balance is important has to do with the limited resources being experienced in health care today. Payers, in an effort to conserve their expenditures, are interested in knowing where their dollars are being spent. They want to know what patients are getting for their money (Hill). This does not mean payers are interested only in the dollar value; they are also interested in the quality of the care. In other words, a balance needs to be achieved between quality and cost of care. If the cost is low but patients are continually being readmitted because they did not receive appropriate care in the beginning, nothing would be gained. Conversely, high cost does not necessarily translate into quality care.

Nurses' Belief Systems Related to Practice

Nurses are no different than most humans when asked to make changes. For many people, change is difficult. Some might react by outright refusal to change. Others will pretend to go along with the change but in reality not be in favor of it. Some will totally embrace the change. Studies indicate that nurses generally have a positive attitude toward research (Thompson, 2001), but they often feel that they do not have the authority to change their practice (Sitzia, 2001). Some nurses, while having been exposed to research in their basic programs, have in the ensuing years done little with the knowledge they gained in school. For others, no formal instruction related to research was required, making the ability to read, understand, and analyze research a skill that was never developed (Polit & Beck, 2004). Creating educational opportunities for nurses to learn about EBP will help to overcome this barrier.

Research-Related Barriers

Research-related barriers make it difficult for the nurse at the point of care to understand, interpret, and/or use the research. Because the ability to replicate a study and achieve the same results means a nurse can have greater confidence in applying the evidence to practice it would seem there is a need to conduct and disseminate research findings in a way that bedside nurses can understand. Unfortunately this is not the case because "complex statistical information and dense research jargon pose barriers to knowledge diffusion to most practicing nurses" (Polit & Beck, 2004, p. 680). The authors suggest that there are no perfect studies, and nurses would be wise to consider research findings as they engage in EBP.

 TEST YOUR KNOWLEDGE 15-1

1. Which of the following described the use of research by RNs?
   a. Stetler model
   b. Iowa model
   c. CURN
   d. Institute of Medicine Report

2. Which of the following are American Nurses Association Nursing Quality Indicators?
   a. pressure ulcers
   b. patient satisfaction with pain management
   c. staffing mix
   d. nurse satisfaction

How did you do? 1. c; 2. a, b, c, d

15.2 Creating Change

At the end of this section, you will be able to:

< Discuss strategies for creating change to support EBP
< Describe strategies for engaging others in change
< List Kotter's eight phases of change

The key to transitioning evidence to practice is to reframe thinking about organizational culture, knowledge about research, attitudes about research, and skills in using research. Change is at the heart of reframing our thinking to make decisions about EBP.

What Is Change?

Change is a process that creates an alteration in a person or the environment. Fullan (2001) defines change as a "double-edged" sword (p. 1). For many people change represents excitement and challenge, while for others change is feared and avoided. Just as we needed to understand the barriers to research utilization, we now need to understand how change can affect EBP. On one hand, if nurses are in organizations that operate from a philosophy of "we have done it this way for years," one can expect change to be painful. On the other hand, it can be equally disturbing if one is in an organization that seems to change with the seasons. So what is the solution? Prepare, prepare, prepare, or as Fullan notes, it is about strategizing. Think of EBP as a process. By using some of the models described in this chapter, nurses can strategize about how to embed evidence into practices, processes, and policies. You can learn more about the change process by reading the works of Beer, Eisenstat, and Spector (1990), Hammel (2002), and Kotter (1996).

> **FYI**
>
> Just as nurses need to understand the barriers to research utilization, they need to understand how change can affect EBP. One place to start when engaging others in transitioning to EBP is to conduct an assessment of the practice environment.

CRITICAL THINKING EXERCISE 15-2

Identify a nurse on your clinical unit who has a skill for creating tables in a computer program. Who would be good at collecting and organizing data? Find another nurse who has a talent for public speaking. Try to include as many colleagues as possible.

Engaging Others in Change

One place to start engaging others in transitioning to EBP is to conduct an assessment of the practice environment. In conducting the assessment, nurses may find it helpful to include as many of their colleagues as possible.

Table 15-1 provides an example of a tool for assessing the practice environment. While this tool is by no means an exhaustive list of questions, it provides the reader with an understanding of the types of questions to be asked to gain a complete picture of a practice environment. After the data are collected, decide if a problem exists. To illustrate this concept, recall the medical surgical unit where the nurses perceived that there had been an increase in patient falls. Suppose when the data were examined, patient falls appeared to have actually

---

TABLE 15-1 Assessment of Practice Environment

Date of Assessment: _____

Practice Environment Being Assessed: _____

Answer as many of the following questions as possible. The more complete the answers, the better the quality of the assessment.

1. What types of patients do you take care of on your unit?
2. What is the average daily census on the unit?
3. What care delivery model do the nurses on the unit use to care for patients?
4. What is the staffing mix on the unit? How many RNs, LPNs, aides?
5. How are practice errors reported?
6. Who is responsible for reporting practice errors?
7. What are the top three practice errors reported on your unit?
8. When errors are identified, what is done to correct the error?
9. Where is the policy and procedure manual on your unit?
10. How easy is it for you to access the policy and procedure manual?
11. How often are policies and procedures updated in your organization?
12. Who is responsible for updating policies and procedures?
13. How much input do staff nurses have related to creating or revising policy and procedure?
14. What are the quality initiatives in place on the unit at present?
15. How well is the unit doing related to the quality initiatives?
16. How are the results of quality initiatives communicated to staff?

decreased. One would have a difficult time convincing colleagues on the unit, much less nursing administrators, that there was a need to change practice, process, or policy. From this scenario it would seem that another important activity to engage others in transitioning evidence to practice is the need to be able to demonstrate that a problem exists.

What if you did not have this skill related to creating and communicating a problem statement? What could you do next? One approach that might be considered would be to develop competencies related to data collection and problem identification. Identify someone on the unit or within the organization who collects, organizes, and presents the data and problem well. You will recognize these colleagues because you will understand the issues and data when listening to their presentations. Another way to develop abilities to gather, organize, and present data would be to volunteer to help a more experienced nurse. Through such collaboration, two things will be accomplished. First, a better understanding of the process can be gained. Second, you will develop a collegial relationship with someone who can assist you in the future.

A *journal club* is another technique to engage others in transitioning evidence to practice (Krugman, 2003). If you do not feel comfortable taking the lead on this, ask a nurse manager, nurse educator, advanced practice nurse (APN), or nursing administrator in your organization for help. In many organizations, journal clubs take the form of brown bag lunches, nursing grand rounds, or unit-based potlucks. These gatherings provide a relaxed atmosphere where nurses can be exposed to practice issues and current evidence and ask questions. For some individuals, it is easier to ask questions and challenge assumptions with those they interact with on a daily basis. For others, a more formal structure to the inquiry and learning process may be necessary. The *disciplined clinical inquiry model* (**Figure 15–3**) is useful for structuring a journal club (Sanares & Heliker, 2002). This model was developed to empower nurses in clinical practice to consider the patient, the clinical setting, resources, and evidence as they transition evidence to practice. Because the model addresses unit problems and relies on the unit staff to be engaged in the process, nurses tend to be more collaborative, thus creating a unit culture of support and accomplishment.

Many of the preceding examples for engaging others in the change process are voluntary. However, at times change is mandatory. For example, the American College of Cardiology (ACC) and the American Heart Association have strong evidence for how to treat patients with heart failure (HF) and myocardial infarcts. The ACC has developed guidelines that have demonstrated improved patient outcomes when the guidelines are followed. Payers are evaluating the effect of these guidelines on patient outcomes. Organizations that have initiated practice, process, and policy changes are recognizing the

KEY TERMS

Journal club:
Disseminating research among nurses by discussing articles in a small group

Disciplined clinical inquiry model:
Model developed to empower nurses to transition evidence to practice

FIGURE 15-3   **Disciplined Clinical Inquiry Model**

The UTMB
Disciplined Clinical Inquiry Model

Source: Sanares, D., & Heliker, D. (2006). A framework for nursing clinical inquiry: Pathway toward EBNP. In K. Malloch & T. Porter-O'Grady (Eds), *Introduction to evidence-based practice in nursing and health care* (p. 37). Sudbury, MA: Jones and Bartlett.

high quality, low cost care that patients receive. Organizations are changing by using standardized order sets where practice guidelines are embedded into physician orders or nursing care plans, care maps, or clinical pathways. Care maps and clinical pathways tend to be multidisciplinary in nature and guide practitioners along a continuum of care for the patient. **Figure 15-4** is an example of a clinical pathway for treating patients with HF. Healthcare providers are expected to follow the guidelines. Care maps or clinical pathways, while not mandatory, are effective means to incorporate EBP.

Making Change Happen

What can we say about change? Because individuals do not view the concept of change in the same manner, identifying strategies to make change less frequent or less frightening for others is desirable. Constant organizational change can be stressful. Think how you would feel if every 6 months the policies related to charting changed. It would be frustrating to learn a new way of charting so frequently. Conversely, never making any changes or making changes very slowly can also be frustrating. Much has been written about the change process. John Kotter (1996) is known for his work on change. He proposes an eight-

FIGURE 15-4   Pathway Population Goals

CORE MEASURE DOCUMENT

☐ SMMC ☐ SMHS ☐ SMDC Medical Center

Pathway Population Goals

1. Four day average length of stay
2. 100% of appropriate HF patients prescribed ACE or ARB and Beta Blockers at discharge or documentation (if contraindicated)
3. Diuretic need assessed at discharge
4. Smoking cessation education is addressed in 100% of smoking patients
5. All HF patients and their appropriate support persons to receive a copy of completed discharge instructions per national quality measures
6. Documented ejection fraction by method and date or plan in place to complete per national quality measures
7. 100% patients with HF and atrial fibrillation are anticoagulated (if not contraindicated)
8. Influenza & pneumonia immunizations status assessed and administered, if required.
9. **All goals must be completed and documented for this pathway**

Consider Heart Failure Pathway if:

☐ Cardiomyopathy, Congestive Heart Failure (CHF), Hypertensive Heart Disease, Valvular Heart Disease (ie: aortic / stenosis insufficiency, mitral regurgitation) Ischemic Cardiomyopathy, Diastolic Heart Failure Biventricular devices and Defibrillators

RN Signature: _____

Pathway Overview

- Etiology of CHF identified on chart
- Breathing symptoms controlled
- Tolerating PO meds
- O2 not needed: or home O2 arranged
- VS / rhythm stable

- WT down from admission
- CHF with A-fib Patients anticoagulated
- Smoking cessation education provided, if indicated
- All Patient / family education components provided by discharge

Day 1	Day 2	Day 3	Day 4
• O2 SATS greater than 93% with or without O2 • Patient tolerating meds / diet • Status of HCD on chart • Lab & diagnostic tests initiated • Education Assessment made & charted • Day 1 Patient education components completed • Pneumococcal Influenza screening completed • Patient smoking status on chart • Discharge plan / needs reviewed • Chaplaincy referral for chronic disease.	• Daily weight less than previous day • Patient tolerating PO meds / diet • Ejection fraction documented on chart • ACE inhibitor or ARB initiated or intolerance on chart • Day 2 patient education components completed • Patient received required vaccination • Discharge plan in progress	• Daily weight stable or less than precious day • Tolerating PO meds / diet • Patient's symptoms improving • ACE inhibitor dose titrated up from admission dose (if applicable) • Patient received required vaccination • Discharge plan in progress	• Breathing signs and symptoms controlled with or without O2 • Tolerating PO meds • VS / rhythm stable • Education R / T daily WT, smoking cessation, meds, diet, activity, follow-up care completed • Daily weight stable or less than previous day • Immunization status up-to-date • Patient received required vaccination • Discharge plans finalized

Date: _____

SMDC HEALTH SYSTEM

PATH.005 Orig. 11/05 Rev. 5/08

Patient Label

HEART FAILURE PATHWAY

Reprinted with permission by SMDC Health System, Duluth, MN, 2007.

(continues)

Content Owners:

	Date:						Date:						Date:						Date:						
Weight																									
Time	24	04	08	12	16	20	24	04	08	12	16	20	24	04	08	12	16	20	24	04	08	12	16	20	VITAL SIGNS
Temperature																									
Pulse																									
Resp																									
BP																									
Oxygen Sat / O₂																									
Intake	23-07		07-15		15-23		24°H	23-07		07-15		15-23		24°H	23-07		07-15		15-23		24°H	23-07	07-15	15-23	24°H	
Oral																									
Tube Feeding / Flush																									
IVF																									INPUT
Drips																									
Periop																									
Blood Prod																									
Total in 8°H																									
Output																									
Urine																									
Emesis																									
NG																									OUTPUT
Stool																									
Drain																									
Other																									
Total in 8°H																									
Time																									
Glucose Meter																									
Glucose																									
Insulin																									
Time																									
Glucose Meter																									LAB, ETC.
Glucose																									
Insulin																									
Time																									
INR																									
Coumadin																									
Time																									
Personal Hygiene																									PATIENT CARE
Hourly Checks																									
Initials																									

* = See Frequent Check Flowsheet

Signature :_____   Signature :_____   Signature :_____

Signature :_____   Signature :_____   Signature :_____

Signature :_____   Signature :_____   Signature :_____

Date : _____

	Day 1 _____ / Date ___/___/___	N	D	E
Consults / Referrals	Cardiology Consult			
	Chaplaincy referral			
	Social Services referral			
Labs / Tests	Basic Metabolic Panel, Magnesium, Hem Profile			
	Cardiac enzymes ordered			
	ECG Ordered			
	Echocardiogram ordered-or result less than 1 year charted			
	CXR obtained			
Assessments / Treatments	Orthostatic BP documented daily			
	Daily weight recorded, daily			
	I&O recording initiated			
	Cardiac telemetry			
	O_2 SAT on room air daily			
	O_2 titrated to keep SpO_2 greater than 93% if required			
	Foley catheter PRN			
	Initiate & maintain IV access / site care as ordered			
	PICC line ordered for IV inotropes			
Core Measures Documentation **DO NOT LEAVE BLANK**	Smoking cessation information given			
	Left Ventricular assessment done or planned			
	ACE / ARB ordered on discharge or documentation to support why both or either not ordered			
	Check the heart failure box on the patient discharge instruction sheet NOW and review with patient			
	Pneumococcal/Influenza screening completed and faxed to pharmacy...			
Nutrition	2 Gm sodium diet tolerated			
	2400 mL day fluid moderation if ordered			
	Fluid restriction / intolerances if ordered			
Activity	Bedrest with BRPs			
	Cardiac Phase I ordered			
Teaching / Discharge Planning MUST INITIAL DO NOT LEAVE BLANK	Educational assessment made			
	Give Cardiac *straight* from the heart education book-include CHF section that addresses, diet, activity, daily weight monitoring, medications, symptoms worsening, and follow up appts.			
	Provide Day 1 Patient / family education:			
	☐ Recognize CHF symptoms			
	☐ Monitor daily weight			
	Explain anticipated LOS / Treatment plan to Patient / family			
	Notes on Teaching:			
	☐ Smoking cessation information given			

Day 1 Outcomes	N	D	E
O_2 SATS greater than 93% with or without O_2	M☐ NM☐	M☐ NM☐	M☐ NM☐
Patient tolerating meds / diet	M☐ NM☐	M☐ NM☐	M☐ NM☐
Status of HCD on chart	M☐ NM☐	M☐ NM☐	M☐ NM☐
Lab & diagnostic tests initiated	M☐ NM☐	M☐ NM☐	M☐ NM☐
Day 1 Patient education components completed	M☐ NM☐	M☐ NM☐	M☐ NM☐
Pneumococcal Influenza screening completed	M☐ NM☐	M☐ NM☐	M☐ NM☐
Medication Reconciliation is checked and completed	M☐ NM☐	M☐ NM☐	M☐ NM☐
Discharge outcomes reviewed	M☐ NM☐	M☐ NM☐	M☐ NM☐
Patient smoking status within the last 12 months on chart: Smoker: ☐ N/A	Y☐ N☐	Y☐ N☐	Y☐ N☐
Diuretics if ordered ☐ N/A	M☐ NM☐	M☐ NM☐	M☐ NM☐
Digoxin if ordered ☐ N/A	M☐ NM☐	M☐ NM☐	M☐ NM☐
ACE inhibitor / ARB <u>or</u> hydralazine / nitrate comb if ordered ☐ N/A	M☐ NM☐	M☐ NM☐	M☐ NM☐
IV inotropes if ordered ☐ N/A	M☐ NM☐	M☐ NM☐	M☐ NM☐
Beta Blocker if ordered ☐ N/A	M☐ NM☐	M☐ NM☐	M☐ NM☐
*= See Progress Note	(Key: M = Met NM = Not Met)		

Review of Systems

Night - Time _____ Initials _____	Day - Time _____ Initials _____	Eve - Time _____ Initials _____
Neurological: Alert oriented to person, place & time; behavior appropriate to situation; verbalization clear & understandable, symmetrical movements arms / legs		
☐ WNL	☐ WNL	☐ WNL
Respiratory: R 12-24 / min at rest, unlabored, breath sounds clear & skin color within norm, cough absent, no sleep apnea		
☐ WNL	☐ WNL	☐ WNL
Cardiovascular: Heart tones regular $S^1 S^2$ @Rate of 50 - 90, pulse present, capillary refill less then 3 sec, no edema present		
☐ WNL	☐ WNL	☐ WNL
GI / GU: Abdomen soft, Active bowel sounds in all 4 quadrants, no N&V / diarrhea, BM every 1-3 days, clear yellow or amber urine, no bladder distention, no dysuria, no vaginal or urethral drainage		
☐ WNL	☐ WNL	☐ WNL
Nutrition: Absence N & V, tolerating prescribed diet, nutritional, intake adequate		
☐ WNL	☐ WNL	☐ WNL
Musculoskeletal: Absence of joint swelling & tissues, normal ROM of all joints, no muscle weakness surrounding tissue with evidence of inflammation		
☐ WNL	☐ WNL	☐ WNL
Skin: Braden score greater than 2 in each category, skin is warm & dry, no pressure areas, skin breakdown or rashes		
☐ WNL Braden Score _____	☐ WNL Braden Score _____	☐ WNL Braden Score _____
Pain: *Patient states pain free or pain controlled with an acceptable level*		
☐ Denies Pain ☐ See Flow Sheet	☐ Denies Pain ☐ See Flow Sheet	☐ Denies Pain ☐ See Flow Sheet
Psychosocial: Patient / Family demonstrates coping with hospitalization / illness / surgery		
☐ WNL	☐ WNL	☐ WNL
Safety: Patient free from injury		
☐ WNL Fall Risk Level 1 ☐ Fall Risk Level 2 ☐ Restraint ☐	☐ WNL Fall Risk Level 1 ☐ Fall Risk Level 2 ☐ Restraint ☐	☐ WNL Fall Risk Level 1 ☐ Fall Risk Level 2 ☐ Restraint ☐
RN _____	RN _____	RN _____

Signature : _____ Signature : _____ Signature : _____

Signature : _____ Signature : _____ Signature : _____

Signature : _____ Signature : _____ Signature : _____

Date : _____

Patient Label

(continues)

	Day 2 _____ / Date ___/___/___	N	D	E
Consults	Registered Dietitian for 2 Gm sodium diet education			
Labs / Test	Daily K+, BUN, Creatinine ordered			
	Report abnormal results to MD / NP			
	Angiogram or stress test ordered for new CHF with multiple			
	risk factors and / or CAD, or signs / symptoms ischemia			
	Echocardiogram result on chart			
	Test results from prior 24H on chart			
Assessments / Treatments	CV & pulmonary assessments completed			
	H&P MD on chart			
	weight recorded daily			
	I&O completed every 8 hours			
	Cardiac telemetry			
	Orthostatic BP documented			
	O₂ SAT on room air & O₂, if required			
	O₂ titrated to keep SpO₂, greater than 93%			
	Foley catheter discontinued			
Core Measures Documentation	Smoking cessation information given			
	Left Ventricular assessment done or planned			
	ACE / ARB ordered on discharge or documentation to			
	support why both or either not ordered			
	Recheck the heart failure box on the patient discharge			
	instruction sheet NOW and review			
DO NOT LEAVE BLANK	Influenza/pneumonia immunizations listed on MAR if required.......			
Nutrition	2 Gm sodium diet tolerated			
	2400 mL day fluid moderation			
	Fluid restriction followed if ordered			
Activity	WT bearing every shift if tolerated			
	Cardiac Rehab Phase 1 initiated			
Teaching / Discharge Planning MUST INITIAL DO NOT LEAVE BLANK	Provide Day 2 Patient / family education:			
	Smoking cessation for current smokers			
	Role of sodium / fluid diet control			
	Caregiver & support services identified			
	Discharge needs identified by RN			
	Patient has copy of Cardiac *straight* from the heart education			
	book that -includes CHF section that addresses, diet, activity,			
	weight monitoring, medications, symptoms worsening, and			
	follow up appts			

Day 2 Outcomes	N	D	E
Daily WT less than previous day	M☐ NM☐	M☐ NM☐	M☐ NM☐
Patient tolerating PO meds / diet	M☐ NM☐	M☐ NM☐	M☐ NM☐
Ejection fraction documented on chart	M☐ NM☐	M☐ NM☐	M☐ NM☐
ACE inhibitor or ARB initiated or intolerance Documented if applicable ☐ N/A	M☐ NM☐	M☐ NM☐	M☐ NM☐
Day 2 Patient education components completed	M☐ NM☐	M☐ NM☐	M☐ NM☐
Recheck Pneumococcal Influenza screening completed	M☐ NM☐	M☐ NM☐	M☐ NM☐
Discharge outcomes reviewed	M☐ NM☐	M☐ NM☐	M☐ NM☐
Patient smoking cessation support offered: ☐ N/A	Y☐ N☐	Y☐ N☐	Y☐ N☐
Patient tolerating increase activity	M☐ NM☐	M☐ NM☐	M☐ NM☐
Patient appropriately vaccinated for flu & pneumonia	M☐ NM☐	M☐ NM☐	M☐ NM☐
	M☐ NM☐	M☐ NM☐	M☐ NM☐
	M☐ NM☐	M☐ NM☐	M☐ NM☐
	M☐ NM☐	M☐ NM☐	M☐ NM☐
	M☐ NM☐	M☐ NM☐	M☐ NM☐
Patient meets pathway outcomes?	Y☐ N☐	Y☐ N☐	Y☐ N☐
= See Progress Note	**(Key: M = Met NM = Not Met)**		

Review of Systems

Night - Time _____ Initials _____	Day - Time _____ Initials _____	Eve - Time _____ Initials _____

Neurological: Alert oriented to person, place & time; behavior appropriate to situation; verbalization clear & understandable, symmetrical movements arms / legs

☐ WNL	☐ WNL	☐ WNL

Respiratory: R 12-24 / min at rest, unlabored, breath sounds clear & skin color within norm, cough absent, no sleep apnea

☐ WNL	☐ WNL	☐ WNL

Cardiovascular: Heart tones regular S¹ S² @Rate of 50 - 90, pulse present, capillary refill less then 3 sec, no edema present

☐ WNL	☐ WNL	☐ WNL

GI / GU: Abdomen soft, Active bowel sounds in all 4 quadrants, no N&V / diarrhea, BM every 1-3 days, clear yellow or amber urine, no bladder distention, no dysuria, no vaginal or urethral drainage

☐ WNL	☐ WNL	☐ WNL

Nutrition: Absence N & V, tolerating prescribed diet, nutritional, intake adequate

☐ WNL	☐ WNL	☐ WNL

Musculoskeletal: Absence of joint swelling & tissues, normal ROM of all joints, no muscle weakness surrounding tissue with evidence of inflammation;

☐ WNL	☐ WNL	☐ WNL

Skin: Braden score greater than 2 in each category, skin is warm & dry, no pressure areas, skin breakdown or rashes

☐ WNL Braden Score _____	☐ WNL Braden Score _____	☐ WNL Braden Score _____

Pain: *Patient states pain free or pain controlled with an acceptable level*

☐ Denies Pain ☐ See Flow Sheet	☐ Denies Pain ☐ See Flow Sheet	☐ Denies Pain ☐ See Flow Sheet

Psychosocial: Patient / Family demonstrates coping with hospitalization / illness / surgery

☐ WNL	☐ WNL	☐ WNL

Safety: Patient free from injury

☐ WNL Fall Risk Level 1 ☐ Fall Risk Level 2 ☐ Restraint ☐ RN _____	☐ WNL Fall Risk Level 1 ☐ Fall Risk Level 2 ☐ Restraint ☐ RN _____	☐ WNL Fall Risk Level 1 ☐ Fall Risk Level 2 ☐ Restraint ☐ RN _____

Signature :_____   Signature :_____   Signature :_____

Signature :_____   Signature :_____   Signature :_____

Signature :_____   Signature :_____   Signature :_____

Date : _____   Patient Label

	Day 3 _____ / Date ___/___/___	N	D	E	Review of Systems		
Consults	SMDC Heart Failure Program offered				**Night - Time _____** Initials _____	**Day - Time _____** Initials _____	**Eve - Time _____** Initials _____
					Neurological: Alert oriented to person, place & time; behavior appropriate to situation; verbalization clear & understandable, symmetrical movements arms / legs		
Labs / Tests	Daily K+, BUN, Creatinine ordered				☐ WNL	☐ WNL	☐ WNL
	Report abnormal results to MD / NP / PA						
	Review test results						
	Patient notified of test results						
Assessments / Treatments	Daily weight recorded, daily				**Respiratory:** R 12-24 / min at rest, unlabored, breath sounds clear & skin color within norm, cough absent, no sleep apnea		
	I&O completed				☐ WNL	☐ WNL	☐ WNL
	Cardiac telemetry						
	Orthostatic BP documented daily						
	O₂ titrated to keep SpO₂ greater than 93%						
Core Measures Documentation	Smoking cessation information given				**Cardiovascular:** Heart tones regular S¹ S² ®Rate of 50 - 90, pulse present, capillary refill less then 3 sec, no edema present		
	Left Ventricular assessment done or planned				☐ WNL	☐ WNL	☐ WNL
	ACE / ARB ordered on discharge or documentation to support why there not						
DO NOT LEAVE BLANK	Check the heart failure box on the patient discharge instruction sheet NOW and review with patient				**GI / GU:** Abdomen soft, Active bowel sounds in all 4 quadrants, no N&V / diarrhea, BM every 1-3 days, clear yellow or amber urine, no bladder distention, no dysuria, no vaginal or urethral drainage		
	If ferile assure required vaccinations are on MAR to be given Prior to discharge..........................				☐ WNL	☐ WNL	☐ WNL
Nutrition	2 GM sodium diet tolerated						
	2400 mL day fluid moderation						
	Fluid restriction followed if ordered						
Activity	WT bearing every shift, if tolerated				**Nutrition:** Absence N & V, tolerating prescribed diet, nutritional, intake adequate		
	Cardiac Rehab Phase 1				☐ WNL	☐ WNL	☐ WNL
	Rest period after meals						
Teaching / Discharge Planning	Provide Day 3 Patient / family education:						
	Medication, dose & side effects RN / Pharmacist						
MUST INITIAL DO NOT LEAVE BLANK	Activity / exercise guidelines per cardiac rehab				**Musculoskeletal:** Absence of joint swelling & tissues, normal ROM of all joints, no muscle weakness surrounding tissue with evidence of inflammation;		
	Discharge needs arrangements made for follow up.						
	Consider home O₂ and other needs				☐ WNL	☐ WNL	☐ WNL
	Patient has copy of Cardiac *straight* from the heart education book that –includes: CHF section that addresses, diet, activity, daily weight monitoring, medications, symptoms worsening, and follow up appts				**Skin:** Braden score greater than 2 in each category, skin is warm & dry, no pressure areas, skin breakdown or rashes		
					☐ WNL Braden Score _____	☐ WNL Braden Score _____	☐ WNL Braden Score _____

Day 3 Outcomes	N	D	E	Pain: Patient states pain free or pain controlled with an acceptable level		
Daily weight stable or less than previous day	M☐ NM☐	M☐ NM☐	M☐ NM☐	☐ Denies Pain ☐ See Flow Sheet	☐ Denies Pain ☐ See Flow Sheet	☐ Denies Pain ☐ See Flow Sheet
Tolerating PO meds / diet.	M☐ NM☐	M☐ NM☐	M☐ NM☐			
Patients symptoms improving	M☐ NM☐	M☐ NM☐	M☐ NM☐			
ACE inhibitor dose titrated up from admission dose	M☐ NM☐	M☐ NM☐	M☐ NM☐	**Psychosocial:** Patient / Family demonstrates coping with hospitalization / illness / surgery		
Discharge outcomes reviewed.	M☐ NM☐	M☐ NM☐	M☐ NM☐	☐ WNL	☐ WNL	☐ WNL
Patient provided with written copy of discharge instructions straight from the Heart Handbook related to diet, activity, daily weight monitoring, symptoms worsening, medications, and follow up appts	M☐ NM☐	M☐ NM☐	M☐ NM☐	**Safety:** Patient free from injury		
RD education on 2GM Na diet for home	M☐ NM☐	M☐ NM☐	M☐ NM☐	☐ WNL	☐ WNL	☐ WNL
Patient appropriately vaccinate for flu & pneumonia	M☐ NM☐	M☐ NM☐	M☐ NM☐			
Social Services / Discharge Specialist. notified for new O₂ needs at home.	M☐ NM☐	M☐ NM☐	M☐ NM☐	Fall Risk Level 1 ☐ Fall Risk Level 2 ☐ Restraint ☐	Fall Risk Level 1 ☐ Fall Risk Level 2 ☐ Restraint ☐	Fall Risk Level 1 ☐ Fall Risk Level 2 ☐ Restraint ☐
	M☐ NM☐	M☐ NM☐	M☐ NM☐	RN _____	RN _____	RN _____
	M☐ NM☐	M☐ NM☐	M☐ NM☐			
*= See Progress Note	**(Key:** M = Met NM = Not Met)					

Signature : _____   Signature : _____   Signature : _____

Signature : _____   Signature : _____   Signature : _____

Signature : _____   Signature : _____   Signature : _____

Date : _____   Patient Label

(continues)

	Day 4 _____ / Date ___/___/___	N	D	E
Consults	SMDC Heart Failure Program (if ordered)			
	Consult notes in chart...			
Labs / Tests	Daily K+, BUN, Creatinine ordered...			
	Report abnormal results to MD / NP / PA...			
	Angiogram or stress test completed during stay if ordered...			
	Patient / family notified of test results...			
Assessments / Treatments	Daily weight recorded, daily...			
	I&O completed...			
	Cardiac telemetry...			
	Orthostatic BP documented daily...			
	O₂ titrated to keep SpO₂ greater than 93%...			
	Rest & exercise SpO₂ documented on chart...			
Core Measure Documentation	Smoking cessation information given...			
	Left Ventricular assessment done or planned...			
	ACE / ARB ordered on discharge or documentation to support			
	why there not...			
	Check the heart failure box on the patient discharge instruction			
DO NOT LEAVE BLANK	sheet NOW and review with patient...			
	If febrile assure required vaccination on MAR to be given before			
	discharge...			
Nutrition	2 Gm sodium diet tolerated...			
	2400 mL day fluid moderation...			
	Fluid restriction followed if ordered...			
Activity	Ambulating...			
	Cardiac Rehab Phase 1 continues...			
Teaching / Discharge Planning	Provide Day 4 Patient / family education completed:			
	Reinforce all education components...			
	Review, complete, and sign discharge instructions sheet NSG.026			
	Provide printed medication schedule before discharge...			
	Follow-up appointment scheduled & Patient notified or pt instructed			
	to call for appointment next business day...			
	Referrals to other care agencies done & sent...			
	Discharge data entered onto discharge order Nsg.026 sheet...			
	Home Equipment ordered if needed...			

Day 4 Outcomes	N	D	E
Daily weight stable or less than previous day	M☐ NM☐	M☐ NM☐	M☐ NM☐
Breathing signs / symptoms controlled with or without O₂	M☐ NM☐	M☐ NM☐	M☐ NM☐
Tolerating PO meds	M☐ NM☐	M☐ NM☐	M☐ NM☐
VS. rhythm stable	M☐ NM☐	M☐ NM☐	M☐ NM☐
Immunization status up-to-date	M☐ NM☐	M☐ NM☐	M☐ NM☐
Patient provided with written discharge instructions			
related to daily weight, diet, activity, symptoms			
worsening, medications, and follow up via Straight From			
the Heart Handbook	M☐ NM☐	M☐ NM☐	M☐ NM☐
Patient appropriately vaccinated for flu & pneumonia	M☐ NM☐	M☐ NM☐	M☐ NM☐
	M☐ NM☐	M☐ NM☐	M☐ NM☐
	M☐ NM☐	M☐ NM☐	M☐ NM☐

* = See Progress Note   (Key: M = Met NM = Not Met)

Review of Systems

	Night - Time _____	Day - Time _____	Eve - Time _____
	Initials _____	Initials _____	Initials _____

Neurological: Alert oriented to person, place & time; behavior appropriate to situation; verbalization clear & understandable, symmetrical movements arms / legs

☐ WNL	☐ WNL	☐ WNL

Respiratory: R 12-24 / min at rest, unlabored, breath sounds clear & skin color within norm, cough absent, no sleep apnea

☐ WNL	☐ WNL	☐ WNL

Cardiovascular: Heart tones regular S¹ S² @Rate of 50 - 90, pulse present, capillary refill less then 3 sec, no edema present

☐ WNL	☐ WNL	☐ WNL

GI / GU: Abdomen soft, Active bowel sounds in all 4 quadrants, no N&V / diarrhea, BM every 1-3 days, clear yellow or amber urine, no bladder distention, no dysuria, no vaginal or urethral drainage

☐ WNL	☐ WNL	☐ WNL

Nutrition: Absence N & V, tolerating prescribed diet, nutritional, intake adequate

☐ WNL	☐ WNL	☐ WNL

Musculoskeletal: Absence of joint swelling & tissues, normal ROM of all joints, no muscle weakness surrounding tissue with evidence of inflammation;

☐ WNL	☐ WNL	☐ WNL

Skin: Braden score greater than 2 in each category, skin is warm & dry, no pressure areas, skin breakdown or rashes

☐ WNL	☐ WNL	☐ WNL
Braden Score _____	Braden Score _____	Braden Score _____

Pain: Patient states pain free or pain controlled with an acceptable level

☐ Denies Pain	☐ Denies Pain	☐ Denies Pain
☐ See Flow Sheet	☐ See Flow Sheet	☐ See Flow Sheet

Psychosocial: Patient / Family demonstrates coping with hospitalization / illness / surgery

☐ WNL	☐ WNL	☐ WNL

Safety: Patient free from injury

☐ WNL	☐ WNL	☐ WNL
Fall Risk Level 1 ☐	Fall Risk Level 1 ☐	Fall Risk Level 1 ☐
Fall Risk Level 2 ☐	Fall Risk Level 2 ☐	Fall Risk Level 2 ☐
Restraint ☐	Restraint ☐	Restraint ☐
RN _____	RN _____	RN _____

Signature :_____   Signature :_____   Signature :_____

Signature :_____   Signature :_____   Signature :_____

Signature :_____   Signature :_____   Signature :_____

Date : _____   Patient Label

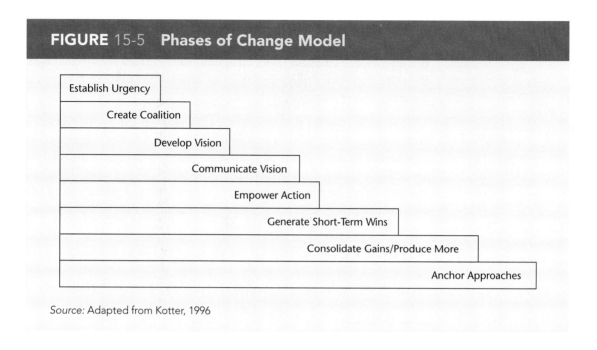

FIGURE 15-5   **Phases of Change Model**

Establish Urgency

Create Coalition

Develop Vision

Communicate Vision

Empower Action

Generate Short-Term Wins

Consolidate Gains/Produce More

Anchor Approaches

Source: Adapted from Kotter, 1996

step process that has been described as a top-down transformation process (Fullan, 2001). While not widely noted in the nursing literature, Kotter's eight *change phases model* is useful here because of its simplicity. The phases of the model are establish urgency, create a coalition, develop a vision and strategy, communicate the vision, empower broad-based action, generate short-term wins, consolidate improvements and produce more change, and anchor new approaches. The "top" of his model is the starting point in any change effort and should not be confused with an administrative top (**Figure 15-5**).

Kotter's model (1996) can be applied to clinical situations. For example, suppose there is a desire to develop a policy about patients leaving the unit to smoke, but a consensus cannot be reached about what the policy should be. Because there is no policy, nurses do not feel that they have the authority to stop patients from leaving the unit. Frustration builds after repeated attempts to create a policy are unsuccessful.

How could this situation be changed? Using Kotter's model of change (Kotter, 1996), the first phase is to create a sense of urgency. One strategy to accomplish this is to collect data about the problem. Data can be a powerful tool for creating a sense of urgency by communicating the scope of an issue. For example, suppose you learn that four patients per month are leaving the unit to smoke. Knowing this begins to give a more concrete picture about what is happening. Four patients per month means 48 patients per year are now

KEY TERM

Change phases model: Eight-phased process to describe organizational change

Because constant organizational change can be stressful, while never making any changes or making changes very slowly can be frustrating. It is essential to identify strategies that make change desirable to others. An effective strategy is to implement change in phases: establish urgency, create a coalition, develop a vision and strategy, communicate the vision, empower broad-based action, generate short-term wins, consolidate improvements and produce more change, and anchor new approaches.

at risk for potential injury as they leave the relative safety of the hospital to smoke. Now consider how much strength could be added to the description of the problem if colleagues from other units were engaged in collecting data. By taking the time to collect data about an issue and presenting it to others, a sense of urgency is created.

Communicating the sense of urgency often results in the development of a coalition, the second phase of Kotter's model (1996). A coalition is a group of colleagues who share similar thoughts and a vision for change. In the example about a no smoking policy for patients, a coalition is created when colleagues recognize the potential safety concerns for patients and participate in the creation of a policy. A benefit of creating a coalition is the collaboration and cooperation that arises.

A cohesive group sharing similar thoughts and ideas can work toward developing a vision and strategy for change, the third phase of Kotter's model (1996). It will be through the process of collaboration and cooperation of the coalition members that a clear vision and strategy have the greatest potential to be developed.

After the vision and strategy for change have been developed, the group will need to communicate the vision to others. Communicating the vision is the fourth phase of the model (Kotter, 1996). Oftentimes, it seems that change is not possible because communication has not been clear. Unclear communication can lead to misunderstandings and misconceptions about the change that is being suggested, resulting in unnecessary resistance. Communication then becomes an important phase of the change process. Good communication contributes to the potential to gain increased support to change the policy.

Creating a sense of urgency, building a coalition, developing a vision and strategy, and communicating a vision will not cause a policy, process, or practice to change. Kotter (1996) describes this fifth phase as empowering broad-based action. The diversity of the coalition should be considered. A diverse group of members from the nursing unit will be able to help develop, communicate, and sustain the vision for a policy, process, or practice change. The sustained support of the group is needed to ensure that the new policy is understood and followed. Empowering broad-based action means that members from all departments have a responsibility and accountability for the success or failure of any policy, practice, or process. To understand this idea further, suppose the proposed no smoking policy has been approved. The policy requires that physicians write recommendations for their patients to not leave the unit to smoke. This means the nurses can now advise patients against leaving the unit. The policy indicates that aides, housekeepers, and any other ancillary staff members have the responsibility to communicate the policy to patients. They also have a responsibility to notify nurses if they become aware of a patient's intent to leave the unit to smoke. If the no smoking policy was considered only a nursing policy, then the needed change would be less likely to occur.

When a variety of healthcare providers are empowered, there is a greater chance for success. Succeeding in some aspect of any proposed change becomes the focus for Kotter's (1996) sixth phase of the change process, which is to generate short-term wins. This could mean recognizing individuals on the unit who embrace the new policy. Tell them how much you appreciate their support of the new policy or practice. For example, a physician begins to routinely write recommendations that patients not go out to smoke. This action represents a short-term win. By acknowledging the physician's effort, the opportunity exists to reinforce the change. Each time someone on the healthcare team role models the desired practice change, a short-term win is created.

Kotter's (1996) seventh phase involves consolidating the improvements. Each time changes can be articulated, there is a greater chance of producing more change. In the no smoking policy, for example, each time that all members of the healthcare team are united in their efforts to enforce the new policy, success has been achieved. Each success builds upon previous successes, perpetuating adherence to the policy. Consolidating improvements that produce more change also creates a sense of teamwork.

The more successes the healthcare team can recognize, the stronger the practice becomes, essentially anchoring the change in practice. The process of anchoring the change is the last, or eighth, phase of the process (Kotter, 1996). Although identified as the last phase, it should not be considered unimportant. If change does not become anchored, thus transforming practice behaviors, then all of our energies have been wasted. The need to consider how change will be anchored is an aspect that needs to be considered and identified early in the change process. You may want to remember this and make sure you think about how you will anchor a practice behavior change.

From this discussion it should be apparent to you how the concepts of engaging others in the change process and Kotter's (1996) strategies for change are intertwined. Depending upon the type of evidence we wish to transition to the bedside, it will be important for you to identify and know who the stakeholders are in the change process.

Stakeholder Involvement

Whenever you consider a practice change, it is important to consider the stakeholders. Identification of stakeholders is important because it allows for clarification of the purpose of the proposed change, decreases misunderstandings

TABLE 15-2 Stakeholder Identification Tool

The following list of questions, when answered, may help to identify many of the stakeholders to any proposed change of practice, process, or policy.

1. What is the proposed change?
2. Does it affect practice, process, or policy?
3. What are the components of the practice, process, or policy?
4. What is the setting and context for the practice, process, or policy?
5. What is the history behind the practice, process, or policy?
6. What is the structure and administrative design of the practice, process, or policy?
7. Who participates in the practice, process, or policy?
8. Who sponsors the practice, process, or policy?
9. Are there any group(s) that will be excluded by the practice, process, or policy?
10. Who are the direct beneficiaries of the practice, process, or policy?
11. Are there any indirect beneficiaries of the practice, process, or policy?
12. Does the proposed change to practice, process, or policy create opportunities for any particular group(s)?
13. Does any particular group(s) stand to lose power as a result of the proposed change to practice, process, or policy?
14. Is there a funding group(s) for the proposed change to practice, process, or policy?

related to the change, and facilitates implementation of the change. **Table 15-2** presents an example of a questionnaire that can be used to identify stakeholders. The following illustrates how implementing a change without collaborating with stakeholders can have negative results. Nurses on a busy medical surgical unit have discovered that many patients are not being assessed in the morning. This is causing some difficulty for patients because physicians need morning assessments completed so they can make treatment changes. Upon further examination it is discovered that the physical therapy department, in an effort to balance their staffing and workload, has changed its routine and staff are now coming to the unit first thing in the morning before the nurses have had a chance to assess the patients. Nurses on the unit voice their concerns, but change does not occur, and the physical therapy staff continues with the new schedule.

What factors contribute to some of the negative outcomes associated with the physical therapy scheduling change? Had the physical therapy staff identified all the stakeholders, they might have discovered that their proposed practice change would impact patient care negatively. Because patients were being taken out of their rooms before breakfast, nurses were unable to complete morning assessments; thus physicians did not have the information to make decisions about treatment options. The only group that benefited from the change was the physical therapy department, which was able to balance its staffing and workload. When input from stakeholders is not solicited, mistrust can develop among healthcare providers, often putting patients in the middle of the feuding disciplines.

TEST YOUR KNOWLEDGE 15-2

1. Which of the following are ways to engage others in transitioning evidence to practice?
   a. journal club
   b. collaborating with an APN
   c. developing care maps
   d. maintaining status quo

2. Put Kotter's eight phases of change in order.
   a. develop a clear vision
   b. anchor the change
   c. create a coalition
   d. empower people to clear obstacles
   e. establish a sense of urgency
   f. consolidate and keep moving
   g. secure short-term wins
   h. share the vision

How did you do? 1. a, b, c; 2. e, c, a, h, d, g, f, b

15.3 Keeping It Ethical

At the end of this section you will be able to:

< Discuss dilemmas that can be encountered during change

KEY TERM

Cost-benefit ratio:
Comparison of
benefits to potential
costs that might result
from change

Dilemmas associated with the change process can be attributed to the *cost-benefit ratio*. This means that one must compare the benefits of any proposed change to the potential cost that might be incurred as a result of that change. Sadly, many individuals in health care think about cost only in terms of dollars and cents. While the financial bottom line cannot be ignored, other kinds of cost must be considered such as time, personnel, patient preferences, and relationships. If changes are made to practice, process, and policy without considering other aspects of cost, change may be inadvertently sabotaged.

To illustrate this point, consider how health care has changed to a system of reimbursement based upon a patient's length of stay (LOS). Suppose a patient is admitted to the hospital with HF, and the insurance will pay $10,000 for his care. It costs the hospital $10,000 to provide 6 days of care for this type of patient. If the patient stays for 6 days, the hospital breaks even. If the patient goes home in less than 6 days, the hospital profits because it still receives $10,000. If the patient stays longer than 6 days, the extra costs of providing care such as salaries, food, and supplies are assumed by the hospital.

Some nurses decide to approach administration and change the care map whereby HF patients are discharged in 4 days. Is this a good idea? Will patients be ready to go home in 4 days? HF patients often need several days for medications to work. They also need education related to diet and activity. Some patients are so weak that they need the services of physical therapy. The proposed decrease in LOS for HF patients means that the physical therapist would need to see patients within 24 hours of admission. Will HF patients be too sick during that time to benefit from a physical therapy evaluation? Patients who are discharged before they are ready are at risk for being readmitted just days after discharge, potentially adding cost and compromising quality of care. Readmissions can result in patient and family dissatisfaction and mistrust of healthcare providers and the healthcare system. This example illustrates how one simple change, discharging HF patients 2 days early, has the potential to increase cost while expected benefits are not realized. To achieve the most positive benefits, it is important to examine all aspects of any proposed change.

APPLY WHAT YOU HAVE LEARNED

Now that the policy has been written and received the necessary administrative approvals, the committee must devise an implementation plan. Use strategies identified in this chapter to create your plan, being sure to consider communication channels, equipment needs, and any education that the staff might need. Include what outcomes you measure to know if the policy reduces medication errors.

RAPID REVIEW

- Three models serve as a foundation for EBP: CURN, Stetler model, and Iowa model.

- Barriers to EBP include organizational culture, nurses' belief systems, and research-related barriers.

- The ANA has developed Nursing Quality Indicators that address patient safety and quality of nursing care.

- Change is a process that results in an alteration. Some individuals adapt well to change, while others resist it.

- Strategies for transitioning evidence to practice include forming a journal club, creating a care map, and collaborating with an APN.

- Kotter's model outlines eight phases of change that can be used to guide the process.

- The cost-benefit ratio must be examined when planning for change because dilemmas can arise when changing practice, process, and policies.

REFERENCES

Agency for Healthcare Research and Quality (AHRQ). (2005). *Hospital fall prevention programs should target certain patient, medication, and care-related factors that increase falling risk.* Retrieved October 9, 2010, from http://www.ahrq.gov/research/aug05/0805RA9.htm

American Nurses Association. (1998). *Nursing-sensitive quality indicators for acute care settings and ANA's safety and quality initiative.* Retrieved September 13, 2007, from http://nursingworld.org/MainMenuCategories/ThePracticeofProfessionalNursing/PatientSafety/Quality/NDNQI/Research/QIforAcuteCareSettings.aspx

Beer, M., Eisenstat, R. A., & Spector, B. (1990). Why change programs don't produce change. *Harvard Business Review, 68,* 158–166.

Fink, R., Thompson, C. J., & Bonnes, D. (2005). Overcoming barriers and promoting the use of research in practice. *Journal of Nursing Administration, 35*(3), 121–129.

French, P. (2002). What is the evidence on evidence-based nursing? An epistemological concern. *Journal of Advanced Nursing, 37*(3), 250–257.

Fullan, M. (2001). *Leading in a culture of change.* San Francisco: Jossey-Bass.

Funk, S. G., Tornquist, E. M., & Champagne, M. T. (1995). Barriers and facilitators of research utilization: An integrative review. *Nursing Clinics of North America, 30*(3), 395–407.

Hammel, G. (2002). *Leading the revolution? How to thrive in turbulent times by making innovation a way of life.* New York: Plume.

Hill, M. (1999). Outcomes measurement requires nursing to shift to outcome-based practice. *Nursing Administration Quarterly, 24*(1), 1–16.

Hommelstad, J., & Ruland, C. (2004). Norwegian nurses' perceived barriers and facilitators to research use. *AORN, 79*(3), 621–634.

Horsely, J. A., Crane, J., & Bingle, J. D. (1978). Research utilization as an organizational process. *Journal of Nursing Administration, 8,* 4–6.

Institute of Medicine. (2004). *Keeping patients safe: Transforming the work environment of nurses.* Washington, DC: National Academies Press.

Kotter, J. (1996). *Leading change.* Boston: Harvard Business School Press.

Krugman, M. (2003). Evidence-based practice: The role of staff development. *Journal for Nurses in Staff Development, 19,* 279–285.

Melnyk, B., & Fineout-Overholt, E. (2005). *Evidence-based practice in nursing and health care: A guide to best practice.* Philadelphia: Lippincott Williams & Wilkins.

Pettengill, M. M., Gillies, D. A., & Clark, C. C. (1994). Factors encouraging the use of nursing research findings. *Image: Journal of Nursing Scholarship, 26,* 143–147.

Polit, D. F., & Beck, C. T. (2004). *Nursing research principles and methods* (7th ed.). Philadelphia: Lippincott Williams & Wilkins.

Retsas, A. (2000). Barriers to using research evidence in nursing practice. *Journal of Advanced Nursing, 31,* 599–606.

Riddle, L. (2006). *Biographies of women mathematicians: Florence Nightingale.* Retrieved October 9, 2010, from http://www.agnesscott.edu/Lriddle/WOMEN/nitegale.htm

Rutledge, D. N., Greene, P., Mooney, K., Nail, L., & Ropka, M. (1998). Barriers to research utilization for oncology staff nurses and nurse managers/clinical nurse specialists. *Oncology Nursing Forum, 25,* 497–506.

Sanares, D., & Heliker, D. (2002). Implementation of an evidence-based nursing practice model. Disciplined clinical inquiry. *Journal for Nurses in Staff Development, 18,* 233–240.

Sitzia, J. (2001). Barriers to research utilization: The clinical setting and nurses themselves. *European Journal of Oncology Nurses, 5,* 154–164.

Stetler, C. B. (2001). Updating the Stetler model of research utilization to facilitate evidence-based practice. *Nursing Outlook, 49,* 272–279.

Thompson, C. J. (2001). The meaning of research utilization: A preliminary typology. *Critical Care Nursing Clinics of North America, 13,* 475–485.

Titler, M. G., Kleiber, C., Steelman, V., Rakel, B., Budreau, G., Everett, L. Q., et al. (2001). The Iowa model of evidence-based practice to promote quality care. *Critical Care Nursing Clinics of North America, 13*(4), 497–509.

University of Minnesota. (2001). *Evidence based nursing.* Retrieved October 9, 2010, from http://evidence.ahc.umn.edu/ebn.htm

U.S. Department of Health and Human Services (USDHHS). (2006). *Reducing tobacco use: A report of the surgeon general.* Retrieved October 9, 2010, from http://www.surgeongeneral.gov/library/tobacco_use

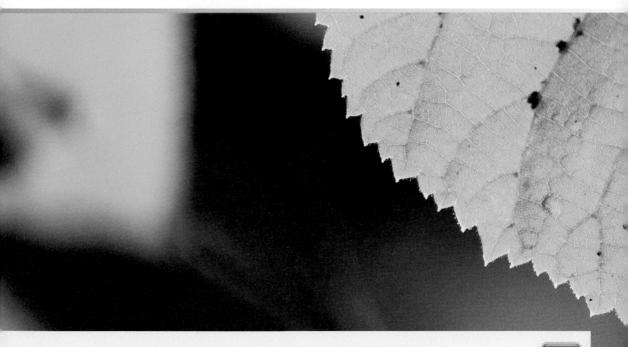

WWW

At the end of this chapter, you will be able to:

< List four characteristics of an innovator
< Provide examples of innovative behaviors in clinical practice
< Establish two goals to develop oneself in a new job
< Explain how to implement at least one characteristic for a team leader as applied to one's job

< Outline a plan to develop your professionalism as a nurse
< List three behaviors important to maintaining professional integrity over the course of your career

awareness
behavioral inventory for professionalism
career development
change agent
communication
critical thinking
developing oneself
flexibility to change

information overload
innovator
ladder program
leader
lifelong learning
mentor
personal development file
preceptors
professionalism

role model
self-awareness
sense of inquiry
socialization
team leadership skills
wheel of professionalism in nursing

CHAPTER 16

Developing Oneself as an Innovator

Diane McNally Forsyth

16.1 Who Is an Innovator?

At the end of this section, you will be able to:

< List four characteristics of an innovator
< Provide examples of innovative behaviors in clinical practice

An *innovator* is one who is willing to try new things in practice, using evidence, to enhance the quality of patient care and to foster nursing knowledge. According to Rogers (2003) "innovativeness is the degree to which an individual . . . is relatively earlier in adopting new ideas than other members of a social system" (p. 18). It is vital that a nurse be an innovator because one's practice is ever evolving. Retaining and using new information is enhanced when one becomes an active participant in change (Chubinski, 1996). Will you be the first to enroll in a new charting class on your unit? Will you wait and see how those who took the class earlier evaluate it before you register? Evolving into an evidence-based practice (EBP) *leader* on one's unit or practice area is a process that occurs with effort and time.

Innovator Characteristics

There are several characteristics of an innovator. These include a) a *sense of inquiry* (Titler, 2001), b) *flexibility to change* (Shaver, 2001), c) *awareness* of self and of the unit (MacIntosh, 2003), and d) good *communication* skills (Rogers, 2003).

KEY TERMS

Innovator: One who is willing to try new things

Leader: One who takes initiative for change and empowers others

Sense of inquiry: Curiosity

Flexibility to change: Being open and positive about change

Awareness: Understanding about oneself and the world

Communication: Process of creating and sharing information with one another to reach mutual understanding

Critical thinking: Skill set that involves critical appraisal of information

Sense of Inquiry

First, an innovator needs a sense of inquiry or curiosity. Maintaining currency in practice is critical. How many journals or nursing articles will a nurse read to stay abreast of changes in practice? When in nursing school, reading is automatic. However, as a graduate nurse, it is not uncommon to dislike opening nursing journals. Because new graduates are prone to focus on technical nursing tasks, "they reflect very little, if at all, on their nursing practice. 'When you first graduate, you think you've finally made it and so you think that you haven't got anything to learn and you know everything'" (MacIntosh, 2003, p. 731). However, reading the latest research, education, and practice in one's field is vital to maintain a fresh practice in the constantly changing nursing world.

Thinking critically about a nursing dilemma is a part of this characteristic. How might a practice problem be solved? What are new resources to improve a procedure? Following one's sense of inquiry can lead to improved patient care. One example is when a nurse noted that a policy about staff accompaniment for patients going off the unit for tests and procedures was flawed. This nurse discussed it with supervisors, gathered input for needed changes, and then moved the policy revisions through the necessary practice committees in that institution to make a change. In this case, both staff and patients benefited from the enhancement.

The decision to be an innovator begins with knowledge. According to Rogers, information-seeking and information processing (2003) are foundational and a means to gain an understanding about a proposed change or problem. Data to support EBP planning, implementation, and evaluation must be "credible and persuasive" (Bradley et al., 2004, p. 6), so practicing one's sense of inquiry should be a daily behavior. A sense of inquiry to continually seek knowledge and critique the evidence is key (Titler, 2001).

Having a sense of inquiry or curiosity is analogous to being a critical thinker. Inherent in obtaining knowledge for an innovator are *critical thinking* strategies. Richard Paul's (1990) theory of critical thinking includes a set of interdependent or micro skills. These skills include (a) identifying the problem for practice; (b) deciphering the purpose by reading critically to understand the why behind the problem; (c) uncovering assumptions that may include personal or institutional biases; (d) recognizing and using different paradigms, such as looking at the evidence in different ways; (e) demonstrating different methods of reasoning by examining values and rationale behind decisions for change; (f) examining data, which entails an understanding of statistical or other methods for critiquing; (g) creating alternate solutions using creativity to invent new options to the problem; and (h) evaluating one's thinking to improve it (Chubinski, 1996). Experienced nurses often use these skills automatically. Because research skills to review and evaluate the evidence and strength of evidence are foundational to EBP, such critical thinking skills will serve the innovator well.

Flexibility

The second innovator characteristic is flexibility to change. In any practice setting, change is constant, so being open to these changes and maintaining a positive attitude about the change makes it easier for oneself and one's peers. A successful change in the practice setting occurs when a skilled *change agent*, an innovator, manages the many feelings associated with change, such as feelings of achievement, loss, pride, and stress (Marquis & Huston, 2006). On one hand, flexibility is being willing to try a new product or implement a new policy; your peers and patients will benefit from trying this change. You will also benefit personally by updating your practice. On the other hand, if nurses do not try the new product or implement the new policy, their practices will stagnate. Flexibility to change also requires openness to failure because sometimes new ideas do not work as planned. One example occurred when a new graduate nurse read a research article about a new procedure and tried to implement it into her unit. Unfortunately, this change was rejected by most staff members on the unit. Reasons for this might have been that implementation of the new procedure worked fine in the research setting but did not carry through to the practice setting, this particular unit was different from the one in the research setting, or the nurse was a novice change agent and therefore unable to understand the process of making policy changes on her unit. Whatever the reason for failure, it is important to keep trying to implement new changes for the benefit of patients. Strive to evaluate why a proposed change did not work and use unit resources to try the new procedure in a different way. Rogers (2003) noted that the innovation-decision process may lead to rejection for a variety of reasons. Think of the many experiments that failed at first, such as Thomas Edison's search for electricity.

Awareness

Awareness is a third characteristic of an innovator. This awareness is about oneself and one's unit or area of work (MacIntosh, 2003). *Self-awareness* is about knowing yourself; how you think, act, use your senses to make decisions, and why you do these things. It entails your ethical, cultural, and spiritual values. Think about the reasons you became a nurse or why you opted to work in a specific practice area. A better understanding of how one thinks leads to knowledge of why one acts in ways that ultimately affect practice decisions.

FYI

An innovator is one who is willing to try new things in practice, using evidence, to enhance the quality of patient care and to foster nursing knowledge. Evolving into an EBP leader on one's unit or practice area is a process that occurs with effort and time.

KEY TERM

Change agent: Individual who leads or champions change

KEY TERMS

Self-awareness:
Knowing yourself

Socialization:
Awareness about
formal and informal
rules of behavior

An example was when a nurse disagreed with an institutional policy change relating to withdrawal of food and fluids for terminally ill patients in specific circumstances because he had different beliefs about life and death. He spoke with his nurse manager and the chaplain assigned to that unit in an effort to alleviate his discomfort. By understanding the ethical rationale behind this institutional policy and devising strategies he could use when faced with such a situation, he was able to continue working on this unit. Because of his self-awareness, he was able to seek resources to make meaning of the new policy and promote his continued job satisfaction.

Awareness of one's unit is also an important component of self-awareness. On one level, knowing the names and some characteristics about coworkers is basic. On a higher level, understanding what motivates certain people or knowing how different people react to changes will assist the innovator when change education is needed. The unit, or social system, is where the staff shares a common culture. It is important to know this culture, because diffusion of innovation occurs within the social system (Rogers, 2003). MacIntosh (2003) notes the importance of realizing one's practice as a part of finding one's professional identity when beginning work as a new graduate. In this stage, she notes that "nurses begin to develop an awareness of their work contexts that enables them to recognize discrepancies, compare competence, experience dissonance, and attempt to balance differences" (p. 732). Having an awareness of one's unit and colleagues increases self-awareness that will enhance one's practice.

Socialization to the unit helps to assimilate the new nurse. Things that will help with unit awareness include uncovering who the formal and informal leaders are, how education occurs, levels of communication for implementing practice changes, and possible motivators that are positive rewards for staff (often this is food). Awareness of both oneself and the unit will assist the innovator to create positive changes that can improve patient care and allow the new nurse to be an effective team member.

Communication Skills

Another characteristic of an innovator is use of good communication skills. Although these are vital skills as a nurse and leader, it is also important as an innovator. Rogers (2003) defines communication as "a process in which participants create and share information with one another in order to reach a mutual understanding" (p. 335). Communication behavior of innovators includes increased social participation and being connected through interpersonal networks (Rogers). There are two parts of communication that are related to being an innovator for EBP. During day-to-day practice, one must communicate clearly to one's peers and patients; this is a natural part of one's professional practice and is learned in your nursing program. Communicating with one's peers is vital when planning and implementing EBP changes (Rogers, 2003; Titler, 2001). The second part of communication as an innovator means communicating to a wider audience. For example, communicating practice changes to others is an important aspect of disseminating EBP. As you lead your peers in unit changes, communicating effectively to others will involve both parts of communication. When planning an EBP change, it is important to discuss proposed changes with peers to gather broader input. Later, communication might mean one-on-one sharing of information or teaching a large group, such as a class about the new topic. This could also entail diffusion of research from your institution at a conference, sharing current research related to a specialty practice, and/or publishing.

Communicating with peers occurs in many ways throughout the EBP process. Creating one's professional network not only assists the development of leadership skills, but it contributes to positive growth as a professional. This might mean belonging to a specialty organization or getting involved in institutional committees. Frequently, these groups provide EBP discussions. Another way to discuss new ideas related to current nursing research and EBP is through a journal club (Luby, Riley, & Towne, 2006). There are many ways to discuss practice changes.

All of these characteristics of an innovator blend to enhance EBP. These are also characteristics of a leader. When one is an innovator, one is also a leader. This does not necessarily mean becoming a nurse manager; rather it means leading your unit or specialty area or hospital in creating positive changes for nursing practice. When innovators manifest these characteristics in a confident manner, they become role models for other nurses, too. Nursing is a team practice. When going solo you are less likely to be successful in creating change. The hospital may have educators or other advanced practice nurses who can assist you in creating changes for EBP. Use of a professional network and institutional resources can be helpful when solving a clinical issue.

CRITICAL THINKING EXERCISE 16-1   (www)

Think of a nurse who you consider to be an innovator. What characteristics does this person have? How might you model these characteristics?

TEST YOUR KNOWLEDGE 16-1

1. Which of the following are characteristics of an innovator?
   a. sense of curiosity
   b. cynical nature
   c. inflexible
   d. self aware

True/False

2. Innovators are critical thinkers.

3. Change keeps nursing practice up to date.

4. All change is positive.

5. The culture of the social system can inhibit change.

How did you do? 1. a, d; 2. T; 3. T; 4. F; 5. T

16.2 Developing Oneself

At the end of this section, you will be able to:

‹ Establish two goals to develop oneself in a new job

‹ Explain how to implement at least one characteristic for a team leader as applied to one's job

Self-development benefits you as well as your employer and your patients. Each time you gain new knowledge, whether from reading or a formal class, your patients will benefit by receiving the latest information. Because this increases the quality of care, your institution benefits, too. Therefore, it is imperative that nursing professionals commit to long-term growth and development (Watson, 2005).

Lifelong Learning

Lifelong learning simply means to continue adding skills and knowledge about the profession as it continues to evolve. Students learn how to do basic nursing in their undergraduate program, but it is imperative to continue to evolve as a professional nurse. Florence Nightingale (1969) recognized this when she stated her reason for writing *Notes on Nursing*, "I do not pretend to teach her [*sic*] how, I ask her to teach herself, and for this purpose I venture to give her some hints" (p. 4). Continued learning is up to each person.

All of the innovator characteristics described previously are developed through lifelong learning. Generally, one learns how to learn in school. The clinical and theory skills gained in college should be applied upon entering the nursing practice world. Just as you are learning to apply theory to patient situations throughout your nursing education, nurses must continue to do the same throughout their nursing careers. MacIntosh (2003) found in her research that as new graduates developed a "reputation for professional expertise" (p. 735), an important stage was pursuing learning and growth.

There are formal and informal ways of gaining knowledge and growing professionally throughout one's career. Explore whether your facility will offer partial payment for this learning. Many facilities provide partial tuition reimbursement for graduate classes or continuing education credits. Many State Boards of Nursing require continuing education credits for registered nurse (RN) license maintenance; hourly classes or daylong conferences provide this continuing education.

Formal means of learning are accomplished by enrolling in a higher degree program, such as a master's or doctoral program of study. Currently, master's in nursing programs offer either a role-related focus (i.e., clinical nurse specialist, nurse practitioner, nurse educator, or nurse administrator) or a clinical focus area (i.e., adult medical-surgical, pediatrics, psychiatric, forensic, etc.). Often other admission requirements include an established undergraduate grade point average, specified scores on the Graduate Record Examination, or another standardized graduate test. Explore possible master's programs that fit your learning style (i.e., online programs or in person classes), your future goals, and the potential job market in your area.

In general, nursing doctoral programs are of two types: doctor of philosophy (PhD) and doctor of nursing practice (DNP). PhD programs focus on generating theory and research whereas DNP programs focus on EBP and clinical practice. In the future, the DNP will be necessary to become certified in advanced practice nursing roles. In the past, admission requirements for doctoral programs meant some practice experience in a specific clinical specialty; however, because of the need for educators and researchers in nursing, more doctoral programs admit new baccalaureate graduates directly into their programs (American Association of Colleges of Nursing, 2005). When exploring prospective doctoral programs, it is important to consider the specific research interests of faculty because doctoral students work closely with faculty on common research topics. Some doctoral programs require that

FYI

Self-development benefits you as well as your employer and your patients. Each time you gain new knowledge, whether from reading or a formal class, your patients, and by extension your institution, will benefit by receiving the latest information and increased quality of care.

KEY TERM

Lifelong learning: Adding skills and knowledge about the profession as it continues to evolve

KEY TERMS

Developing oneself:
Engaging in activities
that promote long-
term professional
growth and
development

Mentor: One
who assists with
professional growth

students are full-time and do not work, so question such requirements at the onset. Ultimately, choose the program that fits you best.

Attending structured learning programs is another formal way of *developing oneself* as a professional. Conferences are excellent opportunities for learning new practices. These have the added advantage of renewing one's spirit and enthusiasm for nursing. They also provide opportunities for networking that improve self-growth. Participating in practice updates or classes offered by your institution is vital. Often these are mandatory.

Informal methods for growth include reading journals or new nursing books, reviewing current literature (i.e., the Cochrane database or Joanna Briggs Institute), attending nursing journal clubs, or talking with peers and advanced practice nurses about innovations in practice. Professional organizations offer another excellent method to promote lifelong learning. Many times, speakers provide reports about current research at meetings. Specialty organizations include a variety of members, many with vast experiences in that specialty. Asking questions of these experts at meetings or via online discussions provides the novice nurse with increased learning. It is also possible to find a *mentor* who will assist with your professional growth at such organizations. A preceptor is an experienced nurse who is familiar with unit practices and who acts as a guide throughout the orientation process.

The timing of lifelong learning is a factor that enters into one's personal and professional life. One must look for opportunities as they happen, even though the timing is not always right. For example, if you have an opportunity to attend a national conference in your specialty area, but you think you cannot afford the time or money to go, think about the professional benefits if you attended. Look for resources to foster attendance, such as institutional funds, community agency scholarships, or grants. Discuss it with your supervisor and your mentor. Many times options open up to enable conference attendance.

It is important not to get into a rut with your work because this can stifle your lifelong learning. "In seeking and responding to stimulation, nurses actively look for and engage in activities to prod their development" (MacIntosh,

CRITICAL THINKING EXERCISE 16-2 www.

Consider a specialty organization that you might consider joining. Find the organization's home page on the web and explore opportunities for networking.

2003, p. 735). Discovering ways for professional stimulation, such as connecting with others in a similar practice at a national or regional conference, tends to bolster current practice.

Developing on the Job

It is a good idea to uncover the ways to move up the ranks in any new job. Maybe it is becoming a charge nurse or volunteering for a unit or institutional committee. Perhaps the institution has steps in a rank or *ladder program* that offer promotion. Try to uncover institutional promotional methods before starting a new job. Ask the human services representative or your supervisor to go over these steps so that you know what they are before taking the job. For example, if your institution has a ladder promotion, ask what types of criteria are needed to move up the ladder. Often peer reviews factor into annual performance reviews, so cultivate peer relationships and get feedback as a routine part of your practice.

Orientation

Take full advantage of the orientation program in any new job and learn from all the classes offered. During orientation, seek out possible mentors. Frequently these knowledgeable nurses do presentations during orientation sessions or act as *preceptors* during clinical orientation. A mentor is a practicing nurse who acts as a competent *role model* and acts as a "safety net as beginning nurses attempt to master their acquired roles" (Brockopp et al., 2003, p. 563). During this time of newness on your unit, be sure to observe other nurses and ask them questions about how they do certain procedures or use various resources. Frequently, resource time is offered to new employees as a part of the orientation process. Use this time to look up resources at your new hospital, such as online manuals or resources, the committee structure (i.e., unit, specialty divisions, or hospital wide), opportunities to volunteer for committees, or other unit activities. Inquire about the research process and how evidence-based changes are implemented on the unit. Ask whether there are journal clubs or similar venues where practice updates are discussed. Many times facilities have interest groups whose purpose is to discuss specific practices. Schedule a time during orientation to meet with any advanced practice nurses (such as clinical nurse specialists, nurse practitioners, or nurse researchers) who may be resources for your unit. Get to know these nurses because they can provide excellent resources and updates for your unit. Inquire whether nursing and/or interdisciplinary rounds or other learning opportunities are provided. If you have a staff educator assigned to your unit, determine his or her role in EBP updates. Talk with your nurse manager or supervisor about

KEY TERMS

Ladder program: Organizational process for promotion and career advancement

Preceptors: Knowledgeable nurses who provide clinical orientation for new employees

Role model: One who demonstrates desired characteristics and skills how he or she sees EBP and how you will receive updates for your practice. Try to understand the level of support from management because this is a key element for a nursing culture that embraces EBP (Krugman, 2003). Locate sources for maintaining practice updates. Some facilities forward a table of contents or website of monthly journals to any staff members who request it. During your orientation, build in time to visit the hospital library or website for the latest practice updates. Frequently, practice or education committees discuss a current research article that is germane to that specialty. Ask your preceptor about such committees or councils and arrange to sit in on one of their meetings to observe how they field questions about practice changes. Try to learn about the process of how changes occur in your facility, such as the route that practice changes take for approval. One example of understanding the EBP change is attending a specialty practice committee as a new employee and being impressed by the excellent debate about updating a practice policy. When the process for change is better understood, it is easier to prepare for new updates because you know where information about EBP changes will come from or where you need to go to initiate practice changes.

Learning from role models is a good way to learn, provided it is positive role modeling. Role modeling can be informally observed by any nurses on the unit, or it may be formalized by having a preceptor or by asking someone to act as a mentor. Any or all of these role models are helpful to enhance *professionalism* for novice nurses. Ask positive role models how they use current evidence in their practice. However, be forewarned that the expert nurse might not be able to provide specifics because that person weaves daily practice and change so inherently in practice that it is difficult for this nurse to share what the novice needs to know (Benner, 1984).

On the down side, there may be practices observed as a new graduate that are not desirable or even safe. A word of caution here: As the new person on the unit, you need to be careful about questioning those practices or your self-development could be stunted. You need to alert someone, especially if what you observe is unsafe. But there are people who remain quite behind in their adoption of new practices. An example of this was when a new employee learned how to use correct body mechanics when moving patients. When she was first on the unit and assisted staff members with moving a patient from a bed to a cart, she commented that the others were not using correct body mechanics, as she had learned. An experienced nurse negated her comments, noting that this was the fastest way to move patients and the way it was always done. The new employee was puzzled by this comment because she understood the statistics behind back injuries, so she discussed this with her nurse educator. As a result, all staff members on the unit needed to relearn proper body mechanics to prevent injuries, thereby enhancing clinical practice for all, not just the new graduate. Talking to a preceptor or another trusted peer can offer insight into these observations. Be careful not to be overly critical of unit practice because there may be reasons behind the observations that are not readily apparent. As a new person on the unit, you need to gain some trust among your peers, and this takes time. Becoming aware of discrepancies between expectations and what actually occurs on the unit is a stage of becoming a professional and feeling comfortable with one's own practice (MacIntosh, 2003). Eventually, new nurses can work to change outdated practices through the proper channels.

After a short time in the orientation process, new employees begin to realize the vast amount that they do not know about their specific practice area. This is the time to read literature in this specialty practice area. Sometimes reviewing nursing texts and past notes is sufficient. Now that specific practices are seen on a daily basis in a new job, theory means more because it is applied. Explore current research about new practices. Glean all that you can as soon as you can to foster self-development in your new specialty area. Having a rationale for making a practice change is helpful both to convince yourself that the change can be effective and to convince others.

As one's formal orientation is completed, new employees frequently experience a time of uncertainty. New nurses might question if this is the right unit or specialty area. They long for their days of classes when they had more guidance as a student, and there are struggles with learning the vast amount of information about quality patient care. Moving from a novice to a competent nurse can be frustrating, such as learning how to organize one's shift with the many tasks, delegating to unlicensed personnel, and managing patient crises. It is so easy to leave work and want to forget about it. Yet this is the time when a true innovator will set goals and strive toward enhanced professionalism. Learn all that you can about this new practice and facility. Enroll in staff development classes or other learning opportunities. Push your comfort zone so that as you feel more confident about one type of patient care diagnosis, you can seek out new opportunities for learning about other nursing interventions. Perhaps this is the time to volunteer for a unit committee, so that you can broaden your horizons and learn more about the inner workings of creating and changing policy, or offer to present a topic for a staff development class. Remind yourself that this is part of developing as a professional.

Performance Appraisals and Reviews

In any job, there will be some type of appraisal and review. Usually it is tied to salary or other promotional mechanisms, so it is important to pay attention to the details applicable for your agency. This process is designed to provide an

Personal development file: A compilation of career accomplishments

Career development: Experience and education that contribute to one's professional growth

opportunity to reflect on your strengths, areas for improvement, what you have done since the last review, and what you plan to accomplish within the next time period. Normally, setting goals is a part of this review process. However, acting in a goal-centered manner provides a framework for practice as well. The goals might be for you, such as seeking a promotion, or for your unit or institution. Goals might include professionalism, such as active work in a nursing organization. Whether you set goals only once per year during your annual performance review with your supervisor or you have daily goals, they serve to offer reflection for your practice and foster increased awareness. All of nursing should be goal oriented, such as how goals are always present in any nurse–patient interaction. Goals should incorporate EBP, such as monthly exploring the use of a new EBP guideline or technique for your practice.

Frequently input from peers or other supervisors is requested as a part of a performance review. This is the time to ask peers who have provided helpful feedback for your development, such as preceptors or mentors. It is also helpful to organize your input, enabling your supervisor to get a full picture of your accomplishments. Watson (2005) suggests a *personal development file* or folder as a means to compile what you accomplish in your career because those "little things . . . [merge] into a substantial amount of additional *career development* activity" (p. 992; emphasis added). Make notes or include documents to remind you to include those items as a part of your review process. If you expended a special effort to teach a nursing student on your unit, make a note about it at the time to include in this self-appraisal. If you assisted with data collection for a research project, try to obtain a study summary to include for your records. Keep an accurate file of your continuing education documents. Organized personal record keeping is important and will provide objective data for the performance review.

Developing Team Leadership Skills

The impact of team effectiveness for one's unit is significant (Disch, 2001). To implement EBP on a unit, all members need to be involved and work together to create the change. A small number of unit leaders can positively influence other unit staff members to enhance patient care with new evidence for practice change. Rogers (2003) notes that the people involved in an innovation decision at a large organization are frequently not the people who implement the change. Although nurses are likely involved in making decisions, the unit staff are directed to implement the changes. This is where awareness about one's unit is important. Use the informal and formal leaders. Strategically organize common groups within the unit, such as those who work similar schedules. An example of this is "communication groups" within the unit where a small number of staff members are assigned to each group, a leader is assigned who acts as

TEST YOUR KNOWLEDGE 16-2

Identify the following as either formal or informal means of developing oneself as a professional.

1. Attending conferences

2. Finding a mentor

3. Enrolling in graduate education

4. Reading a journal

5. Attending a mandatory in-service

How did you do? 1. formal; 2. informal; 3. formal; 4. informal; 5. formal

the communicator to the other members in that group, and the leader provides information, communicates about changes, and/or clarifies questions.

Another strategy suggested by Titler (2006) is a unit change champion. Change champions are staff members on the unit who continually promote new ideas for change and act as role models. Characteristics of successful change champions are the following: a) expert clinician, b) informal leader who is respected among peers, c) positive working relationship with other interdisciplinary team members, d) passionate about the topic of practice, and e) commitment to improving the quality of patient care (Titler). These characteristics are important for any innovator as well. Innovators might be known as change champions or by any other title used by the institution to implement practice changes.

Developing *team leadership skills* occurs over time. This is also where innovator characteristics, a sense of inquiry, flexibility to change, awareness of self and of the unit, and good communication skills are needed. As you develop, your team leadership skills will emerge.

KEY TERM

Team leadership skills: Behaviors that collaboratively engage others while working toward a goal

16.3   Professionalism

At the end of this section, you will be able to:

< Outline a plan to develop your professionalism as a nurse

Models of Professionalism

Professionalism is how one deports oneself within the nursing profession. Miller, Adams, and Beck (1993) developed a *behavioral inventory for professionalism* in nursing to measure the following: a) education and training, including continuing education, b) skill based on theoretical knowledge, c) a code of ethics, d) a professional organization, and e) service. For example, their inventory measures continuing education attendance, the number of journals read, nursing books recently purchased, professional organization memberships, whether nursing theories are applied in one's practice, and participation in organization and community service. These authors surveyed over 500 nurses and found that 92.3% reported reading from 1 to 10 nursing articles per month; however, only 15.9 % belonged to a professional organization.

The *wheel of professionalism in nursing* (**Figure 16-1**) depicts components to enhance professionalism (Miller, 1984). The behaviors included in the wheel indicate degrees of professionalism; these behaviors might also be used as measures in working up a clinical ladder in one's facility. One example is that active participation in a specialty organization could assist with promotions in some institutions where such professional behaviors are a part of that institution's philosophy. Other examples include routinely reading articles related to one's practice to enhance theory application for practice, pursuing continuing education regularly for competence, and making practice changes for one's own practice to enhance professional autonomy.

Perhaps the most important aspect of being a professional is to use what was learned in one's basic nursing program, especially the application of theory to clinical situations. One can innovate; however, one is still obligated to use a theory base for safe patient care. Continuing to apply learning contributes to ongoing EBP as one uses newer research and theory as a part of one's practice.

A difficult component of professionalism for those new to the practice world involves *information overload*. Rogers (2003) defines this as "the state of an individual or system in which excessive communication inputs cannot be processed and utilized, leading to breakdown" (pp. 368–369). With added technology, healthcare professionals must manage an array of communication media, such as volumes of e-mail, numerous websites within and outside of the institution, and evidence for updated practice arriving at breakneck speed. It is complex enough for the new nurse to become proficient with patient care and learn to manage multiple patients, and the additional expectations for keeping up with multiple modes of communication add stress. Learning how to manage technology is vital. Using all of the innovator characteristics can assist a new nurse to become an effective member of the team and provide quality patient care. Incorporating EBP will become a routine part of professional practice.

FIGURE 16-1 **Wheel of Professionalism in Nursing**

Source: Copyright 1984 Barbara Kemp Miller.
Reprinted with permission by Miller, Adams, & Beck.

A Final Word About Developing Oneself as an Innovator

Recognizing a possible gap between experiences in education programs and the actual workplace (Wilson & Hayes, 2000) means that new graduates must seek resources to bridge this gap. Being proactive will ease this transition into practice for new graduates and put them on the road to becoming innovators and leaders in practice. When nurses develop a strong sense of inquiry, are flexible toward change, become aware of self and of the unit, and implement good communication skills, they can be innovators, thus enhancing quality patient care for the facility. It is imperative that innovators continue to learn and assimilate ongoing changes about new evidence into one's practice. Normally practice is incorporated into education programs and initiatives by "what practitioners *do* (and choose not to do) but also what they *are* and the knowledge and thought that underpin their actions" (Coles, 2002, p. 8). In today's ever changing world, knowledge is not always adequate; one must incorporate knowledge gained into one's practice. That can make the difference between being an innovator in one's practice and being a refrigerator nurse (one who works only to acquire money to buy goods, like a refrigerator, and sees nursing as a job rather than a profession). Maintaining an EBP is vital.

16.4   Keeping It Ethical

At the end of this section, you will be able to:

< List three behaviors important to maintaining professional integrity over the course of your career

FYI

Nurses have a duty to give back to the profession. All nurses have a responsibility to assist novice nurses. EBP is more likely to thrive in environments where nurses feel supported and are provided with resources necessary to develop both personally and professionally.

It may not be evident to you at this point in your career, but nursing professionals have an obligation to develop self-awareness. In your nursing program, you are being socialized to become a lifelong learner. Developing yourself is necessary if you are to remain current about practice issues and new technologies. A sense of self-awareness can bring a level of maturity that is necessary for ethical decision making.

Professional nurses need to promote themselves and the profession by making others aware of their accomplishments. There are many ways to achieve this. For example, when you earn a certification, be certain that your accomplishment is recognized in your healthcare organization's newsletter. Make yourself available to promote nursing as a career through interactions with youth. Writing an editorial on a health topic that interests you or that you are passionate about is another way to make nursing more visible. The *Code of Ethics for Nurses with Interpretive Statements* (ANA, 2001) holds nurses accountable for the development of the profession.

At this point in your development, you have begun to build a personal development file. This will be exceptionally important to you as you seek your first position as an RN and apply to graduate school. It is desirable to include a representative picture of your abilities. However, it would be unethical for

TEST YOUR KNOWLEDGE 16-3

1. Which of the following are ethical behaviors?
   a. Reading journal articles for a club meeting.
   b. Skipping the afternoon conference sessions to go shopping.
   c. Providing an accurate and meticulous resume.
   d. Sharing information at a staff meeting about a new innovation that you heard about at a conference.
   e. Ignoring a student assigned to your unit who has a question about a procedure.

How did you do? 1. a, c, d

you to overstate your capabilities. Records should never be falsified and must accurately reflect your work history.

As a nurse, you must take advantage of both formal and informal opportunities for professional growth. For example, your employer might provide educational benefits. Investigate conferences that will help to establish yourself as an expert in your field. If your participation in these types of offerings is paid for by your employer, you are obligated to attend the sessions and maximize your learning while you are there. Willingly accept responsibility for reporting back to your colleagues what you have learned.

Nurses have a duty to give back to the profession. All nurses have a responsibility to assist novice nurses to establish their practices. Recall the characteristics of a preceptor who was particularly helpful to you. Emulate this behavior with students you encounter. As your career progresses, make it a personal goal to always be mentoring at least one person. EBP is more likely to thrive in environments where nurses feel supported and are provided with the resources necessary to develop both personally and professionally.

RAPID REVIEW

 The four characteristics of an innovator are a sense of inquiry, flexibility to change, awareness of self and the unit, and good communication skills.

 A sense of inquiry is one's curiosity and can lead to seeking knowledge that improves patient care. This characteristic is analogous to being a critical thinker.

APPLY WHAT YOU HAVE LEARNED

Do you have what it takes to be an innovator? Complete An Assessment of Leadership Qualities and Skills Part I and Skills of Leadership Part II on the companion website to find out.

⚡ Flexibility is the willingness to try something new, and it requires an openness to failure.

⚡ Self-awareness is knowing yourself, and it helps you understand how you make decisions about practice. Awareness about the unit facilitates change because of understanding the social system.

⚡ Communication skills are vital to leading and being a change agent.

⚡ Lifelong learning takes place in formal and informal ways, both of which can contribute to EBP. Formal ways of learning include enrolling in graduate programs, attending conferences, and participating in in-services. Informal learning can involve reading literature, attending journal clubs, networking at meetings, and mentoring.

⚡ Orientation, ladder programs, and personal development files are ways to develop oneself on the job.

⚡ Setting goals and peer review are components of performance appraisals and employment reviews.

⚡ EBP practice changes are facilitated when a team approach is used.

⚡ The wheel of professionalism in nursing is a model that lists professional behaviors.

⚡ Nurses are obligated to develop themselves as lifelong learners to thrive both personally and professionally.

REFERENCES

American Association of Colleges of Nursing, Washington, DC. Task Force on Future Faculty. (2005). *Faculty shortages in baccalaureate and graduate nursing programs: Scope of the problem and strategies for expanding the supply.* Retrieved October 9, 2010, from http://www.aacn.nche.edu/publications/whitepapers/facultyshortages.htm

American Nurses Association. (2001). *The code of ethics for nurses with interpretative statements.* Washington, DC: ANA Publications.

Benner, P. (1984). *From novice to expert: Excellence and power in clinical nursing practice.* Menlo Park, CA: Addison-Wesley.

Bradley, E. H., Webster, T. R., Baker, D., Schlesinger, M., Inouye, S. K., Barth, M. C., Lapane, K. L., Lipson, D., Stone, R., Koren, M. J. (2004). Translating research into practice: Speeding adoption of innovative health care programs. *The Commonwealth Fund,* (July), 1–12. Retrieved September 13, 2007, from http://www.cmwf.org/programs/elders/bradley_translating_research_724.pdf

Brockopp, D., Schooler, M., Welsh, D., Cassidy, K., Ryan, P. Y., Mueggenberg, K., Chlebowy, D. B. (2003). Sponsored professional seminars: Enhancing professionalism among baccalaureate nursing students. *Journal of Nursing Education, 42,* 562–564.

Chubinski, S. (1996). Creative critical-thinking strategies. *Nurse Educator, 21*(6), 23–27.

Coles, A. (2002). Developing professional judgment. *The Journal of Continuing Education in the Health Professions, 22,* 3–10.

Disch, J. (2001). Creating healthy work environments for nursing practice. In N. L. Chaska (Ed.), *The nursing profession: Tomorrow and beyond* (pp. 735–749). Thousand Oaks, CA: Sage.

Krugman, M. (2003). Evidence-based practice: The role of staff development. *Journal for Nurses in Staff Development, 19,* 279–285.

Luby, M., Riley, J. K., & Towne, G. (2006). Nursing research journal clubs: Bridging the gap between practice and research. *MEDSURG Nursing, 15,* 100–102.

MacIntosh, J. (2003). Reworking professional nursing identity. *Western Journal of Nursing Research, 25,* 725–741.

Marquis, B. L., & Huston, C. J. (2006). *Leadership roles and management functions in nursing: Theory and application* (5th ed.). Philadelphia: Lippincott Williams & Wilkins.

Miller, B. K. (1984). Professionalism in nursing in nurse educators in baccalaureate and associate degree programs in Texas (Doctoral dissertation, The University of Texas at Austin, 1984). *Dissertation Abstracts International, 46,* 1118B.

Miller, B. K., Adams, D., & Beck, L. (1993). A behavioral inventory for professionalism in nursing. *Journal of Professional Nursing, 9,* 290–295.

Nightingale, F. (1969). *Notes on nursing: What it is, and what it is not.* New York: Dover.

Paul, R. (1990). *Critical thinking: What every person needs to survive in a rapidly changing world.* Rohnert Park, CA: Center for Critical Thinking and Moral Critique.

Rogers, E. M. (2003). *Diffusion of innovations* (5th ed.). New York: Free Press.

Shaver, J. L. F. (2001). Looking to the future of academic administrative leadership. In N. L. Chaska (Ed.), *The nursing profession: Tomorrow and beyond* (pp. 931–943). Thousand Oaks, CA: Sage.

Titler, M. (2001). Research utilization and evidence based practice. In N. L. Chaska (Ed.) *The nursing profession: Tomorrow and beyond* (pp. 423–437). Thousand Oaks, CA: Sage.

Titler, M. (2006). Developing an evidence-based practice. In G. LoBiondo-Wood & J. Haber (Eds.), *Nursing research: Methods and critical appraisal for evidence-based practice* (pp. 439–481). St. Louis, MO: Mosby.

Watson, R. (2005). Self-development and self-appraisal. In L. Caputi & L. Engelmann (Eds.), *Teaching nursing: The art and science* (Vol. 2.) Glen Ellyn, IL: College of DuPage Press.

Wilson, A. L., & Hayes, E. R. (2000). On thought and action in adult and continuing education. In A. L. Wilson & E. R. Hayes (Eds.), *Handbook of adult and continuing education* (pp. 15–32). San Francisco: Jossey-Bass.

Confirmation

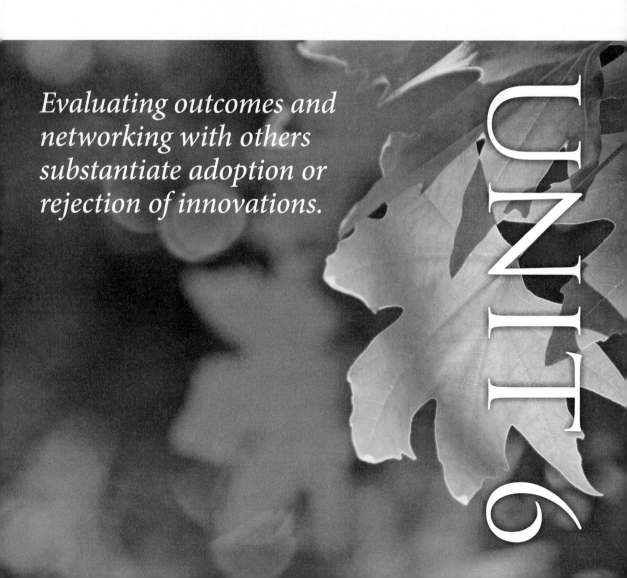

Evaluating outcomes and networking with others substantiate adoption or rejection of innovations.

UNIT 6

CHAPTER OBJECTIVES

At the end of this chapter, you will be able to:

< Define outcome

< Discuss ways outcomes can be classified

< Discuss factors that should be considered when selecting outcomes

< Discuss how data are used to evaluate outcomes

< List three dilemmas that can arise when nurses are involved in testing protocols

KEY TERMS

benchmarking
care-related outcome
continuous quality
   improvement
Forces of Magnetism
indicator
intermediate outcome

long-term outcome
mandated reporting
nursing outcome
nursing-sensitive outcome
organizational priorities
outcome
outcomes research

patient populations
patient-related outcome
performance-related
   outcome
short-term outcome
team membership

CHAPTER 17

Evaluating Outcomes of Innovations

Kathleen A. Rich

17.1 What Is an Outcome?

At the end of this section, you will be able to:

< Define outcome
< Discuss ways outcomes can be classified

Implementing an innovation, policy or procedure does not necessarily guarantee that it will become the standard of care. Ongoing evaluation of an innovation through *outcome* measurements is necessary to ensure successful incorporation into clinical practice. An outcome is defined as the consequence or visible result (Webster, 2001). *Nursing outcomes* measure states, behaviors, or perceptions of individuals, families, or communities (Moorehead, Johnson, & Maas, 2004). *Outcomes research* examines the effects of care and treatments on individuals and populations (Rubenfeld et al., 1999). In nursing research, the outcome is frequently known as the dependent variable (Polit & Hungler, 2006).

Outcomes may be classified by several different methods. One way outcomes can be classified is by focusing on who is being measured. Nurses may measure outcomes for individuals, groups, or organizations.

Another way that outcomes can be grouped is by type: *care-related*, *patient-related*, and *performance-related outcomes* (Kleinpell, 2001). An example of a care-related outcome is the rate of pressure ulcer formation in patients on bed rest for more than 24 hours. Patient knowledge related to fluid restriction is an

KEY TERMS

Outcome:
Consequence or
visible result

Nursing outcomes:
Measures of
states, behaviors,
or perceptions of
individuals, families,
or communities

Outcomes research:
Studies about the
effects of care
and treatments
on individuals and
populations

**Care-related
outcomes:** Category
of outcomes that
measures the effect of
nursing interventions

**Patient-related
outcomes:** Type of
outcome related to
patient behaviors or
actions

**Performance-related
outcomes:** Type of
outcome related to
how nurses perform
their jobs

**Short-term
outcomes:** Results
achieved in a brief
period of time

example of a patient-related outcome. Nursing staff adherence to best practice guidelines when providing discharge education to a heart failure patient is an example of a performance-related outcome.

Time is another way of classifying outcomes. *Short-term outcomes* are results achieved in a relatively brief period of time that usually involve a change in condition, such as absence of postoperative pain, or an increase in knowledge or skills, such as a patient's ability to draw up insulin. Another category of outcome classified by time is *intermediate outcomes*. They exist when changes occur after an innovation is introduced. Lifestyle modifications, such as weight loss and smoking cessation after enrolling in a wellness program, can be examples of intermediate outcomes. *Long-term outcomes* are primary changes in patients' behaviors or status, such as a reduction in blood cholesterol levels (Plantz, Greenway, & Hendricks, 1996).

Nursing administrators are responsible for reporting *nursing-sensitive outcomes* at their institutions to demonstrate effectiveness of nursing care. Outcomes of nursing care should be measurable. These measurements can assist in determining responsibility in patient care (Krau, 2001). One nursing-sensitive outcome considered a National Patient Safety Goal mandated by The Joint Commission (JC) is to reduce the risk of patient harm resulting from falls (Joint Commission, 2007a). The Joint Commission requires healthcare organizations to have fall reduction programs. Two desirable outcomes that may result from an evidence-based fall prevention protocol are a reduction in the number of patient falls and fewer fall-related injuries.

Outcome-based measurements are a means used to establish evidence-based practice (EBP) and to evaluate the care delivered. In healthcare organizations, many activities are outcome driven. The rising costs of health care, increasingly stringent accreditation standards, and public reporting are several reasons why outcomes are closely scrutinized and are integral to ensuring the successful implementation of an innovation. In health care, outcomes are typically quantitative, not qualitative.

CRITICAL THINKING EXERCISE 17-1

Consider your last clinical experience. Are you aware of any outcomes that are being monitored on the unit or in the facility? If so, what are they and how would you classify them?

TEST YOUR KNOWLEDGE 17-1

Match the type of outcome with the indicator

1. system-related outcome

2. patient-related outcome

3. care-related outcome

4. long-term outcome

5. short-term outcome

a. Patient will not hemorrhage after delivery

b. Patient will maintain weight loss over two years

c. Patient will be afebrile after surgery

d. The rate of hospital-acquired infections

e. Patient satisfaction will be 90% or greater

How did you do? 1. d, e; 2. a, b, c; 3. d; 4. b; 5. a, c

Evaluating outcomes is not static, but rather an ongoing process. Outcomes must be well defined for the evaluation to be meaningful. The effectiveness of any innovation is measured by the outcomes that result. These results are compared to baseline data in order to draw conclusions about the effectiveness of the innovation. The process continues as the innovation becomes standard practice.

17.2   Choosing Outcomes

At the end of this section, you will be able to:

‹ Discuss factors that should be considered when selecting outcomes

Choosing outcomes that appropriately fit an innovation is vital. This allows for an accurate evaluation of practice changes. During the selection process, outcomes should be considered for their significance and scope. Considerations may include morbidity, quality of life, and appropriate use of resources (Ciliska, DiCenso, & Guyatt, 2005). Outcomes should be measured using specific quantitative criteria, sometimes referred to as *indicators*. For example, if postoperative pain control is of interest, then pain should be quantified

KEY TERMS

Intermediate outcomes: Changes that occur after an innovation is introduced

Long-term outcomes: Primary changes in patient behaviors or status over time

Nursing-sensitive outcomes: Results that demonstrate the effectiveness of nursing care

 FYI

Outcome-based measurements are a means used to establish EBP and to evaluate the care delivered. The effectiveness of any innovation is measured by the outcomes that result.

KEY TERMS

Indicators: Quantitative criteria used to measure outcomes

Patient populations:
A group of patients
with similar
characteristics

Team membership:
The composition of
a team with respect
to expertise and
leadership

**Organizational
priorities:** Situations
of high importance
because of volume of
patients or costs

**Mandated
reporting:** Data
that must be shared
with supervising
or governmental
agencies by a
specified timeline

through a recognized indicator such as the numeric rating scale. If focusing on an outcome such as quality of life, then using an established instrument, such as the SF-36 published by Ware and Sherbourne, is preferred over the use of a self-developed instrument (Padilla, Frank-Stromborg, & Koresawa, 2004). Instruments that have been tested for reliability and validity will improve credibility of the evaluation process. **Table 17-1** lists examples of outcomes and associated indicators.

When determining outcomes to be measured, there are four major factors to consider: *patient populations*, *team membership*, *organizational priorities*, and *mandated reporting*. It is best when the selected outcomes address multiple factors. Journals, books, and websites are available to assist. **Table 17-2** lists selected organizations with their associated websites that contain health outcome information.

Patient Population

It is necessary to select outcomes that reflect the patient population served by the healthcare facility. Use of a generic patient outcome is a good strategy to measure outcomes when populations are diverse. For example, measuring symptom control or increased knowledge may apply to many disease conditions (Whitman, 2003). The nursing outcomes classification (NOC), developed at the University of Iowa College of Nursing, is a standardized list of generic patient outcome classifications that can be used to evaluate the efficacy of nursing interventions (Moorehead et al., 2004). There are currently 330 outcomes in the NOC system that are associated with the North American Nursing Diagnosis Association and the nursing interventions classification. Each outcome is coded and consists of several components: a definition, a list of numeric indicators from which the nurse selects to evaluate the patient's status, a target

TABLE 17-1 Outcomes and Indicators

Outcome	Indicator
Dyspnea reduction	Dyspnea rating scale
Decrease in postoperative pain	Pain numeric rating scale
Absence of skin ulcers	Pressure sore staging
Fluid restriction compliance	Daily weight
Knowledge: blood pressure medication	Blood pressure

TABLE 17-2 Selected Health Outcome Information Websites	
Organization	**Website**
AcademyHealth	http://www.academyhealth.org
Agency for Healthcare Research and Quality	http://www.ahrq.gov/clinic/outcomix.htm
Centers for Medicare and Medicaid Services	http://www.hce.org
Harvard College Library Health Data Resources	http://hcl.harvard.edu/research/guides/health_us/
Institute for Healthcare Improvement	http://www.ihi.org
Joint Commission on Accreditation of Healthcare Organizations	http://www.jointcommission.org
National Cancer Institute	http://outcomes.cancer.gov/
National Committee for Quality Assurance	http://www.ncqa.org/
United Way	http://liveunited.org/our-work/health/
University of Iowa College of Nursing	http://www.uihealthcare.com/depts/nursing/rqom/index.html

outcome rating, and a five-point Likert-type scale for measuring the status. "Knowledge: diet" is an example of an NOC patient outcome and is defined as the extent of understanding conveyed about the recommended diet. The outcome may be applied to a diverse group of patients in a wide spectrum of healthcare settings. Included in this outcome are 15 indicators that the nurse may choose for evaluation purposes, such as description of diet and description of potential for food and medication interaction (Moorehead et al., 2004). The Likert-type scale yields data ranging from none (1) to extensive (5) for each indicator.

Team Membership

When selecting an outcome, consideration should be given to the composition of members who form the team responsible for monitoring the outcome (Whitman, 2003). This includes the personnel members and capabilities that would be involved in implementing the innovation and outcome measurements. Utilizing an interdisciplinary approach including nursing, education, ancillary support services, and quality improvement allows for incorporation of different viewpoints and knowledge. It may also result in recommendation of new outcomes that were not previously considered. The creation of interdisciplinary relationships in the formulation and approval of policies and protocols is required to achieve American Nurses Credentialing Center (ANCC) Magnet

KEY TERM

Continuous quality improvement: Participatory process involving indicators that measure quality

Recognition (ANCC, 2005). Advanced practice nurses (APNs) are integral members of interdisciplinary teams. The APN has expert clinical knowledge about rapidly occurring changes in the healthcare environment. APNs are familiar with institutional data and are able to assist with comparison to national benchmarks. APNs can assist with selecting realistic outcomes. An outcome that is realistic has a base definition that is true to life (Minnick, 2001). For example, selecting an outcome such as "improved quality of life in heart failure patients" is vague and has a multitude of meanings dependent upon the individual and the severity of the associated disease condition. People with slight limitation of physical activities might have a different perception of quality of life than individuals who are unable to carry out physical activities without discomfort or symptoms at rest. Therefore, the vaguely written outcome cannot be realistically evaluated. APNs can assist to narrow the focus, thus making an outcome more measurable. Staff nurses may be involved at several different levels during outcome selection and subsequent measurements. Nurses are familiar with the *continuous quality improvement* (CQI) process through participation with internal quality improvement measures. Staff nurses are often members of the interdisciplinary team involved in protocol development. They frequently provide insightful suggestions on approaches that can be used in the clinical setting to obtain outcome measurements. Staff nurses can identify patients who meet criteria for inclusion in the protocol. They can also collect data such as reviewing charts for compliance in documentation.

Organizational Priorities

A second consideration is selecting outcomes that address organizational priorities (Whitman, 2003). Sometimes outcomes can be linked to the mission of the healthcare organization. For example, a faith-based hospital may focus attention on ensuring that all patients receive a spiritual assessment. Organizations may also use outcomes to evaluate specific areas that need improvement. CQI activities are an evaluation of existing practices that involve delivery of services to the people (Reinhardt & Ray, 2003). The goal of CQI is to improve service. CQI measures can be generic indicators or narrowed into disease-specific outcomes.

CRITICAL THINKING EXERCISE 17-2

Your nurse manager selects you to represent the unit on a team monitoring patient safety. What outcomes would you suggest the team monitor?

Mandated Reports

There are multiple publicly reported nursing indicators that can be used to measure outcomes of EBP protocols. Hospitals and other healthcare agencies are required to gather data on specific disease entities and to report their findings to public agencies. Outcome data, available on State Boards of Health and the Centers for Medicare and Medicaid Services (CMS) websites, are published to make comparisons among healthcare facilities. Organizations use these data to gain a picture of how they compare to similar facilities. This is known as *benchmarking*. Clinical practice guidelines or standards of care recommended by professional organizations can also drive outcome selection. There is often overlap among the various organizations that mandate reporting. For example, consider when a healthcare organization implements a smoking cessation program for patients with cardiac disease. The American College of Cardiology (ACC) and American Heart Association (AHA) have issued joint guidelines delineating the expected standards of care for patients experiencing an ST-elevation myocardial infarction (MI) (AHA, 2004). These guidelines recommend offering smoking cessation counseling to all patients who either currently smoke or have quit smoking within the past year (AHA, 2004). The Joint Commission requires hospitals to report on two of the four core measures that include MI (Joint Commission, 2007b). The CMS has eight MI quality care measures that hospitals must report about, one of which measures smoking cessation counseling (CMS, n.d.).

In addition to reporting mandatory CMS and JC data, many healthcare facilities are members of not-for-profit organizations to benchmark indicators. For example, hospitals can subscribe to databases maintained by the ACC and The Society of Thoracic Surgeons (STS). The ACC (2007) has four databases that include cardiac catheterization/percutaneous coronary intervention, implantable cardioverter defibrillator, carotid revascularization, and acute coronary syndrome. The STS (2007) provides statistics on adult and congenital heart surgery and for thoracic surgery patients. Organizations such as these provide EBP guidelines for various disease entities, allowing subscribers to review the latest information for protocol development and implementation within the facility.

Another such organization is the Institute for Healthcare Improvement (IHI). The IHI (n.d.) initially developed a program known as the 100,000 Lives Campaign, now known as the 5 Million Lives Campaign. This initiative targets saving 100,000 lives through instituting six major hospital programs: a rapid response team, MI care, prevention of adverse drug effects, reduction of central line infection, reduction of surgical site infection, and ventilator-associated pneumonia (VAP). For example, a reduction in the incidence of VAP was proposed through implementation of five interventions grouped together known

KEY TERM

Benchmarking:
Comparison of organizational outcome data to other organizations or national databases

KEY TERM

Forces of Magnetism: Qualities that exhibit nursing excellence

as the "ventilator bundle" (Resar et al., 2005). VAP is defined as a nosocomial pneumonia that develops 48 hours or longer after a patient has an artificial airway such as a tracheostomy or endotracheal tube inserted (De Rosa & Craven, 2003). The mortality rate for patients diagnosed with VAP ranges from 25% to 40%, and the diagnosis adds an estimated cost of $40 thousand to a hospital admission (Tablan, Anderson, & Besser, 2004). The ventilator bundle consists of these strategies: keeping the head of the bed elevated at least 30 degrees at all times unless clinically contraindicated, daily sedation vacations, assessments of weaning readiness, peptic ulcer prevention, and deep vein thrombosis prophylaxis. To evaluate VAP protocol, based upon the ventilator bundle, an outcome could be to reduce the incidence of VAP by 75%.

In the Magnet Recognition Program (ANCC, 2005), healthcare organizations are required to provide examples of nurse-sensitive quality indicators as part of the application process or to maintain Magnet Recognition. There are 14 components, known as *Forces of Magnetism*, that exhibit nursing excellence. **Table 17-3** lists these forces. For example, for a healthcare organization to meet force seven, quality improvement, evidence must show that nursing staff members participate in CQI activities and that CQI is perceived to im-

TABLE 17-3 Fourteen Forces of Magnetism

Force 1	Quality of Nursing Leadership
Force 2	Organizational Structure
Force 3	Management Style
Force 4	Personnel Policies and Programs
Force 5	Professional Models of Care
Force 6	Quality of Care
Force 7	Quality Improvement
Force 8	Consultation and Resources
Force 9	Autonomy
Force 10	Community and the Healthcare Organization
Force 11	Nurses as Teachers
Force 12	Image of Nursing
Force 13	Interdisciplinary Relationships
Force 14	Professional Development

Source: Adapted from American Nurses Credentialing Center. 2005. *Magnet recognition program* (pp. 2–3). Silver Springs, MD: Author.

prove care within the facility (ANCC). In addition, the organization must provide examples of a change in nursing practice that occurred as a result of data originating from fiscal, satisfaction, or clinical outcomes. The following scenario demonstrates how one outcome can be used to address mandates from the Joint Commission, IHI, and the Magnet Recognition Program.

Continuing with VAP as an example, suppose the infection control nurse in your facility reports that, despite implementing the ventilator bundle, the VAP rate has not decreased in the last two quarters.

A multidisciplinary committee consisting of nursing, respiratory therapy, infection control, quality improvement, and staff education examines the evidence. The committee determines that regularly scheduled oral hygiene, including teeth brushing, while on the ventilator has been linked with a reduction of plaque and oropharyngeal colonization.

The committee decides to change oral care products currently used in your facility and recommends a change in protocol. The new ventilator oral care protocol is developed and presented to the staff along with a review of related infection control findings related to VAP. The staff are enthusiastic about the change in oral care products and the new protocol. Over the next few months, follow-up reporting will be provided to the nursing staff. The quarterly VAP rate will be compared to the rate prior to the implementation of the new protocol to determine the effectiveness of the practice change.

TEST YOUR KNOWLEDGE 17-2

1. Which of the following are considerations when selecting outcomes?
   a. organizational mission
   b. publicly reported benchmarks
   c. type of patients served at healthcare facility
   d. expertise of team members

2. Which of the following statements is false?
   a. Journals, books, and websites are available to assist nurses in selecting outcomes.
   b. NOC outcomes could be used in evaluation plans.
   c. Benchmarking is a way to compare facility with national data.
   d. Clinical guidelines are only suggestions and are not evidence based.

How did you do? 1. a, b, c, d; 2. d

17.3 Evaluating the Outcomes

At the end of this section, you will be able to:

< Discuss how data are used to evaluate outcomes

After an outcome has been selected and measured, data are compiled and evaluated to draw conclusions. Demonstrating the effectiveness of an innovation is a challenge, and conclusions must not extend beyond the scope of the data. Evaluation is facilitated when appropriate outcomes and associated indicators are chosen. If the outcome is not clearly defined, then the measurements and subsequent evaluation will be flawed. For example, suppose that

CRITICAL THINKING EXERCISE 17-3

You are asked to join an interdisciplinary committee being formed to examine glucose management in intensive care unit (ICU) patients. You note that the current ICU practice is to administer a sliding scale subcutaneous insulin dose based upon the bedside glucose obtained at 6-hour time intervals. A retrospective chart review on 50 ICU patients receiving the sliding scale insulin dosage for 24 hours reveals that glycemic control in ICU patients is not present. Consequently, the committee develops an evidence-based intravenous (IV) insulin protocol based upon hourly glucose measurements. Glycemic control in ICU patients is the outcome selected and you are going to use a blood sugar result between 80–110 mg/dL within 8 hours of instituting the IV protocol as a measurement indicator. Staff nurses collect data on 50 patients over a 3-month time period and compared that to the baseline data as shown here:

	Mean Blood Glucose Level Before Change	Mean Blood Glucose Level After Change
On admission	250	248
8 hours after admit	235	122
12 hours after admit	230	110
24 hours after admit	212	111

While these reductions were statistically significant ($p = .02$), the outcome was not met. What other variables could be accounting for the fact that the outcome was not met? Would you continue to use the IV insulin protocol?

you are a member of an interdisciplinary team that has developed a nursing protocol that reduces the amount of time the patient remains on bed rest after a cardiac catheterization procedure from 6 hours to 4 hours. The outcome selected is absence of bleeding from the femoral arterial puncture site. No other indicators are measured. The results obtained after implementing the protocol revealed that there was an increase in bleeding at the femoral arterial site in the 4-hour bed rest patients compared to the 6-hour bed rest patients. Before concluding that a shorter bed rest time leads to an increase in femoral bleeding, a few additional questions need to be considered. First, was absence of bleeding defined in a measurable way? Because bleeding might be interpreted in several different ways, a precise definition of bleeding should have been provided to ensure consistency in reporting. Second, when should patients be assessed for absence of bleeding? Is the absence of bleeding to be assessed when the patient first ambulates or at a later time? Input from the staff prior to changing the nursing protocol could have clarified these questions resulting in more reliable results.

Another consideration in outcome evaluation is to obtain data relative to current practice for comparison purposes. To document the need for a practice change and to support a new protocol, baseline data might need to be collected to demonstrate limitations of the current standard of care. Consideration must be given to all extraneous variables that may be influencing the outcome, such as time, equipment, safety, and costs. It could be helpful to involve a statistician to perform complex analyses.

FYI

After an outcome has been selected and measured, data are compiled and evaluated to draw conclusions. Evaluation is facilitated when appropriate outcomes and associated indicators are chosen—conversely, if the outcome is not clearly defined, then the measurements and subsequent evaluation will be flawed.

TEST YOUR KNOWLEDGE 17-3

True/False

1. Baseline data are unimportant in outcome measurement.

2. Precise description of indicators is essential.

3. For complex analyses, the assistance of a statistician may be needed.

4. Input from staff can help clarify outcome measurement.

1. F; 2. T; 3. T; 4. T

17.4   Keeping It Ethical

At the end of this section, you will be able to:

< List three dilemmas that can arise when nurses are involved in testing protocols

FYI

When nurses are involved in testing protocols, there are ethical dilemmas that can arise. Issues can concern the selection of the sample, data collection, and reporting.

As a staff nurse, it is likely that you will be involved at some point in evaluating patient care outcomes. At the very least, your documentation will be a source of data. There are other ways for you to become involved in evaluation. When nurses are involved in testing protocols, there are ethical dilemmas that can arise. Issues can concern the selection of the sample, data collection, and reporting. When considering the recruitment of patients to participate in protocol testing, you must make certain that they fit the criteria and are not included simply to reach the sample size needed. You are obligated to collect data as directed by the protocol. Reflect back to the example of reducing the number of hours on bed rest following cardiac catheterization. Suppose you were to assess for bleeding in one of your patients but were unable to do that assessment because of an emergency on the unit. You might be tempted to guess or enter data collected at a later time. But for the integrity of the process, it would be preferable to indicate that the data are missing. Another issue that can arise is that sometimes nurses have a tendency to change behaviors when they are aware that data are being collected. For example, a hospital is implementing a smoking cessation program. Because the nursing staff knows that their unit is being compared to other units in the facility, they are very careful to follow the program exactly as outlined. However, after data collection is concluded and the protocol is found to be effective, it would not be in the best interest of patients for nurses to return to using former protocols.

TEST YOUR KNOWLEDGE 17-4

1. Which of the following behaviors is unethical?
   a. ensuring patients enrolled in a protocol meet criteria
   b. filling in all missing data at the conclusion of your shift
   c. refusing to participate in outcome measurement
   d. continuing to follow protocols after data collection ends

How did you do? 1. b, c

RAPID REVIEW

 An outcome is a consequence or a visible result. Nursing outcomes measure states, behaviors, or perceptions of individuals, families, or communities.

 Outcomes research examines the effect of care on individuals and populations.

 Outcomes can be classified by focusing on who is to be measured: individuals, groups, or organizations. They can also be grouped as care related, patient related, and performance related. They also may be classified according to time: short term, intermediate, and long term.

 Outcomes that demonstrate the effectiveness of nursing care are known as nursing-sensitive outcomes.

 Indicators specify how the outcome should be measured. Usually, quantitative measures are used.

 Four major factors should be considered when considering outcomes: patient populations, team selection, organizational priorities, and mandated reporting.

 Outcomes may be derived from a variety of sources such as NOC, clinical practice guidelines, standards of care, and Forces of Magnetism. CQI and benchmarking are processes that involve outcome evaluation.

 Conclusions are best drawn when outcomes are clearly defined, data are carefully collected, and findings are compared to baseline data. Considerations should be given to possible extraneous variables.

APPLY WHAT YOU HAVE LEARNED

It has been 6 months since the medication policy was implemented throughout your facility. Now it is time to evaluate if the desired outcomes have been met. You invite the chair of the Quality Assurance Committee to attend the next meeting of the EBP Committee. You ask her to report on the monthly incidence of medication errors for the past 6 months and the errors from the same months in the previous year. This will allow committee members to compare error rates before and after implementation of the policy. Review her report on the companion website. What conclusions can you draw about the effectiveness of the policy?

⚡ Ethical issues can concern selection of the sample, data collection, and reporting.

REFERENCES

American College of Cardiology. (2007). *National cardiovascular data registry.* Retrieved September 7, 2007, from http://www.accncdr.com/WebNCDR/Common/

American Heart Association. (2004). ACC/AHA guidelines for the management of patients with ST-elevation myocardial infarction. *Circulation, 110,* 82–292.

American Nurses Credentialing Center. (2005). *Magnet recognition program.* Silver Spring, MD: Author.

Centers for Medicare and Medicaid Systems. (n.d.) *Acute myocardial infarction.* Retrieved November 12, 2010, from http://www.guideline.gov/content.aspx?id=11074

Ciliska, D., DiCenso, A., & Guyatt, G. (2005). Summarizing the evidence through systematic reviews. In A. DiCenso, D. Ciliska, & G. Guyatt (Eds.), *Evidence-based nursing: A guide to clinical practice* (pp. 151–168). St. Louis, MO: Mosby.

De Rosa, F., & Craven, D. (2003). Ventilator-associated pneumonia: Current management strategies. *Infectious Medicine, 20,* 248–259.

Institute for Healthcare Improvement. (n.d.). *Campaign.* Retrieved October 9, 2010, from http://www.ihi.org/IHI/Programs/Campaign/Campaign.htm

Kleinpell, R. (2001). Measuring outcomes in advanced practice nursing. In R. Kleinpell (Ed.), *Outcome assessment in advanced practice nursing* (pp. 1–50). New York: Springer.

Krau, S. (2001). Using nurse-sensitive outcomes to improve clinical practice. *Critical Care Nursing Clinics of North America, 13,* 487–495.

Minnick, A. (2001). General design and implementation challenges in outcomes assessment. In R. Kleinpell (Ed.), *Outcome assessment in advanced practice nursing* (pp. 91–101). New York: Springer.

Moorehead, S., Johnson, M., & Maas, M. (Eds.) (2004). *Nursing outcomes classification (NOC)* (3rd ed.). St. Louis, MO: Mosby.

Padilla, G., Frank-Stromborg, M., & Koresawa, S. (2004). Single instruments for measuring quality of life. In M. Frank-Stromborg & S. Olsen (Eds.), *Instruments for clinical health-care research* (3rd ed., pp. 128–139). Sudbury, MA: Jones and Bartlett.

Plantz, M., Greenway, M., & Hendricks, M.(1996). *Measuring program outcomes: A practical approach.* Alexandria, VA: United Way of America.

Polit, D., & Hungler, B. (2006). *Essentials of nursing research* (5th ed.). Philadelphia: Lippincott.

Reinhardt, A., & Ray, L. (2003). Differentiating quality improvement from research. *Applied Nursing Research, 16*, 2–8.

Resar, R., Pronovost, P., Haraden, C., Simmonds, T., Rainey, T., & Nolan, T. (2005). Using a bundle approach to improve ventilator care processes and reduce ventilator-associated pneumonia. *Joint Commission Journal Quality Patient Safety, 31*, 243–248.

Rubenfeld, G., Angus, D., Pinsky, M., Randall, C., Connors, A., & Bernard, G. (1999). Outcomes research in critical care. *American Journal of Respiratory Critical Care Medicine, 160*, 358–367.

Tablan, O., Anderson, L., & Besser, R. (2004). CDC healthcare infection control practices advisory committee. Guidelines for preventing health care-associated pneumonia, 2003: Recommendations of CDC and the healthcare infection control practices advisory committee. *MMWR, 26*, 1–36.

The Joint Commission. (2007a). *Hospital accreditation standards.* Oakbrook Terrace, IL: Author.

The Joint Commission. (2007b). *ORYX non-core measure information.* Retrieved October 9, 2010, from http://www.jointcommission.org/PerformanceMeasurement/PerformanceMeasurement/ORYX+Non-Core+Measure+Information.htm

The Society of Thoracic Surgeons. (2007). *Executive summaries.* Retrieved September 7, 2007, from http://www.sts.org/sections/stsnationaldatabase/publications/executive/article.html.

Webster Comprehensive Dictionary. (2001). Chicago, IL: Ferguson.

Whitman, G. (2003). What patient outcomes should our outcomes-management team measure? *Outcomes Management, 7*(3), 94–96.

CHAPTER OBJECTIVES

At the end of this chapter, you will be able to:

< Discuss the importance of dissemination of research findings to building evidence-based practice

< Recognize the importance of dissemination in the cycle of science

< Explain how poster presentations are useful to disseminate new knowledge

< List the essential components of a well constructed poster

< List elements that must be considered when preparing a manuscript

< Discuss the process for submitting a manuscript for publication

< Describe strategies that make oral presentations successful

< Demonstrate professional behaviors when attending conferences

< List strategies to get the most out of conference attendance

< Discuss why nurses are obligated to participate in the process of dissemination

KEY TERMS

authorship
call for abstracts
dissemination

manuscript
networking
papers

posters
presentations

CHAPTER 18

Sharing the Insights With Others

Janet M. Brown and Nola A. Schmidt

18.1 Dissemination: What Is My Role?

At the end of this section, you will be able to:

- ‹ Discuss the importance of dissemination of research findings to building EBP
- ‹ Recognize the importance of dissemination in the cycle of science

EBP cannot be successful if nurses fail to read or hear about new knowledge. Evidence must be made available in accessible and comprehensible ways so that innovations are adopted. *Dissemination* is the communication of clinical, research, and theoretical findings for the purpose of transitioning new knowledge to the point of care. EBP cannot evolve unless communication channels in the societal system are used effectively to bring about change. Dissemination of findings is most successful if multiple methods are used over time. In the profession of nursing, there are three major ways that new knowledge is disseminated: posters, papers, and presentations. These are often referred to as the 3 Ps of dissemination.

Every healthcare discipline faces the challenge of conveying research findings to clinicians in a timely manner. Cronenwett (1995) notes that most nurses are not familiar with research methods and that because they are busy providing patient care, they have little time to keep up with new knowledge. She suggests that attention be given to: a) what information should be disseminated, b) the most effective way for nurses to access the information, and c) to whom the information should be targeted.

Recall the four phases of the cycle of scientific development: theory development, research, dissemination, and application to practice. All nurses must be accountable for professional activities that facilitate dissemi-

FYI

Dissemination is the communication of clinical, research, and theoretical findings for the purpose of transitioning new knowledge to the point of care. EBP cannot evolve unless communication channels in the societal system are used effectively to bring about change.

KEY TERM

Dissemination: Communication of clinical research and theoretical findings to transition new knowledge to the point of care

TEST YOUR KNOWLEDGE 18-1

1. New knowledge is effectively disseminated through
   a. papers
   b. posters
   c. proclamations
   d. presentations

2. Dissemination is important for which of the following reasons?
   a. Publishers need to make a profit.
   b. Most research grants require reporting.
   c. New knowledge is transmitted to patient care.
   d. Theorists and researchers need something to do.

3. Dissemination is an important phase in
   a. the cycle of scientific development
   b. the Krebs cycle
   c. the cycle of life
   d. the cycle of professional nursing

How did you do? 1. a, b, d; 2. c; 3. a

nation. Just as theorists and researchers have responsibilities to communicate findings, nurses have responsibilities to actively seek and apply new knowledge. Without dissemination, there is no reason to develop theories and conduct research because nurses would not read and hear about the latest findings.

18.2 The 3 Ps of Dissemination

At the end of this section, you will be able to:

< Explain how poster presentations are useful to disseminate new knowledge
< List the essential components of a well constructed poster
< List elements that must be considered when preparing a manuscript
< Discuss the process for submitting a manuscript for publication
< Describe strategies that make oral presentations successful

Posters

Posters are an important scholarly venue for disseminating evidence (Horne, Kosper, & Carpenter, 1993). A major advantage of poster presentations over other methods is that opportunities for *networking* exist. Poster sessions allow for interactions among professionals. Presenters receive immediate feedback from a variety of individuals who attend the poster session. Interactions allow for the exchange of ideas about areas of common interest (Moneyham, Ura, Ellwood, & Bruno, 1996). The versatility of the poster as a medium for dissemination makes it effective in a variety of situations. Posters are often used in the clinical arena to convey innovations or describe EBP. At professional conferences, research studies are often summarized in a poster display. Nurses may have opportunities to display posters at their places of employment. A poster could be displayed on a unit or in an area where staff members are likely to gather, such as the cafeteria or hallway. Because dissemination from individuals in clinical practice is essential to building nursing knowledge, unit-based posters are an excellent opportunity for nurses to disseminate the unique knowledge they possess. Evidence-based projects, quality improvement, and interesting patient case studies lend themselves to poster presentations. For example, a nurse notes that a better way is needed for securing scalp needles used with infants. Over time, he devises a technique that is superior to other taping methods. A poster presentation would be an ideal way to share his innovation with other nurses. Poster presentations are a mainstay of professional conferences. Most all major conferences include at least one poster session, and such sessions are growing in popularity to the point that it is not uncommon to have several sessions throughout a conference. Because poster submissions are usually competitive, it is an honor to have a poster selected for display.

How to Be a Poster Presenter

There is a typical process for selecting individuals to present at poster presentations. To be considered for presentation, individuals are required to submit an abstract summarizing the project. Abstracts are peer reviewed using stringent criteria. To increase the likelihood of having an abstract selected, attention to poster guidelines when writing an abstract for submission is critical. For example, it would be expected that the abstract contain the exact headings as specified in the guidelines. Another way to increase the chances of having an abstract accepted for presentation is to consider whether the poster would be appropriate for the audience expected at the conference. Notices, also known as a *call for abstracts*, publicize that submissions for abstracts are being sought. Calls for abstracts typically include information about submission and provide clues about the intended audience. Information in the call for abstracts can help one decide if a topic is congruent with the conference objectives. For

FYI

The three Ps of dissemination are: posters, papers, and presentations. Nurses have an obligation to facilitate dissemination, and can best participate in this by learning the proper processes and methods of the three Ps of dissemination.

KEY TERMS

Poster: Scholarly venue for disseminating evidence

Networking: Interacting with colleagues to exchange information and build relationships

Call for abstracts: Notices publicizing the desire for posters or presentations at conferences

TABLE 18-1 Tips on How to Write a Good Abstract

< Target appropriate audience and conference aim
< Ensure abstract is submitted by the deadline
< Carefully follow directions for formatting
  < Use appropriate font and font size (Arial and Times New Roman 10 and 12 allow maximum wordage in a limited space)
  < Adhere to the word limit specified
  < Provide biographical and contact information as requested
< Keep title clear and concise using less than 10 words
< Write in past tense
< Provide key information in a succinct manner
< Correct errors
  < Ask a colleague to provide feedback
  < Check for spelling mistakes
  < Take 5 minutes to conduct a final check

Source: Adapted from Coad & Devitt (2005) and Duchin & Sherwood (1990).

example, if childhood obesity is the focus of a conference, it is unlikely that a poster about obesity in older adults would be selected. Carefully matching one's scholarly work to the appropriate conference can reduce wasted effort and disappointment. See **Table 18-1** for tips on how to write a good abstract.

Individuals who submit abstracts for consideration at a conference are notified about the outcome of the review. With the acceptance of an abstract come several professional obligations. It is important to indicate acceptance of the invitation. If circumstances have changed and it is necessary to decline, doing so in a timely manner will allow the selection committee to fill the spot. When a commitment to present is made, it is essential to fulfill that commitment. Conference attendees become disgruntled if presenters are absent. If circumstances warrant an absence, having a colleague present is an acceptable alternative. Registration and payment of conference fees is required of most presenters but, sometimes a reduced fee is available.

When at the conference, presenters have a responsibility to fulfill the obligations of being a presenter. There are designated times for setting up and taking down posters. Presenters should adhere to these scheduled times. Presenters should make themselves available next to their posters during poster sessions to answer questions and convey excitement about the topic (Ellerbee, 2006). It is not unusual for attendees to seek out specific presenters who have similar interests. This type of networking is invaluable. Poster sessions provide an excellent forum for nurses from different settings to meet and exchange information (Botter, Giardino, & Wolf, 1990). Having handouts containing information not included in the abstract promotes dissemination. It is often helpful to offer business cards to individuals who are interested in your work (Ellerbee). If your organization does not provide business cards, it is easy to make your own (**Figure 18-1**).

Tips for Creating Effective Posters

Regardless of the environment or setting in which posters will be displayed, they should be created to effectively communicate ideas. Attention to both content and appearance is necessary. Creating posters requires more skill and effort than is usually anticipated, but while it is time consuming, most nurses find the process to be rewarding (Botter et al., 1990). There are many strategies that can be used to enhance delivery of the message. No matter how attractive a poster appears, if attention is not given to content, dissemination of information is diminished. It is helpful to ask, "What is it that viewers should know after reading this poster?" Having this outcome in mind focuses the scope of the content to be presented. The message should be straightforward, and the text should be written in a common and meaningful language. Complete sentences are not needed, and content can be mixed with charts and graphs. Staggering bullets in an outline format is an effective way to present content

FIGURE 18-1   **Example of Self-designed Business Card**

Suzanne Smith, BSN, RN
Critical Care Staff Nurse
123 Main Street
Springfield, IN 11111
555-454-6789
Suzy.Smith@yahoo.com

and avoid redundancy. Jargon, abbreviations, and symbols should be avoided unless it is certain that the intended audience will recognize them. The goal is to be succinct yet deliver a complete message (Duchin & Sherwood, 1990). It should take viewers no longer than 5 minutes to read a poster (Ryan, 1989).

Specific content to be included on a poster is often outlined in the call for abstracts. Every poster should have a title and indicate the authors and their affiliations. It is acceptable to include a logo of the affiliation. Most posters will also include a purpose statement. Other content is determined by the type of information that is being presented. See **Table 18-2** for a listing of content typically included in posters. Acknowledgment should be given to organizations that provided funding for the project. It is also acceptable to acknowledge individuals who provided assistance for the project.

TABLE 18-2 Content Typically Included in Posters

Research	EBP	Clinical Case Study	Quality Management Project
Title/Author/ Affiliation	Title/Author/ Affiliation	Title/Author/ Affiliation	Title/Author/ Affiliation
Research Aim, Question, Hypothesis	PICO Question	Clinical Problem	Clinical Issue
Review of Literature	Review of Literature	Background Information	Description of Team
Conceptual Model	Method	Assessment	Preparation
Research Design	Synthesis of Findings	Nursing Diagnosis	Planning
Sample	Decision About Practice	Plan	Assessment
Results	Implementation	Implementation	Implementation
Limitations	Evaluation	Evaluation	Diversification
Discussion of Findings	Discussion	Discussion	Discussion
Implications			

Source: Adapted from Small Business Encyclopedia (n.d.)

No matter how well content is articulated in a poster, if the display is not visually appealing, individuals will not be enticed to read it. Consideration should be given to the layout, font, color, and graphics.

Arranging poster elements in a logical sequence allows the viewer to move easily from one section to another through the material. Title, author, and affiliation are usually centered at the top of the poster. Layout of the poster should be balanced with content flowing from top to bottom of each section. Typically, displays are divided into three sections. For example, 6 by 4 feet is a common poster size. The center section should be 4 feet wide, leaving a 1-foot section on each side (see **Figure 18-2**). Important information should be placed at eye level at the center of the poster. Arrows can be used to direct viewers, and it is acceptable to vary the orientation of the pages (Ellerbee, 2006; Moneyham et al., 1996). Layouts should appear scholarly and professional. Presenters should avoid cluttering layouts with items such as ribbons, lace, and flowers because these items distract from the information being presented.

It is important to select fonts that make the content easy to read (Ellerbee, 2006). Titles and headings should be easily visible from 3 to 6 feet away. This means that letters should have a font size of 96 points or more (2–3 inches high). Other text should be visible from 2 to 4 feet away; therefore, font sizes of 24 to 36 points (about 1 inch high) are recommended. A simple way to test

FIGURE 18-2   **Logical Layout for EBP Posters**

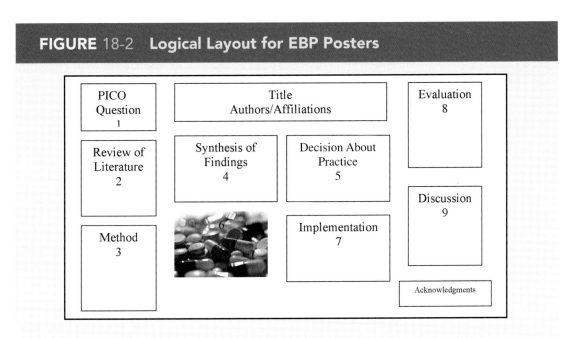

Source: Image © Photos.com

if the font is large enough is to place the poster on the ground. If it can be read while standing over it, the font size is sufficiently large. Fonts should be limited to one or two different styles. A roman-style font with a serif type is recommended. It is easier to differentiate similar looking letters and numbers because serif typefaces have tails or feet. By limiting each line to no more than 30 characters and having no more than six lines of text per heading, content can be kept organized and succinct. Consistency in the use of capitalization and punctuation should be maintained. Capital letters are usually used for titles and headings.

While selecting colors for posters is fun, choices should make material more attractive and emphasize important content (Duchin & Sherwood, 1990). Sometimes easels are provided for poster displays. If this is the case, background colors are not easily altered and will usually be brown, dark blue, or dark gray (Ellerbee, 2006). Selecting colors that compliment standard backgrounds is advised. Dark-colored fonts on lighter backgrounds are the easiest to read. Bright colors attract while complementary colors provide the greatest contrast (Duchin & Sherwood). Red and green are often used to highlight critical information; however, use of these two colors should be limited because some individuals have difficulty distinguishing them (Ellerbee). Sometimes presenters select colors because they represent a particular topic. For example, a poster on breast cancer may include pink as an accent color because this color is associated with breast cancer. Construction paper, color-coded art paper, or commercial paper with preprinted designs are inexpensive ways to add color (Duchin & Sherwood). Picture mattes, another way to add color, add dimension and provide distinct boundaries for content sections. Preformed letters or stencils are sometimes used on picture mattes for the title, author, and affiliation. Although mattes can be more costly than construction paper, they can be reused over a number of years. Because color choices have both scientific and artistic implications, presenters can make color choices based on evidence from the literature.

Including graphics is an effective way to present content in a parsimonious manner. Bar charts, line graphs, pie charts, diagrams, and scatter plots can communicate a wealth of information in a limited space. They are also an effective way to integrate color into the display. Clip art is another kind of graphic that can add interest to posters. For example, if the topic is about infant care, then a border showing babies would be appropriate. Overuse of clip art is discouraged. Clip art of nurses' caps and the medical caduceus are not suitable to include in scholarly nursing presentations.

There are several alternatives available for printing and assembling posters. The most cost-effective approach is to create PowerPoint slides. Printing slides on higher grade paper conveys a sense of quality and professionalism.

Some presenters laminate their slides to protect them; however, glare may result, making reading more difficult. Office supply companies can print and laminate PowerPoint slides, but it is wise to obtain price quotes before engaging in these services. Some presenters have access to large printers capable of printing on paper up to 4 feet wide. Entire posters are printed on a single sheet of paper that can be rolled and placed in a tube for easy transport to conferences. There are some disadvantages to this approach. Because large printers are slow and require skill to use, printing ahead of time is advisable. If typographical errors are found and revisions are needed, the entire poster, rather than a single slide, could require reprinting. Another drawback to using large printers is that presenters have a tendency to include too much information, making it difficult to read the posters. Regardless of the method selected to print materials, it is never acceptable to handwrite posters for a professional presentation. Presenters often use Velcro, push pins, or staples to attach their posters to display boards. Regardless of the method used, it is important to securely anchor the poster. Coming prepared with extra supplies is helpful because it is not uncommon to encounter problems when hanging posters. If traveling to conferences by air, it is wise to carry aboard posters to ensure that materials arrive with you.

No matter how many times presenters proofread their posters, it is still possible for an error to be overlooked. Completing posters with sufficient time for obtaining feedback from colleagues is invaluable. For feedback to be constructive, colleagues must be comfortable offering criticism and suggestions. It is recommended that after assembling posters, presenters step back and critically appraise their work. Referring back to submission criteria while appraising can ensure that posters meet conference goals.

Papers

Scholarly *papers* are published in a variety of venues and are essential for disseminating knowledge. Nurses in clinical areas are in an excellent position to write and submit papers about case studies, EBP, and quality management projects. Researchers, theorists, and nurse educators also publish papers for the purpose of extending nursing's body of knowledge. While there are many types of scholarly papers, the process of submission tends to be the same and is similar to the process of submitting a poster abstract. There are several helpful strategies that can assist novice writers to get started. One strategy is to submit a paper based on an already presented poster because the abstract and outline are already prepared. Gray (2005) recommends writing daily for 15–30 minutes and provides some tips for accomplishing this (see **Table 18-3**). Writing daily helps to form good habits about writing and leads to feelings of accomplishment. Another strategy is to recruit a colleague and have standing

TABLE 18-3 **Tips for Writing for 15–30 Minutes a Day**
‹ Write in the same place every day.
‹ Write at the same time every day, preferably in the morning.
‹ Put your writing time in your calendar as an appointment.
‹ Start your writing session in the same way each day.
‹ Learn to stop internal and external interruptions.
Source: Adapted from Gray, 2005.

KEY TERMS

Papers: Manuscripts published in professional journals

Authorship: List of authors in order that reflects the amount of their contributions

Manuscript: A scholarly paper prior to its publication

appointment times designated for writing. Collaborating with others creates accountability and can also be fun. It can be productive when novice writers collaborate with more seasoned writers.

When collaborating with others, it is important to determine *authorship* at the onset. Authors are listed in terms of their contribution to the paper. Usually the idea for the paper was generated by the first author. Other authors are listed in an order reflecting the amount of their contributions. When writing teams have good collegial relationships, authorship may be rotated among members of the team. Early in one's career, it is advisable to give consideration to the way one's name will appear in publications. For example, some authors include a middle name or initial. Consistently using the same format builds publication recognition and facilitates citation chasing.

After the decision to publish has been made, the next decision is to determine where the *manuscript* will be submitted. A manuscript is the term used for a scholarly paper prior to its publication. Just as with poster abstracts, consideration should be given to matching the topic and the intended audience with the purpose of the publication. Reading articles in journals to get a feel for their styles can help in determining if the manuscript would be a good fit. Query letters can be sent to journal editors to receive feedback about their

CRITICAL THINKING EXERCISE 18-1

When you publish an article, how will you want your name to appear?

interest in publishing the manuscript. It is accepted practice to send query letters to several editors simultaneously because the letter does not obligate the author to publish in that particular journal. See **Box 18-1** for an example of a query letter.

When a decision is made about where the manuscript will be submitted, reviewing author guidelines is necessary. Adhering to the guidelines from the beginning saves time by eliminating the need to adjust a manuscript later. Journals specify the type of style to be used for preparation of manuscripts and expect that authors adhere strictly (Sigsby, 1992). For example, some journals require American Psychological Association style, while others may require Modern Language Association style. Guidelines will also specify the number of words in an abstract, page limits, font, headings, and other criteria. It is es-

BOX 18-1

Example of Query Letter

September 1, 2010
Ms. Amy Sibley
Acquisitions Editor
Jones & Bartlett Learning
40 Tall Pine Drive
Sudbury, MA 01776

Dear Ms. Sibley:

I am in the process of preparing a manuscript entitled "How to Publish for Nursing: Tips for Getting it Done." The intended audience is staff nurses, and it will be about 15 pages in length. Would you be interested in reviewing this manuscript for *Hot Issues in Nursing*? Please contact me regarding your interest as indicated below.

Cordially,

Suzanne Smith, BSN, RN
Critical Care Staff Nurse
123 Main Street
Springfield, IN 11111
555-454-6789
Suzy.Smith@yahoo.com

sential that the guidelines be followed meticulously because manuscripts can be rejected when authors fail to follow the criteria. Familiarity with the language and tone used in the journal will also facilitate writing. For example, it is preferred in some journals to use the term "nurses" while the term "clinicians" is used in other journals. There are resources available, such as Pyrczak and Bruce (2007), that provide suggestions for writing effective research reports or other types of articles.

Obtaining feedback from colleagues during the writing process can be invaluable. Gray (2005) suggests sharing early drafts with nonexperts and later drafts with experts. Nonexperts can include family members, students, or colleagues in other disciplines. Because these individuals are less likely to understand the content, problems with organization and clarity are more likely to be identified. Experts are individuals with advanced degrees in nursing. Such individuals can provide reviews about the content as well as organization and clarity. Another way to obtain feedback is to join a writing circle (Gray, 2005). In writing circles, writers convene weekly, giving feedback on only a few manuscript pages. The group is given 5 minutes to read the work of one member. Discussion follows during which members indicate for each paragraph the topic sentence, providing rationales for their choices. If the writing is clear and organized, there will be agreement about the topic sentences. For nurses affiliated with universities, writing centers offer another resource for obtaining feedback. Just as with submission of poster abstracts, it is essential to review manuscripts many times prior to actually submitting them for publication.

There are many similarities between the process of submitting an abstract for presentation at a conference and submitting a manuscript for publication. It is important to review the author guidelines for instructions about submission. Many journals only accept submissions online. Editors of peer-reviewed journals will send blinded copies of manuscripts to several experts for review. Peer reviewers may be selected because of their expertise about the topic, the research method, method of analysis, or theory. For journals not using a peer review process, manuscripts are reviewed by the editor. The length of time it takes for the review varies among journals, but one can expect to wait 3–6 months for a response. It may be tempting to submit manuscripts to multiple journals at the same time, but this is absolutely unacceptable practice. A manuscript cannot be submitted to a second journal unless it is rejected by the first or the author withdraws the manuscript submission. Eventually, authors receive notice about the status of manuscripts. Editorial decisions about manuscripts usually fall into one of four categories: accept, accept with minor revisions, accept with major revisions, and not accepted for publication. Feedback from peer reviewers is usually included with notification of the decision. It is rare for a manuscript to be accepted for publication outright. Most often, minor or major revisions are required. Using feedback from peer reviewers to make revisions is often an effective way to ensure acceptance of the manuscript on a second submission. While it is natural for authors to be disappointed when manuscripts are rejected, they should immediately investigate other opportunities for submission. Feedback from peer reviewers can be used to make revisions, and another journal can be targeted.

KEY TERM

Presentations:
Scholarly oral presentations to disseminate new knowledge

Oral Presentations

Like posters and papers, oral *presentations* are an effective way to disseminate new knowledge. The submission process is very similar to poster abstract submissions. In fact, nurses must often decide whether to deliver a poster or presentation when submitting an abstract to a conference. Authors elect to present orally when the topic is too complex to present in the space of a poster. Philosophical and theoretical work is best suited for oral presentations. While posters work especially well for disseminating information about pilots and work in progress, completed work may be disseminated best through oral presentations.

There are professional responsibilities, similar to poster presentations, which must be fulfilled when accepting invitations to present papers. Many times presenters must submit their PowerPoint slides and handouts in advance of the conference. Objectives for presentations are often requested so that conference planners can apply for continuing education credits. Late fees might be assessed to presenters failing to meet deadlines. Should presenters find themselves unable to attend a conference, sending colleagues to substitute is preferable to canceling.

Successful oral presentations are a result of careful preparation and attention to detail. Principles related to layout, font, color, and graphics of poster preparation are applicable to the preparation of slides that accompany oral presentations. Presentations begin by showing a title slide followed by a slide acknowledging funding sources and contributors. It is recommended to have one slide for every 30–60 seconds. Novice presenters are advised to read papers from typed scripts rather than ad-libbing. Without experience, ad-libbing frequently results in a disorganized presentation that goes beyond the time limits. One can expect that one double-spaced typed page with 1-inch margins using an average sized font equals 2 minutes of speaking time. The best way to gauge the length of the presentation, however, is to rehearse the presentation aloud while using the visual aids. Typically, people speak faster when presenting than when rehearsing. Inserting visual cues into the script, such as "slow down" or "breathe," serves as a reminder for maintaining an appropriate speaking pace. Another helpful strategy to aid delivery is to enlarge the font

CRITICAL THINKING EXERCISE 18-2

You have been asked by a professor at your college to collaborate on a paper for publication in a peer-reviewed nursing journal. The professor expects you to do all of the research and writing, and stated that you will be acknowledged for your assistance, but that your name will not appear as an author on the article. What ethical issues need to be discussed in this situation? What action, if any, would you take?

so that the script is easier to read. Time should be allotted for questions at the end of the presentation.

It is smart to avoid the two most common mistakes made by presenters. First, the audience can become disengaged from the presentation when pre-

TEST YOUR KNOWLEDGE 18-2

1. When making a poster, which of the following should you do?
   a. Use full sentences and avoid using bullets.
   b. Use color to emphasize important points.
   c. Fancy or script font is desirable because viewers find them attractive.
   d. Acknowledgment of funding sources is not included because of space limitations.

2. Which of the following are strategies that are helpful when beginning to write a paper?
   a. Writing 15–30 minutes a week
   b. Collaborating with others
   c. Selecting a journal for submission
   d. Adapting a poster presentation

3. When delivering oral presentations, presenters should do which of the following?
   a. Respect time constraints
   b. Remain to the end of the paper session to network
   c. Read from the PowerPoint slides
   d. Ad-lib to make the presentation more conversational

How did you do? 1. b; 2. b, c, d; 3. a, b

senters read directly from slides. Keeping PowerPoint slides bulleted with phrases discourages this practice. Presenters should strive to present more depth and detail about the topic through speaking rather than through visual aids. The second most common mistake occurs when presenters disregard time constraints. It is expected that presenters adhere to the time limitations for their presentations. It is inconsiderate to continue speaking after room moderators have indicated that the time has expired. Another way presenters disregard time constraints is by failing to be present during the entire paper session. Four to six papers are typically grouped together over 90 minutes. Presenters should arrive well before paper sessions begin and confirm their presence with room moderators and confirm that last-minute scheduling changes have not been made. Arriving early also allows an opportunity to test audiovisual aids. Presenters are expected to make themselves available at the conclusion of paper sessions because attendees might wish to network. Having business cards to share with colleagues during this time is advisable.

18.3   Making the Most of Conferences

At the end of this section, you will be able to:

< Demonstrate professional behaviors when attending conferences
< List strategies to get the most out of conference attendance

Not only are conferences excellent venues for dissemination of new knowledge, but they also provide opportunities for developing connections with colleagues having similar interests, meeting experts in the field, and exploring career opportunities. Conference participants should take full advantage of networking opportunities to make the most of their experiences (French, 2000).

Maintaining a professional demeanor at all times is advantageous because you never know who you might meet or what opportunities could arise. For example, it is possible to be offered the opportunity to interview for a position with a leading expert in your specialty. Invitations to collaborate on papers and research studies are not uncommon. For individuals considering graduate study, networking with students and faculty from programs under consideration can be helpful. Questions about various programs can be answered when conversing with these individuals. It pays to be professional at all times. For example, individuals may find themselves sitting next to the dean of the graduate program under consideration. It would be quite uncomfortable to have an admission interview with this dean if the image portrayed is unfavorable.

FYI

Not only are conferences excellent venues for dissemination of new knowledge, but they also provide opportunities for developing connections with colleagues having similar interests, meeting experts in the field, and exploring career opportunities. Professional behaviors always make favorable impressions and should be practiced when attending conferences.

Professional behaviors always make favorable impressions and should be practiced when attending conferences. Participants should dress professionally. While attending a conference is a day away from work, it should not be considered a day off. Wearing sweatpants or jeans to be comfortable is not acceptable. It is customary for individuals to wear business suits or skirts or trousers that are paired with conservative blouses, sweaters, or jackets. Layering clothing is always wise because presentation rooms can vary in temperature. Arriving on time, introducing yourself to others, and offering a handshake make excellent first impressions. Inquiring where someone is from or why they chose to attend this conference are good ways to begin a conversation. If individuals find areas of common interest, having a business card to share facilitates networking. Allowing cell phones to ring during presentations shows disrespect for both presenters and members of the audience. Phones should be either turned off or silenced. It is also rude to converse with other attendees during presentations.

It is best to take full advantage of conferences because they can be costly to attend. Reviewing conference programs in their entirety allows participants to select sessions that pertain to their interests. Abstracts contain valuable information that helps identify presentations and posters of interest. Highlighting or writing out a schedule of preferred sessions ensures that time is maximized. It can be disappointing to overlook a scheduled session of interest. When planning a schedule, keep in mind that it is acceptable to change rooms

TEST YOUR KNOWLEDGE 18-3

1. When attending a conference, which of the following behaviors are acceptable?
   a. Wear business attire.
   b. Keep cell phones on silent or vibrate.
   c. Feel free to come in and out of sessions at will.
   d. Share business cards with other attendees.

2. Which of the following strategies help make the most of conferences?
   a. Attending receptions.
   b. Attending all sessions with your friends.
   c. Planning a schedule in advance.
   d. Talking with experts.

How did you do? 1. a, b, d; 2. a, c, d

between presentations during the same session time. If attending conferences with colleagues, it can be tempting to attend all sessions together. However, to maximize exposure to new ideas, it is wise to split up and share information later.

In addition to the sessions, conferences offer many other opportunities for networking. Some of the most important exchanges of information occur during conversations in hallways or at receptions. Viewing poster sessions, visiting vendor exhibits, and attending meals and breaks provide opportunities to meet new people or renew friendships. If there is a respected authority you would like to meet, introduce yourself. Most experts are eager to discuss their work. Networking, like dissemination, is vital to building the discipline of nursing.

18.4   Keeping It Ethical

At the end of this section, you will be able to:

‹ Discuss why nurses are obligated to participate in the process of dissemination

"The overall purpose of research dissemination is to begin the process of getting new knowledge used for the good of society" (Cronenwett, 1995, p. 430). There are increased demands for healthcare providers and systems to be efficient and effective in providing patient care. Nurses can no longer plead ignorance of new knowledge. They must be accountable for creating best practice by rapidly moving new information to the point of care (Cronenwett).

FYI

Nurses have a responsibility to actively participate in the process of dissemination. Reading articles, attending conferences, presenting posters and papers, and networking with other professionals are expected activities.

Having accountability means that nurses must use their resources wisely. Opportunities for dissemination are limited; space in journals and presentation times at conferences must be allocated fairly. Authors should never simply tweak a manuscript that has already been published to resubmit to another journal for publication as original work. Furthermore, it is a waste of time and money for nurses to attend conferences but not participate fully. Nurses are obligated to fulfill expectations placed on them by employers who sponsor attendance at conferences.

Nurses have a responsibility to actively participate in the process of dissemination. Reading articles, attending conferences, presenting posters and papers, and networking with other professionals are expected activities. Nurses can organize scholarly events in their facilities such as research days where posters about unit-based projects are presented. It is ethical practice to acknowledge authorship on all scholarly works. The power of sharing information about unit-based activities should not be underestimated. The discipline of nursing

TEST YOUR KNOWLEDGE 18-4

True/False

1. Because information is growing at a rapid pace, it is acceptable for nurses to plead ignorance about new knowledge.

2. All nurses are obligated to participate in the process of dissemination.

How did you do? 1. F; 2. T

is lacking dissemination from individuals in clinical practice. Dissemination of knowledge within nursing also raises the visibility of nursing to the public. To support these types of activities, nurses must advocate for budget dollars and release time from employers.

By concluding the journey through this textbook, it is hoped that an appreciation for nursing research and its importance to EBP has ensued. With the knowledge and skills acquired through the content and application exercises, you are equipped to be an innovator by engaging in the process of moving evidence over time through the communication channels of social systems to improve patient care.

 ## *RAPID* REVIEW

 Dissemination is the communication of clinical, research, and theoretical findings for the purpose of transitioning new knowledge to the point of care. It is an important step of the cycle of scientific development.

 The 3 P's of dissemination are posters, papers, and presentations.

 Posters are an excellent medium for disseminating information in a succinct and visually interesting manner. A mainstay of professional conferences, they can also be used at places of employment to communicate unit-based projects.

 A manuscript is a scholarly paper prior to its publication. Like posters, many papers undergo a rigorous peer review process before being accepted for publication.

 Oral presentations are an effective way to disseminate new knowledge when the topic is too complex to present in the space of a poster. Present-

APPLY WHAT YOU HAVE LEARNED

Because the process that the EBP Committee used was effective in creating a policy that reduced medication errors, several members submitted an abstract to a professional conference. You have just received notification that the abstract was accepted as a poster presentation. On the companion website, you will find the acceptance letter and guidelines for presentation of posters at this conference. While being certain to follow these guidelines, use the ideas in this chapter to create a poster that effectively disseminates your information.

ers have professional responsibilities, such as adhering to the time allotted and making themselves available for networking.

 Maintaining a professional demeanor at conferences is advantageous. There are many strategies for making the most of conference attendance such as writing out a schedule and talking with experts.

 Nurses have a responsibility to actively participate in dissemination by reading articles, attending conferences, presenting posters and papers, and networking with other professionals.

REFERENCES

Botter, M. L., Giardino, E. R., & Wolf, Z. R. (1990). University/community poster sessions. *NursingConnections, 3*, 49–53.

Coad, J., & Devitt, P. (2005). Research dissemination: The art of writing an abstract for conferences. *Nurse Education in Practice, 6*, 112–116.

Cronenwett, L. R. (1995). Effective methods for disseminating research findings to nurses in practice. *Nursing Clinics of North America, 30*, 429–438.

Duchin, S., & Sherwood, G. (1990). Posters as an educational strategy. *The Journal of Continuing Education in Nursing, 21*, 205–208.

Ellerbee, S. M. (2006). Posters with an artistic flair. *Nurse Educator, 31*(4), 166–169.

French, B. (2000). Networking for research dissemination: Collaboration and mentorship. *Nurse Researcher, 7*(3), 13–24.

Gray, T. (2005). *Publish & flourish: Become a prolific scholar*. Las Cruces, NM: Teaching Academy, New Mexico State University.

Horne, P. B., Kosper, K. G., & Carpenter, A. D. (1993). A systematic evaluation of a poster presentation. *The Journal of Continuing Education in Nursing, 24*, 232–233.

Moneyham, L., Ura, D., Ellwood, S., & Bruno, B. (1996). The poster presentation as an educational tool. *Nurse Educator, 21*(4), 45–47.

Pyrczak, F., & Bruce, R. R. (2007). *Writing empirical research reports: A basic guide for students of the social and behavioral sciences* (6th ed.). Glendale, CA: Pyrczak Publishing.

Ryan, N. M. (1989). Developing and presenting a research poster. *Applied Nursing Research, 2,* 52–55.

Sigsby, L. M. (1992). The importance of writing style. *Nurse Educator, 17*(3), 23.

Small Business Encyclopedia. (n.d.). *Total quality management (TQM).* Retrieved June 6, 2007, from http://answers.com/topic/tqm

GLOSSARY

Abstract The first section of a research article that provides an overview of the study

Accessible population The group of elements to which the researcher has reasonable access

Active rejection Purposefully deciding not to adopt an innovation

Adoption Applying an innovation to practice

AGREE II Appraisal of Guidelines Research and Evaluation; internationally developed instrument to evaluate clinical practice guidelines

Alpha level Probability of making a Type I error; typically designated as 0.05 or 0.01 at the end of the tail in a distribution

Alternate form A test for instrument reliability where new instruments are given in two different versions. Scores are correlated. Strong positive correlations indicate good reliability; also known as parallel form

Amodal A data set that does not have a mode

Analysis of variance (ANOVA) An inferential statistical test used when the level of measurement is interval or ratio and more than two groups are being compared

Anonymity Keeping the names of subjects separate from data so that no one, not even the researcher, knows their identities

Applied research Research to discover knowledge that will solve a clinical problem

Assent Permission given by children to participate in research

Associative relationship A type of relationship such that when one variable changes the other variable changes

Attrition rate Drop out rate; loss of subjects before the study is completed; threat of mortality

Auditability The degree to which the examination of qualitative data can be shown to be consistent over time and to support the findings

Audit trail The documentation of the research process in qualitative studies

Authorship A listing of authors in an order reflecting the amount of their contributions

Autonomous Having the ability to make decisions

Awareness Understanding about oneself and the world

Axial coding   The analysis of categories and labels after open coding has been completed

Barriers   Factors that limit or prevent change

Basic research   Research to gain knowledge for the sake of gaining knowledge; bench research

Behavioral inventory for professionalism   A measure of education and training, skill, ethics, professional organization, and service

Belmont Report   A report outlining three major principles (respect for persons, beneficence, and justice) foundational for the conduct of ethical research with human subjects

Benchmarking   Comparison of organizational outcome data to other organizations or national databases

Beneficence   The principle of doing good

Between-groups design   Study design where two groups of subjects can be compared

Bias   A result when extraneous variables influence or distort the relationship between the independent and dependent variables

Bimodal   A data set with two modes

Bivariate analysis   The use of statistics to describe the relationship between two variables

Boolean operators   Words, such as *and*, *or*, or *not*, used when searching for literature that specify the relationship between two or more search terms

Bracketing   A strategy used by qualitative researchers to set aside personal interpretations to avoid bias

Call for abstracts   Notices publicizing the desire for posters or presentations at conferences

Call number   Identification number assigned to documents specifying where they are located in a library collection

Career development   Experience and education that contribute to one's professional growth

Care-related outcomes   A category of outcomes that measures the effect of nursing interventions

Case-control   A type of retrospective study in which researchers begin with a group of people who already had the disease

Case control studies   Studies that compare two groups: those who have a specific condition and those who do not have the condition

Case studies   A description of a single or novel event

Categorical data   The lowest level of measurement whereby data are categorized simply into groups; nominal data

Causal relationship   When one variable determines the presence or change in another variable

Causality   The relationship that exists between a cause and its effect

Change   A process that creates an alteration in a person or environment

Change agent   Individual who leads or champions change

Change phases model   An eight-phase process to describe organizational change

Chi square   A common statistic used to analyze nominal and ordinal data to find differences between groups

CINAHL   *Cumulative Index to Nursing and Allied Health Literature*; index or database for nursing and health-related literature

Citation chasing   Using a reference list to identify sources of evidence

Clinical practice guidelines   Recommendations based on evidence that serve as useful tools to direct clinical practice

Cluster sampling   Random sampling method selecting elements from larger to smaller subsets of an accessible population; multistaging sampling

Coding   Assignment of labels to each line of transcript in qualitative analysis

Coefficient of variation   A percentage used to compare standard deviations when the units of measure are different or when the means of the distributions being compared are far apart

Coercion   The threat of harm or the offer of an excessive reward with the intent to force an individual to participate in a research study

Cohort comparison   Nonexperimental crosssectional design in which more than one group of subjects is studied at the same time so that conclusions about variable(s) over time can be drawn even though data were collected at only one point in time

Cohort studies   Quasi-experimental studies using two or more groups

Communication   A process of creating and sharing information with one another to reach mutual understanding

Community-based participatory action research   Active involvement of community members throughout the research process

Comparative design   A descriptive design to study phenomena by comparing two or more groups or two or more variables

Complex hypothesis   A hypothesis describing the relationships among three or more variables

Concept analyses   Scholarly papers providing an exploration of the attributes and characteristics of a concept

Concepts   Words or phrases that convey a unique idea or mental image that is relevant to a theory

Conceptual definitions   Definitions of concepts contained in a theory that sound like dictionary definitions

Concurrent validity   A test for criterion-related validity when a new instrument is administered at the same time as an instrument known to be valid. Scores of the two instruments are compared. Strong positive correlations indicate good validity.

Conduct and utilization of research in nursing (CURN)   Early study conducted about how nurses transition research findings into practice

Confessionist tales   Personalized accounts by qualitative researchers that provide insight about data collection and scientific rigor

Confidence intervals   Ranges established around means that estimate the probability of being correct

Confidentiality   The protection of subjects' identities from everyone except the researcher

Confirmability   One of four criteria for a trustworthy qualitative study related to the rigorous attempts to be objective and the maintenance of audit trails to document the research process

Confounding variable   Factor that interferes with the relationship between the independent and dependent variables; extraneous variable; *Z* variable

Construct   A word or phrase used to communicate a specific key idea to others

Construct validity   A threat to external validity when the instrument does not accurately measure the theoretical concepts

Content validity   A kind of validity to ensure that the instrument measures the concept; a test in which experts on the topic are asked to judge each item on an instrument by assigning a rating to determine its fit with the concept being measured

Continuous data   Interval- or ratio-level data that use a continuum of numeric values with equal intervals

Continuous quality improvement   A participatory process involving indicators that measure quality

Control   Ability to manipulate, regulate, or statistically adjust for factors that can affect the dependent variable

Controlled vocabularies   Standardized hierarchical lists that have been designated to represent major subject concepts contained in a database

Convenience sampling   Nonprobability sampling method in which elements are selected because they are easy to access

Convergent testing   A test for construct validity in which new instruments are administered at the same time as an instrument known to be valid. Scores of the two instruments are compared. Strong, positive correlations indicate good validity

Correlated t *test*   A variation of the *t* test used when there is only one group or when the groups are related; paired *t* test

Correlation coefficient   An estimate, ranging from 0.00 to +1.00, that indicates the reliability of an instrument; a statistic used to describe the relationship between two variables

Correlational   Nonexperimental designs used to study relationships between two or more variables

Cost-benefit ratio   A comparison of the benefits to the potential costs that might occur as a result of change

Covary   When change in one variable is associated with change in another variable

Credibility   One of four criteria for establishing a trustworthy qualitative study referring to the truth or believability of findings

Criterion-related validity   Degree to which the observed score and the true score are related

Critical thinking   A skill set that involves critical appraisal of information

Cronbach's alpha   A test for instrument reliability used with interval or ratio items; using a computer, all items are simultaneously compared

Crossover design   Experimental design using two or more treatments, and subjects receive both treatments in a random order

Cross-sectional   Nonexperimental designs used to gather data from a group of subjects at only one point in time

Cycle of scientific development   A model of the scientific process

Data reduction   The simplification of large amounts of data obtained from qualitative interviews or other sources

Data saturation   In qualitative research the time when no new information is being obtained and repetition of information is consistently heard

Declaration of Helsinki   An international standard providing physicians with guidelines for conducting biomedical research

Deductive reasoning   Thinking that moves from the general to the particular

Degrees of freedom   A statistical concept used to refer to the number of sample values that are free to vary

Dependability One of four criteria for a trustworthy qualitative study related to consistency in the findings over time; auditability

Dependent variable Outcome or variable that is influenced by the independent variable; *Y* variable

Descriptive correlational design Correlational design used to explain the degree and characteristics of relationships that exist among the variables or groups using a nondirectional hypothesis

Descriptive design A design used to describe a phenomenon

Descriptive research A category of research that is concerned with providing accurate descriptions about phenomena

Descriptive statistics Collection and presentation of data used to explain characteristics of variables found in the sample

Descriptive studies Nonexperimental studies used to provide information about phenomena

Developing oneself Engaging in activities that promote long-term professional growth and development

Dichotomous Nominal measurement when only two possible fixed responses exist such as yes or no

Direct observation Observing phenomena using the five senses

Direction The way two variables covary

Directional hypothesis A hypothesis describing the direction of a relationship between two or more variables

Disciplined clinical inquiry model A model developed to empower nurses, at the unit level, to transition evidence to practice

Discussion section Portion of a research article where interpretation of the results and how the findings extend the body of knowledge are discussed

Dissemination Communication of clinical research and theoretical findings for the purpose of transitioning new knowledge to the point of care

Divergent testing A test for construct validity in which new instruments are administered at the same time as an instrument measuring the opposite of the concept. Scores of the two instruments are compared. Strong negative correlations indicate good validity.

Double-blind experimental designs Studies in which subjects and individuals administering the treatments do not know if subjects are receiving experimental interventions or standard of care

Early adopters Individuals who are the first to embrace an innovation

Effect size An estimate of how large a difference will be observed between the groups

Effects of selection Threats to external validity when the sample does not represent the population

Electronic indexes A list of publications that can be obtained using a computer

Elements Basic unit of the population such as individuals, events, experiences, or behaviors

Emic The insider's or participant's perspective

Empirical evidence Verifiable by experience through the five senses or experiment

Empirical indicators Measures of the variables being studied

Empirical testing Collection of objectively measurable data that are gathered through the five senses to confirm or refute a hypothesis; hypothesis testing

Equivalence An attribute of reliability in which there is agreement between alternate forms of an instrument or alternate raters

Ethnography A type of qualitative research that describes a culture

Ethnonursing Systematic study and classification of nursing care beliefs, values, and practices in a particular culture

Ethnoscience A method used in anthropology to discover new knowledge

Etic The outsider's view

Evidence Ground for belief; something that makes plain or clear

Evidence-based practice (EBP) Practice based on the best available evidence, patient preferences, and clinical judgment

Evidence hierarchies Predetermined scales that guide decisions for ranking evidence; Levels of Evidence

Exclusion criteria Characteristics of elements that will not be included in the sample

Exempt A category of research whereby researchers do not have to obtain consent from subjects

Expedited review A type of review by an institutional review board that can occur quickly

Experimental design Research design involving random assignment to groups and manipulation of the independent variable

Explanatory research A category of research that is concerned with identifying relationships among phenomena

Exploding Technique for searching subject headings where all records indexed to that term, as well as any terms that are in a related narrower category, are identified

Exploratory design Nonexperimental design used when little is known about a phenomenon

Ex post facto Research design in which researchers look back in time to determine possible causative factors; retrospective

External validity The degree to which the results of the study can be generalized to other subjects, settings, and times

Extraneous variable Factor that interferes with the relationship between the independent and dependent variables; confounding variable; Z variable

Face validity A test for content validity when colleagues or subjects examine an instrument and are asked whether it appears to measure the concept

Factor analysis A test for construct validity that is a statistical approach to identify items that group together

Factorial Experimental design allowing researchers to manipulate more than one intervention during the same experiment

Fieldwork Time researchers spend interacting with participants through interviews, observations, and detailed records

Flexibility to change Being open and positive about change

Focus groups A strategy to obtain data from a small group of people using interview questions

Follow-up design A longitudinal design used to follow subjects, selected for a specific characteristic or condition, into the future

Forces of Magnetism Qualities that exhibit nursing excellence

Full review   A type of review by an institutional review board that requires all members of the board to participate

Gatekeeper   Person who facilitates or hinders the entry of the researcher into a particular group or setting

Generalize   Applying findings from a sample to a wider population

GRADE   Grades of Recommendations, Assessment, Development, and Evaluation; an international, universal system for evaluating evidence

Grey literature   Unpublished reports, conference papers, and grant proposals

Grounded theory   A type of qualitative research that examines the process of a phenomenon and culminates in the generation of a theory

Hawthorne effect   Behaviors of subjects in a study that are affected by personal values or desires to please the experimenter; reactivity

Health services research   Research involving phenomena, such as cost, political factors, and culture, related to the delivery of health care

Heterogeneous   The degree to which elements are diverse or not alike

Historical   A type of qualitative method used to examine events or people to explain and understand the past with the hope of guiding the present and future

History   A threat to internal validity when the dependent variable has been influenced by some event that occurred during the study

Homogeneity   The degree to which elements are similar or homogenous

Homogeneous   Elements that share many common characteristics

Hypotheses   Formal statements regarding the expected or predicted relationship between two or more variables

Hypothesis testing   Collection of objectively measurable data that are gathered through the five senses to confirm or refute a hypothesis; empirical testing; a test for construct validity

Human rights   Freedoms to which all humans are entitled

Impressionist tales   Chronicles by qualitative researchers using storytelling and more personal descriptions about the experience of conducting the study

Inclusion criteria   Characteristics that each element must possess to be included in the sample

Independent t *test*   A variation of the *t* test used when data values vary independently from one another

Independent variable   Variable that influences the dependent variable or outcome; intervention or treatment that is manipulated by the researcher; *X* variable

Indexes   A listing of electronic or print resources

Indicators   Quantitative criteria used to measure outcomes

Individual nurse level   Practice changes that can be implemented by an individual nurse

Inductive reasoning   Thinking that moves from the particular to the general

Inferential statistics   Analysis of data as the basis for prediction related to the phenomenon of interest

Informant   Individual in a qualitative study; participant

Information overload State of an individual in which excessive communication cannot be processed or used

Informed consent An ethical practice requiring researchers to obtain voluntary participation by subjects after they have been informed of possible risks and benefits

Innovation Introducing something new or novel

Innovator One who is willing to try new things

Institutional review boards A committee that reviews research proposals to determine that research is ethical

Instrumentation Threat to internal validity when changes are made in the way variables are measured or when data collectors obtain data in an inconsistent manner

Integrative review Scholarly papers that synthesize published studies and articles to answer questions about phenomena of interest

Interaction of treatment and history A threat to external validity concerning how the effects from the intervention might be changed by events occurring in the past or future

Interaction of treatment with selection of subjects A threat to external validity that concerns whether the independent variable will affect other individuals in the same way

Interaction of treatment and setting A threat to external validity when an intervention conducted in one setting cannot be generalized to another setting where the same intervention is used

Interlibrary loan A service whereby libraries provide items in their collections to each other upon request

Intermediate outcomes Changes that occur after an innovation is introduced

Internal consistency An attribute of reliability when all items on an instrument measure the same concept

Internal validity The degree to which one can conclude that the independent variable, not extraneous variables, produced changes in the dependent variable

International level Changes that result from collaboration among nurses from different countries

Interrater reliability A test for instrument reliability when two observers measure the same event. Scores are correlated. Strong positive correlations indicate good reliability

Interval A continuum of numeric values with equal intervals but lacks an absolute zero

Interview A method for collecting data in person or over the telephone

Introduction Component part of a research article that contains a statement of the problem and a purpose statement

Iowa model for EBP to promote quality care A systematic method explaining how organizations change practice

Item to total correlation A test for instrument reliability when each item is correlated to the total score; reliable items have strong correlations with the total score

Jewish Chronic Diseases Hospital Unethical study involving injection of cancer cells to subjects without their consent

Journal A scholarly or professional resource

Journal club A strategy for disseminating research among nurses by discussing articles in a small group

Justice The principle of equity or fairness in the distribution of burdens and benefits

Key informants　Individuals who have intimate knowledge of a subject and are willing to share it with the researcher

Keyword　Words use to search electronic data bases

Known group testing　A test for construct validity in which new instruments are administered to individuals known to be high or low on the characteristic being measured

Kuder-Richardson coefficient　A test for instrument reliability for use with dichotomous items; using a computer, all items are simultaneously compared

Kurtosis　The peakedness or flatness of a distribution of data

Ladder program　An organizational process for promotion and career advancement

Laggards　Individuals who are slow or fail to adopt an innovation

Leader　One who takes initiative for change and empowers others

Levels of evidence　Predetermined scales that guide decisions for ranking evidence; evidence hierarchies

Levels of measurement　A system of classifying measurements according to a hierarchy of measurement and the type of statistical tests that are appropriate; levels are nominal, ordinal, interval, and ratio

Lifelong learning　Adding skills and knowledge about the profession as it continues to evolve

Likert scales　Ordinal level scale containing seven points on an agree or disagree continuum

List of references　Information for each article cited in a research report

Lived experiences　The perspective of an individual who has experienced the phenomenon

Longitudinal design　Design used to gather data about subjects at more than one point in time

Long-term outcomes　Primary changes in patient behaviors or status

Magazine　A resource targeted to the general reading audience

Magnitude　The strength of the relationship existing between two variables

Mandated reporting　Data that must be shared with supervising or governmental agencies according to a specified timeline

Manipulation　The ability of researchers to control the independent variable

Manuscript　A scholarly paper prior to its publication

Maturation　A threat to internal validity when subjects change by growing or becoming more mature

Mean　The mathematical average calculated by adding all of the data values and then dividing by the total number of values

Measurement error　The difference between the true score and the observed score

Measures of central tendency　Measures, such as the mean, median, and mode, that provide information about the typical case found in the data

Measures of variability　Measures providing information about how different data are within a set; measures of dispersion

Median　The point at the center of a data set

Member checks　A strategy for qualitative studies in which the researcher goes back to participants and shares the results with them to ensure the findings reflect what participants said

Memoing   A technique used in qualitative research to record ideas that come to researchers as they live with the data

Mentor   One who assists with professional growth

Meta-analyses   Scholarly papers that combine results of studies, both published and unpublished, into a measurable format and statistically estimate the effects of proposed interventions

Meta-synthesis   Scholarly papers that combine results from qualitative studies

Metaparadigm   Four broad concepts core to nursing: person, environment, health, and nursing

Methodological   Studies for the purpose of creating and testing new instruments

Methods section   Major portion of a research article describing the study design, sample, and data collection

Minimal risk   The probability and magnitude of harm from participating in a research study is not greater than what is ordinarily encountered in daily life

Modality   The number of modes found in a data distribution

Mode   The most frequently occurring value in a data set

Model   Pictorial representation of concepts and their interrelationships

Model of diffusion of innovations   A model describing how new ideas become accepted

Model of EBP levels of collaboration   A model explaining how five levels are intertwined to contribute to EBP

Model-testing   Correlational design to test a hypothesized theoretical model; causal modeling or path analysis

Mortality   A threat to internal validity when there is a loss of subjects before the study is completed; attrition rate

Multiple experimental groups   Experimental design using two or more experimental groups with one control group

Multiple regression   An inferential statistical test used to describe the relationship of three or more variables

Multitrait-multimethod   Test for construct validity in which a new instrument, established instrument of same concept, and established instrument of opposite concept are given at the same time; strong positive and negative correlations indicate good validity

Narrative reviews   Article based on only the very common or uncommon elements of works with little concern for research methods, designs, or settings; traditional literature review

National level   Collaboration among nurses throughout the country to affect practice changes

Nazi experiments   Unethical studies conducted during World War II

Negative case analysis   A qualitative strategy involving the analysis of cases that do not fit patterns or categories

Negatively skewed   A distribution when the mean is less than the median and the mode; the longer tail is pointing to the left

Nesting   A strategy used to search databases when using two or more Boolean operators

Networking   Interacting with professional colleagues to exchange information and build relationships

Nominal The lowest level of measurement whereby data are categorized simply into groups; categorical data

Nondirectional hypothesis A hypothesis stating that a relationship exists between two variabled but it does not predict the direction of the relationship

Nonequivalent control group pretest-posttest A quasi-experimental design where two groups are measured before and after an intervention

Nonequivalent groups posttest only A quasi-experimental design involving two groups who are measured after an intervention with little control for extraneous variables

Nonexperimental A research design that lacks manipulation of the independent variable and random assignment to groups

Nonparametric Inferential statistics involving nominal or ordinal level data to infer to the population

Nonprobability sampling Sampling methods that do not require random selection of elements

Nonpropositional knowledge The art of nursing or knowledge that is obtained through practice

Nonsignificant When critical values fall within three standard deviations of the mean; findings do not support the research hypothesis; findings that support the null hypothesis

Normal distribution A representation of data having a distinctive bell-shaped curve and is symmetric about the mean

Null hypothesis A hypothesis stating that there is no relationship between the variables; the statistical hypothesis

Nuremberg Code Ethical code of conduct to guide investigators when conducting research using human subjects

Nursing outcomes Measures of states, behaviors, or perceptions of individuals, families, or communities as they relate to nursing and health

Nursing-sensitive outcomes Results that demonstrate the effectiveness of nursing care

Nursing quality indicators Outcomes of nursing care, identified by the American Nurses Association, meant to address patient safety and quality of care

Obligations Requirements to act in particular ways

Observation A technique to gather data

One group posttest only A preexperimental design involving one group and a posttest with little control for extraneous variables

Open coding The grouping of qualitative data into categories that seem logical

Operational definitions Definitions that explicitly state how the variable will be measured or operationalized; empirical definitions

Ordinal A continuum of numeric values where the intervals are not meant to be equal

Organizational level When nurses in an organization affect practice changes

Organizational priorities Situations of high importance because of volume of patients or costs

Outcome Consequence or visible result

Outcomes research Studies about the effects of care and treatments on individuals and populations

Panel Design A type of longitudinal design in which the same subjects, drawn from the general population, provide data at multiple points in time

Papers Manuscripts published in professional journals

Parallel form   A test for instrument reliability where new instruments are given in two different versions. Scores are correlated. Strong positive correlations indicate good reliability; also known as alternate form

Parametric   Inferential statistical tests involving interval- or ratio-level data to infer to the population

Participant observation   Role of the researcher in qualitative methods when the researcher is not merely an observer but also a participant during data collection

Participants   Individuals in a qualitative study; informants

Passive rejection   Lack of consideration given to adopting an innovation; hence old practices are continued

Patient populations   A group of patients with similar characteristics

Patient-related outcomes   A type of outcome related to patient behaviors or actions

Pearson's r   An inferential statistic used when two variables are measured at the interval or ratio level; Pearson product-moment correlation

Peer debriefing   A technique used in qualitative research when the researcher enlists the help of another person, who is a peer, to discuss the data and findings

Peer review   A process whereby experts and editors rigorously evaluate a manuscript submitted for publication

Percentage distributions   A descriptive statistic used to group data to make results more comprehensible; calculated by dividing the frequency of an event by the total number of events

Percentile   A measure or rank representing the percentage of cases that a given value exceeds

Performance-related outcomes   A type of outcome related to how nurses perform their job

Periodical   A resource that is published on a set schedule

Persistent observation   When the researcher has spent sufficient quality time with participants attempting to describe and capture the essence of the phenomenon

Personal development file   A compilation of career accomplishments

Personal narrative   A way of conveying the meaning of experiences through a storytelling approach

Phenomenology   A type of qualitative research that describes the lived experience to achieve understanding of an experience from the perspective of the participants

Physiological measures   Data obtained from the measurement of biological, chemical, and microbiological phenomena

PICO model   A model in EBP used to formulate EBP questions; acronym stands for patient population, intervention of interest, comparison of interest, and outcome of interest

Pilot   A small study to test a new intervention with a small number of subjects before testing with larger samples; adopting an innovation on a trial basis

Plagiarism   The use of another's work without giving proper credit

Popular literature   Written to inform or entertain the general public

Population   The entire group of elements that meet study inclusion criteria

Population parameters Characteristics of a population that are inferred from characteristics of a sample

Positional operators Using search terms to specify the number of words that can appear between search terms

Position of the median Calculated by using the formula $(n + 1)/2$, where n is the number of data values in the set

Positively skewed A distribution in which the mean is greater than the median and the mode; longer tail is pointing to the right

Poster A scholarly venue for disseminating evidence

Power analysis A statistical method used to determine the acceptable sample size to detect the true effect of the independent variable

Practice guidelines Systematically developed statements to assist healthcare providers with making appropriate decisions about health care for specific clinical circumstances

Preceptors Knowledgeable nurses who provide clinical orientation for new employees

Precision A strategy used to narrow the parameters of a literature search

Predictive correlational Correlational design in which researchers hypothesize which variables are predictors and which are outcomes

Predictive research A category of research concerned with forecasting precise relationships between dimensions of phenomena or differences between groups

Predictive validity A test for criterion-related validity where a new instrument is given at two different times and scores are correlated. Strong positive correlations indicate good validity

Preexperimental A posttest only design that involves manipulation of the independent variable but lacks control for extraneous variables

Presentations Scholarly oral presentations to disseminate new knowledge

Primary sources Original information presented by the person or people responsible for creating them

Print Index Printed listing of electronic or print resources

Probability Likelihood or chance that an event will occur in a situation

Probability sampling Sampling method in which elements in the accessible population have an equal chance of being selected for inclusion in the study

Problem statement A formal statement describing the problem addressed in the study

Professionalism A set of behaviors that exemplify the role of the professional nurse

Proposition A statement about the relationship between two or more concepts

Propositional knowledge The science of nursing or knowledge that is obtained from research and scholarship

Prospective Designs Studies that begin in the present by identifying presumed causes and then follow subjects into the future to determine if the hypothesized effects actually occur

Psychometrics The development of instruments to measure psychological attributes

Purpose statement A statement indicating the aim of the study

Purposive sampling Nonprobability sampling method used in qualitative studies to select a distinct group of individuals that either have lived the experience or have expertise in the event or experience being studied

Pyramid of evidence   A model showing how evidence can be categorized from strong to weak

Qualification   Limiting fields of search, commonly using limits such as author, title, or subject

Qualitative data analysis   The production of knowledge that results from analysis of words

Qualitative research   A type of research where words are used to describe human behaviors

Quantitative research   A type of research where researchers use numbers to obtain precise measurements

Quasi-experimental   Research designs involving the manipulation of the independent variable but lack either random assignment to groups or a control group

Questionnaires   A printed instrument used to gather data

Quota sampling   Nonprobability sampling method involving selection of elements from an accessible population that has been divided into groups or strata

Random assignment   Assignment of subjects whereby each has an equal chance of being in either the treatment or the control group

Random error   Error that occurs by chance during measurement

Random sampling   Technique for selecting elements whereby each has the same chance of being selected

Randomization   The selection, assignment, or arrangement of elements by chance

Randomized controlled trial   Experimental studies typically involving large samples and conducted in multiple sites

Range   The difference between the maximum and minimum values in a data set

Ratio   The highest level of measurement that involves numeric values that begin with an absolute zero and have equal intervals

Reactivity   The influence of participating in a study on the responses of subjects; Hawthorne Effect

Realist tales   A real-life account of the culture being studied presented in a third person voice clearly separating researchers from participants

Research   Systematic study that leads to new knowledge and/or solutions to problems or questions

Research utilization   Changing practice based on the results of a single research study

Recall   A strategy used to search for the number of records retrieved with a keyword

Record   The basic building block in an electronic or print database

Referential adequacy   A technique used in qualitative research when multiple sources of data are compared and the findings hold true

Regional level   When nurses from a large geographic location collaborate to change practice

Rejection   Making a decision not to adopt an innovation

Reliability   Obtainment of consistent measurements over time

Replicated   When another researcher has findings similar to a previous study

Replication   Repeating studies to obtain similar results

Representativeness   The degree to which elements of the sample are like elements in the population

Research   Planned and systematic activity leading to new knowledge and/or the discovery of solutions to problems or questions

Research hypothesis   A hypothesis statement indicating that a relationship between two or more variables exists

Research imperative   An ethical rule stating that nurses should conduct research

Research problem   Area of concern when there is a gap in knowledge that requires a solution

Research question   An interrogatory statement describing the variables and population of the research study

Research topic   A clinical problem of interest

Research utilization   Changing practice based on the results of a single research study

Respect for persons   Principle based on ethical conviction that individuals should be treated as autonomous and that individuals with diminished autonomy are entitled to protection

Results section   Component of a research article where the methods used to analyze data and characteristics of the sample are reported

Retrospective   Research design in which researchers look back in time to determine possible causative factors; ex post facto

Review of literature   A section of a research article that contains an unbiased, comprehensive, synthesized description of relevant previously published studies

Role model   One who demonstrates desired characteristics and skills

Rule of 68-95-99.7   Rule stating that for every sample 68% of the data will fall within one standard deviation of the mean; 95% will fall within two standard deviations of the mean; 99.7% of the data will fall within three standard deviations of the mean

Sample   A select group of elements that is representative of all eligible elements

Sample statistics   Numerical data describing characteristics of the sample

Sampling bias   A threat to external validity when a sample includes elements that over- or underrepresent characteristics when compared to elements in the target population

Sampling distribution   A theoretical distribution representing an infinite number of samples that can be drawn from a population

Sampling error   Error resulting when elements in the sample do not adequately represent the population

Sampling frame   A list of all possible elements in the accessible population

Sampling interval   The interval (k) between each element selected when using systematic random sampling

Sampling plan   Plan to determine how the sample will be selected and recruited

Scales   Used to assign a numeric value or score on a continuum

Scholarly literature   Works written and edited by professionals in the discipline for other colleagues

Scientific literature publication cycle   A model describing how research becomes disseminated in publications

Search field   Where each piece of information contained in the record is entered

Secondary sources   Commentaries, summaries, reviews, or interpretation of primary sources; often written by those not involved in the original work

Selection bias   A threat to internal validity that occurs when the change in the dependent variable is a result of differences in the characteristics of the subjects before they entered a study

Self-awareness   Knowing yourself

Semiquartile range   The range of the middle 50% of the data

Sense of inquiry   Curiosity

Short-term outcomes   Results achieved in a brief period of time

Significance level   The alpha level established prior to the beginning of a study

Simple hypothesis   A hypothesis describing the relationship between two variables

Simple random sampling   Randomly selecting elements from the accessible population

Skewed   An asymmetrical distribution of data

Snowball sampling   Recruitment of participants based on word of mouth or referrals from other participants

Socialization   Awareness about formal and informal rules of behavior

Solomon four group design   An experimental design involving four groups, some of which receive the intervention and others that serve as controls. Some groups are measured before and after the intervention while others are measured only after the intervention.

Split-half reliability   A test for instrument reliability in which the items are divided to form two instruments. Give both instruments and compare the halves using the Spearman-Brown formula.

Stability   An attribute of reliability when instruments render the same scores with repeated measures under the same circumstances

Standard deviation   A measure of variability used to determine the number of data values falling within a specific interval in a normal distribution

Statistical conclusion validity   The confidence one has that the results of the statistical analysis accurately reflect the true relationship between the independent and dependent variables

Statistical hypothesis   The hypothesis stating that there is no relationship among the variables; null hypothesis

Statistically significant   When critical values fall in the tails of normal distributions; when findings did not happen by chance

Statistics   Used to described the branch of mathematics that collects, analyzes, interprets, and presents numerical data in terms of samples and populations; used to describe the numerical outcomes and probabilities derived from calculations on raw data

Stetler model   Step-by-step instructions for integrating research into practice

Stopwords   Words, such as *a*, *the*, and *in*, that are so commonly used in records that they are a hindrance to accurate record retrieval

Strategic sampling   A unique type of sampling in historical research to locate a small group of people who were either witnesses or participants to the phenomenon being studied

Stratified random sampling   Selecting elements from an accessible population that has been divided into groups or strata

Studies   A level in the pyramid of evidence that contains quantitative and qualitative studies, case studies, and concept analyses

Study   A systematic plan for generating new knowledge to answer a research question

Study validity   Ability to accept results as logical, reasonable, and justifiable based on the evidence presented

Subject headings   Organization of databases according to topic

Subject searching   Searching databases using controlled vocabulary

Subjects   Individuals who participate in studies, typically those using a quantitative design

Summaries   A level in the pyramid of evidence containing detailed descriptions of evidence

Survey design   A descriptive design involving data obtained through subjects' self-report

Synopses   A level in the pyramid of evidence containing synopses that are brief descriptions of evidence

Syntheses   A level in the pyramid of evidence containing evidence to present a whole depiction of a phenomenon

Systematic error   Error that occurs in the same way with each measurement

Systematic random sampling   Sampling method in which every kth element is selected from a numbered list of all elements in the accessible population, using a randomly selected starting point

Systematic reviews   A rigorous and systematic synthesis of research findings about a clinical problem

Systems   A level in the pyramid of evidence involving an electronic medical record that is integrated with practice guidelines

t statistics   Inferential statistical test to determine if a statistically significant difference between the groups exists

Tailedness   The degree to which a tail in a distribution is pulled to the left or to the right

Target population   All elements that meet the study inclusion criteria

Team leadership skills   Behaviors that collaboratively engage others while working toward a goal

Team membership   Composition of a team with respect to expertise and leadership

Testing   A threat to internal validity when a pretest influences the way subjects respond on a posttest

Test-retest reliability   A test for instrument reliability when new instruments are given at two different times under the same conditions. Scores are correlated. Strong positive correlations indicate good reliability.

Theoretical framework   The structure of a study that links the theory concepts to the study variables; a section of a research article that describes the theory used

Theoretical sampling   Nonprobability sampling method used in grounded theory to collect data from an initial group of participants

Theory   A set of concepts linked through propositions to provide an explanation of a phenomenon

Therapeutic imperative   An ethical rule stating that nurses should perform actions that benefit the patient

Time series   A quasi-experimental design where one group is measured prior to administering the intervention and then multiple times after the intervention is concluded

Trade literature   Written for professionals in a discipline using a more casual tone than scholarly literature

Traditional literature review   Article based on only the very common or uncommon elements of works with little concern for research methods, designs, or settings; narrative literature review

Transferability   One of four criteria for a trustworthy qualitative study relating to whether findings from one study can be transferred to a similar context

Translational research   Research for the purpose of linking research findings to the point of care

Translational research model   A model that provides specific strategies that organizations can use to improve adoption of an evidence-based innovation

Trend   A type of longitudinal design to gather data from different samples across time

Truncation   A search strategy involving the use of a symbol at the end of a group of letters forming the root search term

Trustworthiness   The quality, authenticity, and truthfulness of findings from qualitative research

Tuskegee study   An unethical study about syphilis during which subjects were denied treatment so the effects of the disease could be studied

Two group posttest only   An experimental design in which subjects are randomly assigned either an experimental or control group and measured after the intervention is completed

Two group pretest-posttest   A research design in which subjects are randomly assigned to either the experimental or control group and measured before and after the intervention is implemented; classic or true experiment

Type I error   Occurs when the researcher rejects the null hypothesis when it should have been accepted

Type II error   Occurs when researchers inaccurately conclude that there is no relationship between the independent and dependent variables when an actual relationship does exist

Uncertainty   Degree to which alternatives are perceived relative to the occurrence of an event and the probability of these alternatives

Unimodal   A dataset with one mode, such as a normal distribution

Univariate analysis   The use of statistical tests to provide information about one variable

Unstructured observation   A method of data collection associated with qualitative research

Validity   The degree that an instrument measures what it is supposed to measure

Visual analog scale (VAS)   Ratio level scale of a 100 mm line anchored on each end with words or symbols

Vulnerable population   Special groups of people needing special protection because of their limited ability to provide informed consent or their risk for being coerced

Wheel of professionalism in nursing   A model depicting behaviors of the professional nurse

Wildcards   Symbols substituted for one or more letters in a search term

Willowbrook studies   An unethical study involving coercion of parents to allow their children to participate in the study in exchange for admission to a long-term care facility

Within groups   Study design where comparisons are made about the same subjects at two or more points in time or on two or more measures

z scores   Standardized units used to compare data gathered using different measurement scales

INDEX

Questions to Consider When Appraising Nursing Studies

Introduction

1. Does the introduction demonstrate the need for the study?
2. Is the problem clearly and concisely identified?
3. Is the problem presented with enough background material to acquaint the reader with the importance of the problem?
4. Is the purpose of the study clearly stated?
5. Are the terms and variables relevant to the study clearly defined?
6. Are the assumptions clearly and simply stated?
7. If appropriate to the design, are hypotheses stated?
8. Does the study use a theoretical framework to guide its design?

Review of the Literature

1. Is the ROL relevant to the problem?
2. Is the review adequate in terms of the range and scope of ideas, opinions, and points of view relevant to the problem?
3. Is the review well organized and synthesized?
4. Does the review provide for critical appraisal of the contribution of each of the major references?
5. Does the review conclude with a summary of the literature with implications for the study?
6. Is the ROL adequately and correctly documented?

Methods

1. Is the research approach appropriate?
2. Was the protection of human subjects considered?
3. Are the details of data collection clearly and logically presented?
4. Are the instrument(s) appropriate for the study both in terms of the problem and the approach?
5. Are the instrument(s) described sufficiently in terms of content, structure, validity and reliability?
6. Is the population and the method for selecting the sample adequately described?
7. Is the method for selection of the sample appropriate?
8. Is the sample size sufficient?
9. Is attrition of sample reported and explained?
10. Does the design have controls at an acceptable level for the threats to internal validity?
11. What are the limits to generalizability in terms of external validity?

Results

1. Is the presentation of data clear?
2. Are the characteristics of the sample described?
3. Was the best method(s) of analysis selected?
4. Are the tables, charts, and graphs pertinent?

Discussion

1. Are the results based on the data presented?
2. Is the evidence sufficient to draw conclusions?
3. Are the results interpreted in the context of the problem/purpose, hypothesis, and theoretical framework/literature reviewed?
4. Are the conclusions and generalizations clearly stated?
5. Are the limitations of the findings clearly delineated?
6. Are the generalizations within the scope of the findings or beyond the findings?
7. Does the study contribute to nursing knowledge?